Selected References
in Trauma and Orthopaedics

Gavin Bowyer • Andrew Cole
Editors

Selected References in Trauma and Orthopaedics

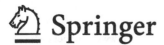 Springer

Editors
Gavin Bowyer, MA, MChir,
FRCS (Orth)
Department of Trauma
and Orthopaedics
University Hospital
Southampton, NHS Trust
Southampton
UK

Andrew Cole, BSc (Hons),
MBBS, FRCS (Tr and Orth)
Department of Trauma
and Orthopaedics
University Hospital
Southampton, NHS Trust
Southampton
UK

ISBN 978-1-4471-4675-9   ISBN 978-1-4471-4676-6   (eBook)
DOI 10.1007/978-1-4471-4676-6
Springer London Heidelberg New York Dordrecht

Library of Congress Control Number: 2013948875

Printed on acid-free paper

Springer is part of Springer Science+Business Media (www.springer.com)

To our wives, who supported us as we trained and continue to support us as we ourselves train, teach and practice trauma & orthopaedics.

Foreword

It is a pleasure to write a foreword for this important book, which will be of interest to those who want to stay up to date with the evidence underlying orthopaedic practice, and will be of great help to those preparing for the Intercollegiate Specialty Examination in Trauma and Orthopaedics. The authors have sought out papers and publications which explain or support our practice, or, indeed, show that further research and evidence is needed.

In choosing to donate all their proceeds from this book to Joint Action, the authors have recognized the importance of research to trauma and orthopaedic practice. Joint Action is the fundraising research arm of the British Orthopaedic Association. This charity specialises in supporting and raising funds for all areas of Orthopaedic research.

London, UK

Timothy Briggs,
MChOrth, FRCS (Ed), FRCS,
Vice President of the British
Orthopaedic Association

Preface

This book is intended as an aid to preparation for the UK's Intercollegiate Examination in Trauma and Orthopaedics, the FRCS (Tr & Orth) examination, and similar end-of-training examinations in other countries. This work provides a selection of references from the trauma and orthopaedic literature, which will be useful to those preparing for the examination. It will be of interest to examiners and trainers who are preparing their trainees for the test, as well as providing a literature basis for their own practice.

As part of the Intercollegiate Examination there are written papers, clinical cases and viva's; the candidates who score well in these sections will have an awareness of the literature and an ability to quote key papers, accurately and appropriately. An awareness of the literature will also aid candidates who are preparing for the examination, as it can be a useful learning strategy; read the essentials of a topic and then examine the background and supporting literature – how do we know what we think we know, and why should we do what we think we should do?

The book aims to present some classic papers underlying current practice as well as recent publications which have brought about innovation, given clarity to a pathological process or treatment rationale, or shown what outcomes can be expected. The references are presented with a brief summary.

The format of the book follows the topic grouping which pertains in the FRCS (Tr & Orth) examination:

- Adult Elective Orthopaedics: spine, shoulder, hip, knee, foot and ankle
- Trauma: spine, shoulder, elbow, pelvic and lower limb, foot and ankle
- Children's Orthopaedics, including paediatric orthopaedic trauma
- Hand and Upper Limb: elective elbow practice, elective hand and wrist practice, hand and wrist trauma
- Applied Basic Sciences

The lead author for each section has been chosen because they are, or have recently been, a senior examiner. The authors know the standards required, and have an awareness of the literature and the topics that are likely to be of interest in the FRCS (Tr & Orth) examination.

The authors have a commitment to orthopaedic training, and appreciate the value of quality orthopaedic research which can underpin practice. For this reason, the authors have all agreed to contribute to this work without fee, so that all the editors' and contributors' royalties can be donated to Joint Action, the charitable organization which contributes so much to research in trauma and orthopaedics.

Southampton, UK   Gavin Bowyer, MA, MChir, FRCS (Orth)
Southampton, UK   Andrew Cole, BSc (Hons), MBBS,
FRCS (Tr and Orth)

Acknowledgements

We gratefully acknowledge those who have trained and taught us, including the trainees from whom we continue to learn.

Contents

Contributors

Stephen Bendall, MBBS, FRCS (Orth) Department of
Orthopaedics, Brighton and Sussex University Hospitals,
Princess Royal Hospital, West Sussex, UK

Gavin Bowyer, MA, MChir, FRCS (Orth) Department of
Trauma and Orthopaedics, University Hospital
Southampton, NHS Trust, Southampton, Hampshire, UK

Andrew Cole, BSc (Hons), MBBS, FRCS (Tr and Orth)
Department of Trauma and Orthopaedics,
University Hospital Southampton, NHS Trust, Southampton,
Hampshire, UK

James Gibbs, MBBS, MSc, FRCS (Tr & Orth) Department
of Trauma and Orthopaedics, Brighton and Sussex
University Hospitals, NHS Trust, Brighton, UK

Martin L. Grover, MB, FRCS Department of Orthopaedics,
Queen Alexandra Hospital, Portsmouth, Hampshire, UK

David Hargreaves, MBBS, FRCS (Orth) Department
of Orthopaedics, University Hospital Southampton Trust,
Southampton, UK

Timothy Kane, MBBS, BSc, FRCS (T&O) Department
of Orthopaedics, Queen Alexandra Hospital, Portsmouth,
Hampshire, UK

Christopher J. Kershaw, MBCHB, FRCS (Ed), FRCS
Department of Trauma and Orthopaedics, Leicester Royal
Infirmary, Leicester, UK

Jayanth Paniker, MBBS, MRCS, MSc (T&O), FRCS (T&O)
Department of Trauma and Orthopaedics, Countess of Chester
Hospital, Chester, Cheshire, UK

**Janardhan Rao, BSc (Hons), MB ChB, FRCS (Ed), FRCS
(Tr & Orth)** Department of Orthopaedics, Countess of
Chester Hospital, Chester, Cheshire, UK

Guy Selmon, MBBS, FRCS, FRCS (Tr and Orth)
Department of Trauma and Orthopaedics, The Conquest
Hospital, St. Leonards on Sea, East Sussex, UK

David J. Shewring, FRCSEd (Orth), Dip Hand Surg (Eur)
Department of Orthopaedic Surgery, University Hospital of
Wales, Cardiff, UK

Ryan Trickett, MBBCh, MRCS, MSc, FRCS (Tr & Orth)
Department of Orthopaedic Surgery, University Hospital of
Wales, Cardiff, UK

Graeme R. Wilson, MBChB Department of Accident
and Emergency, Royal Liverpool University Hospital,
Merseyside, Liverpool, UK

Abbreviations

AC	Acromioclavicular
ACI	Autologous chondrocyte implantation
ACI-C	Autologous chondrocyte implantation with the use of porcine-derived type I/type III collagen as a cover
ACJ	Acromioclavicular joint
ACL	Anterior cruciate ligament
ACR	American College of Rheumatology
ACS	Acute compartment syndrome
AIS	Adolescent idiopathic scoliosis
AKA	Above knee amputations
AKP	Anterior knee pain
AOFAS	American Orthopedic Foot & Ankle Society
AP	Anterior posterior
APL	Abductor polliculongus
ARDS	Adult respiratory distress syndrome
ASA	American Society of Anesthesiologists
ASES	American Shoulder and Elbow Surgeons
ATLS	Advanced trauma and life support
ATT	Anterior tibial tendon
AVN	Avascular necrosis
BAPRAS	British Association of Plastic, Reconstructive and Aesthetic Surgeons
BKA	Below knee amputation
BMD	Bone mineral density
BMI	Body Mass Index
BMP	Bone morphogenic proteins
BOA	British Orthopaedic Association
CA	Coracoacromial

CAI	Chronic ankle instability
CC	Coracoclavicular
CCT	Controlled clinical trial
CI	Confidence interval
CMC OA	Carpometacarpal osteoarthritis
CMT	Charcot-Marie-Tooth disease
CN	Charcot neuroarthropathy
COPD	Chronic obstructive pulmonary disease
CP	Cerebral palsy
CPN	Common peroneal nerve
CR	Cruciate retaining
CRP	C-reactive protein
CRPS	Complex regional pain syndrome
CRRR	Cumulative rerevision rate
CTS	Carpal tunnel syndrome
DASH score	Disabilities of the Arm, Shoulder, and Hand score
DDH	Developmental dysplasia of the hip
DFI	Diabetic foot infections
DHS	Dynamic hip screw
DIACF	Displaced intra-articular calcaneal fractures
DIPJ	Distal interphalangeal joint
DMD	Duchenne muscular dystrophy
DVT	Deep vein thrombosis
ECRB	Extensor carpi radialisbrevis
ECU	Extensor carpi ulnaris
EMG	Electromyography
EPL	Extensor pollicislongus
EQ-5D	Descriptive system of health-related quality of life states consisting of five dimensions (mobility, self-care, usual activities, pain/discomfort, anxiety/depression) each of which can take one of three responses. The responses record three levels of severity (no problems/some or moderate problems/extreme problems) within a particular EQ-5D dimension.
ESR	Erythrocyte sedimentation rate
ESWT	Extracorporeal shock wave therapy
FAI	Femoroacetabular impingement

FAI	Functional ankle instability
FCR	Flexor carpi radialis
FCU	Flexor carpi ulnaris
FDS	Flexor digitorumsuperficialis
FHL	Flexor hallucislongus
fnof	Fractured neck of femur
FRAX	Fracture risk assessment
FTR	Flexor tendon repair
GPA	Glenopolar angle
GUI	Genitourinary injury
HA	Hemiarthroplasty
HA	Hyaluronic acid
HA	Hydroxyapatite
HAD	Hospital Anxiety and Depression
HFS-97	Hannover Fracture Scale-97
HFS-98	Hannover Fracture Scale-98
HHR	Humeral head replacement
HMSN/CMT	Hereditary motor sensory neuropathy/ Charcot-Marie-Tooth
HS	Hamstring
HSS	Hospital for Special Surgery
HT	Hamstring tendon
HXLPE	Highly cross-linked polyethylene
IKDC	International Knee Documentation Committee
IM	Intramedullary
IMHS	Intramedullary hip screw
IMN	Intramedullary nailing
ISS	Injury Severity Score
KSCS	Knee Society Clinical Score
LAF	Laminar air flow
LATN	Lengthening and then nailing
LCL	Lateral collateral ligament
LCPD	Legg-Calve-Perthes disease
LEAP	Lower Extremity Assessment Project
LHB	Long Head of Biceps
LISS	Less Invasive Stabilization System
LRTI	Ligament reconstruction and tendon interposition

LSI	Limb Salvage Index
M/L	Medial/lateral
MACI	Matrix-induced autologous chondrocyte implantation
MCL	Medial collateral ligament
MCP	Metacarpophalangeal
MCPJ	Metacarpophalangeal joint
MESS	Mangled Extremity Severity Score
MFA	Musculoskeletal Function Assessment
MLL	Morel-Lavallee lesion
MOF	Multi-organ failure
MTP	Metatarsophalangeal
MTPJ	Metatarsophalangeal joint
MUA	Manipulation under anesthesia
NAP	Nerve action potentials
NCS	Nerve conduction study
NF	Necrotizing fasciitis
NISSSA	Nerve Injury, Ischemia, Soft-Tissue Injury, Skeletal Injury, Shock, and Age of Patient Score
NSAID	Non-steroidal anti-inflammatory drug
OA	Osteoarthritis
OR	Odds ratio
ORIF	Open reduction and internal fixation
OSS	Oxford Shoulder Score
PBPCs	Peripheral blood progenitor cells
PE	Pulmonary embolism
PEM	Patient Evaluation Measure
PFN	Proximal femoral nail
PFPS	Patellofemoral pain syndrome
PIN	Posterior interosseous nerve
PIP	Proximal interphalangeal
PIPJ	Proximal interphalangeal joint
PLC	Posterolateral corner
PMMA	Polymethylmethacrylate
PPC	Partial physeal closure
PRP	Platelet-rich plasma
PS	Posterior stabilized
PSI	Predictive Salvage Index

PT	Palmaris tendon
PT	Patellar tendon
PTT	Posterior tibial tendon
PTTR	Posterior tibial tendon rupture
RA	Rheumatoid arthritis
RC	Rotator cuff
RCR	Rotator cuff repair
RCT	Randomized controlled trials
RLD	Radial longitudinal deficiency
ROM	Range of motion
RPT	Randomised prospective trial
RRR	Relative risk reduction
RSA	Radio stereometric analysis
RSR	Reverse shoulder replacement
RSWT	Radial shockwave therapy
RTSA	Reverse total shoulder arthroplasty
SAD	Subacromial decompression
SF-36	Short Form-36
SHS	Sliding hip screw
SIP	Sickness Impact Profile
SLAP	Superior labral tear from anterior to posterior
SLE	Systemic lupus erythematosus
SMILE	Staged Multilevel Interventions in the Lower Extremity
SSI	Shoulder Strength Index
SWT	Shock-wave therapy
TAR	Total ankle replacements
TER	Total elbow replacement
THA	Total hip arthroplasty
THR	Total hip replacement
TKA	Total knee arthroplasty
TKR	Total knee replacement
TNF	Tumour necrosis factor
T-POD	Trauma pelvic orthotic device
TSA	Total shoulder arthroplasties
TSR	Total shoulder replacement
UCLA	University of California, Los Angeles
UHMWPE	Ultra high molecular weight polyethylene

UKA	Unicompartmental knee arthroplasty
UKR	Unicompartmental knee replacement
UVL	Ultraviolet light
VAS	Visual analog scale
VISA-A	Victorian Institute of Sports Assessment-Achilles
WOMAC	Western Ontario and McMaster Universities Osteoarthritis Index (?)
WORC	Western Ontario Rotator Cuff Index
WOSI (as in "WOSI score")	Western Ontario Shoulder Instability Score

Part I
Adult Elective Orthopaedics

Spine

Guy Selmon

Abstract This chapter deals with the spinal emergency of cauda equine syndrome and the urgent condition of discitis. It covers the pathology and presentation of these conditions and presents references which give an up-to-date view on the management of these conditions. The very common problem of low back pain is covered with references giving current thoughts on the diagnosis and treatment of this condition. The inflammatory condition, ankylosing spondylitis, is also dealt with as references set out the current management of this disease.

Keywords Lumbar disc protrusions • Spondylolisthesis • Spinal stenosis • Low back pain • Ankylosing spondylitis • Infections of the spine • Cauda equina syndrome

G. Selmon, MBBS, FRCS, FRCS (Tr and Orth)
Department of Trauma and Orthopaedics,
The Conquest Hospital, The Ridge,
St. Leonards on Sea, East Sussex TN37 7RD, UK
e-mail: guyselmon@hotmail.com

G. Bowyer, A. Cole (eds.), *Selected References in Trauma and Orthopaedics*, DOI 10.1007/978-1-4471-4676-6_1,
© Springer-Verlag London 2014

Lumbar Disc Protrusions

Weinstein JN, Tosteson TD, Lurie JD, Tosteson AN, Hanscom B, Skinner JS, et al. Surgical vs non-operative treatment for lumbar disk herniation: the Spine Patient Outcomes Research Trial (SPORT): a randomized trial. JAMA. 2006;296(20):2441–50.

This multicentre randomized trial enrolled 501 patients with persistent (>6 weeks) sciatica secondary to MRI confirmed prolapsed intervertebral disc. Adherence to initially assigned treatment was poor: 30 % of those assigned to non surgical treatment underwent surgery. Both groups of patients improved over a 2 year period but due to the large crossover of patients, firm conclusions could not be made.

Weber H. Lumbar disc herniation. A controlled, prospective study with ten years of observation. Spine (Phila Pa 1976). 1983;8(2):131–40.

This classic paper has remained central to the treatment of patients with sciatica over nearly 30 years. The study comprised three groups of patients with sciatica. The main study group was randomized to surgical and non-surgical treatment. The surgical group showed significantly better results at 1 year. At 4 years the results were still better but not statistically so. There was little difference between the groups at 10 years.

Atlas SJ, Keller RB, Wu YA, Deyo RA, Singer DE. Long-term outcomes of surgical and nonsurgical management of sciatica secondary to a lumbar disc herniation: 10 year results from the maine lumbar spine study. Spine (Phila Pa 1976). 2005;30(8):927–35.

A prospective cohort study that assessed the 10 year outcomes of patients with sciatica treated surgically and non surgically. The surgically treated group had more relief of leg pain and better function and satisfaction than the non surgical group. Work and disability outcomes however were similar in both groups. 25 % of the nonsurgical group had had a spinal operation by 10 years follow-up.

Gibson JN, Waddell G. Surgical interventions for lumbar disc prolapse. Cochrane Database Syst Rev. 2007;(2):CD001350.

This review identified only four trials that compared surgical to non surgical treatment for the lumbar disc prolapse. These trials give suggestive but not conclusive results. The authors concluded that surgery in selected patients resulted in faster relief of symptoms, however the longer term effects are unclear. Microdiscectomy and open discectomy have broadly comparable results.

Ng LC, Sell P. Predictive value of the duration of sciatica for lumbar discectomy. A prospective cohort study. J Bone Joint Surg Br. 2004;86(4):546–9.

In this paper the authors attempt to identify whether timing of surgery affected the clinical outcome. Patients with uncontained disc herniations had shorter duration of symptoms and better functional outcomes than those with contained herniations. Patients with symptoms present for more than 12 months had a less favourable outcome.

Spondylolisthesis

Wiltse LL, Newman PH, Macnab I. Classification of spondylolysis and spondylolisthesis. Clin Orthop Relat Res. 1976;(117):23–9.

This collaborative work provided the classic five category classification of spondylolisthesis. It was expanded to six by Wiltse and Rothman. The classification was based on anatomic variations of the neural arch and acquired pathological conditions. The categories are: Dysplastic (Congenital), Isthmic, Degenerative, Traumatic and Pathologic. The sixth category is Postsurgical.

Beutler WJ, Fredrickson BE, Murtland A, Sweeney CA, Grant WD, Baker D. The natural history of spondylolysis and spondylolisthesis: 45-year follow-up evaluation. Spine (Phila Pa 1976). 2003;28(10):1027–35; discussion 1035.

A prospective study that followed 500 first grade children and identified 30 children with pars defects in this group. No unilateral defects progressed to slip. There was no correlation between slip progression and back pain. There was no statistical difference in SF-36 scores between the study group and the general population of the same age. There was marked slip slowing with each decade and no slip reached 40 %.

Ekman P, Möller H, Hedlund R. The long-term effect of posterolateral fusion in adult isthmic spondylolisthesis: a randomized controlled study. Spine J. 2005;5(1):36–44.

The authors compared the outcome of fusion (either instrumented or non-instrumented) to an exercise programme. With an average follow-up of 9 years, pain and functional disability were significantly better than before treatment in the surgically treated groups (regardless of whether instrumentation was used). Pain was significantly reduced in the exercise group but not functional disability.

Spinal Stenosis

Ragab AA, Fye MA, Bohlman HH. Surgery of the lumbar spine for spinal stenosis in 118 patients 70 years of age or older. Spine (Phila Pa 1976). 2003;28(4):348–53.

A retrospective study that reviewed 118 consecutive patients who underwent simple decompressive surgery for lumbar stenosis. Short follow-up only of average 2 years. 109 patients expressed satisfaction and increasing age did not increase the morbidity of surgery.

Sengupta DK, Herkowitz HN. Lumbar spinal stenosis. Treatment strategies and indications for surgery. Orthop Clin North Am. 2003;34(2):281–95.

This review describes the natural history of lumbar spinal stenosis as well as the surgical treatments available. Rapid deterioration is uncommon. The majority of patients may improve or remain clinically unchanged over time. Patients should be considered for surgery if they fail conservative treatment. Decompression alone is usually all that is needed if there is no segmental instability. Fusion should be considered in the presence of "instability".

Low Back Pain

Fritzell P, Hägg O, Wessberg P, Nordwall A; Swedish Lumbar Spine Study Group. 2001 Volvo Award Winner in Clinical Studies: Lumbar fusion versus nonsurgical treatment for chronic low back pain: a multicenter randomized controlled trial from the Swedish Lumbar Spine Study Group. Spine (Phila Pa 1976). 2001;26(23):2521–32; discussion 2532–4.

This classic paper aimed to establish whether fusion surgery could more effectively improve pain and function compared to nonsurgical treatment. 222 patients were assigned to the surgical group with 72 in the nonsurgical group. At 2 year follow-up, back pain was improved in 33 % of the surgically treated group compared with 7 % in the nonsurgical group. The "back to work rate" was significantly higher in the surgically treated group. The early complication rate in the surgical group was 17 %.

Chou R, Baisden J, Carragee EJ, Resnick DK, Shaffer WO, Loeser JD. Surgery for low back pain: a review of the evidence for an American Pain Society Clinical Practice Guideline. Spine (Phila Pa 1976). 2009;34(10):1094–109.

This systematic review searched all the appropriate databases looking to identify randomized control trials and reviews on the surgical treatment of non radicular back pain (amongst other diagnoses). The overall conclusions were: fusion is no more effective than intensive rehabilitation with an emphasis on cognitive-behavioural treatment. Fusion surgery is slightly to moderately better than standard nonsurgical treatment.

Carreon LY, Glassman SD, Howard J. Fusion and nonsurgical treatment for symptomatic lumbar degenerative disease: a systematic review of Oswestry Disability Index and MOS Short Form-36 outcomes. Spine J. 2008;8(5): 747–55.

The purpose of this study was to evaluate lumbar fusion vs non-surgical treatments for the management of various degenerative spinal conditions. Databases were searched for prospective randomized trials comparing surgical and nonsurgical treatments for chronic low back pain, degenerative disc disease and spondylolisthesis. Oswestry scores were compared. The fusion group improved substantially in spondylolisthesis and degenerative disc disease and less so in the chronic low back pain patients.

Ankylosing Spondylitis

Chen IH, Chien JT, Yu TC. Transpedicular wedge osteotomy for correction of thoracolumbar kyphosis in ankylosing spondylitis: experience with 78 patients. Spine (Phila Pa 1976). 2001;26(16):E354–60.

The authors summarized their experience of this procedure in 78 patients with average 46 month follow-up. Most osteotomies were carried out at L2 and L3 and average correction was 34°. Good to excellent results were seen in 90 % of patients with no evidence of major neurovascular complication.

Infections of the Spine

Rezai AR, Woo HH, Errico TJ, Cooper PR. Contemporary management of spinal osteomyelitis. Neurosurgery. 1999;44(5): 1018–25; discussion 1025–6.

A retrospective review of 57 patients with pyogenic spinal osteomyelitis treated over an 8 year period. 33 patients underwent immediate surgery and 6 underwent surgery after failure of medical management. Anterior alone, posterior alone and combined procedures were all used. Early surgical intervention improved pain outcomes and reduced kyphotic deformity.

Olsen MA, Mayfield J, Lauryssen C, Polish LB, Jones M, Vest J, et al. Risk factors for surgical site infection in spinal surgery. J Neurosurg. 2003;98(2 Suppl):149–55.

This was a retrospective case-control study trying to identify risk factors for surgical site infections following decompression and fusion surgery. Postoperative incontinence, the posterior approach, tumour resection procedures and morbid obesity were all identified as independent risk factors.

Cauda Equina Syndrome

Qureshi A, Sell P. Cauda equina syndrome treated by surgical decompression: the influence of timing on surgical outcome. Eur Spine J. 2007;16(12):2143–51.

A prospective cohort study of 33 patients undergoing surgery for large central disc protrusion causing cauda equina syndrome. The authors were trying to correlate clinical outcome and urinary function to timing of decompression surgery. Timing of surgery did not affect clinical outcome. Severity of bladder dysfunction at the time of surgery seemed to be the dominant factor in deciding recovery of bladder function postoperatively.

Ahn UM, Ahn NU, Buchowski JM, Garrett ES, Sieber AN, Kostuik JP. Cauda equina syndrome secondary to lumbar disc herniation: a meta-analysis of surgical outcomes. Spine (Phila Pa 1976). 2000;25(12):1515–22.

This large meta-analysis looked at 322 patients who underwent surgery for cauda equina syndrome secondary to lumbar disc herniation. They found significant advantages in treating patients within 48 h of onset of symptoms compared to after 48 h in respect of improvements in motor and sensory function. The same applied to urinary and rectal function.

Gleave JR, Macfarlane R. Cauda equina syndrome: what is the relationship between timing of surgery and outcome? Br J Neurosurg. 2002;16(4):325–8.

This review article differentiated incomplete from complete cauda equina syndromes. In the presence of an incomplete lesion (altered urinary sensation, loss of desire to void, poor stream) urgent surgery may prevent patients progressing to a complete lesion (painless urinary retention and overflow incontinence). Patients with complete lesions are unlikely to recover whenever surgery is performed.

Shoulder

Andrew Cole

Abstract This chapter covers the degenerative conditions of shoulder arthritis and cuff pathology. The current understanding of the pathology of these conditions, and of frozen shoulder, is covered in the references, as well as the treatment options. The causes of shoulder instability are discussed, with the potential non-operative and operative treatment options. For all surgical options around the shoulder, particular attention is given to the literature showing the comparative merits of open and arthroscopic surgery and their outcomes.

Keywords Subacromial impingement • Subacromial decompression • Rotator cuff tear • Rotator cuff repair • Anterior shoulder instability • SLAP lesions • Osteoarthritis of the shoulder • Hemiarthroplasty versus total shoulder replacement • Rotator cuff arthropathy • Reverse shoulder replacement • Calcific tendonitis • Frozen shoulder

A. Cole, BSc (Hons), MBBS, FRCS (Tr and Orth)
Department of Trauma and Orthopaedics,
University Hospital Southampton, NHS Trust,
Southampton, Hampshire SO16 6YD, UK
e-mail: andrew.cole@uhs.nhs.uk, andycole34@btopenworld.com

G. Bowyer, A. Cole (eds.), *Selected References in Trauma and Orthopaedics*, DOI 10.1007/978-1-4471-4676-6_2,
© Springer-Verlag London 2014

Impingement and Subacromial Decompression

Ellman H. Arthroscopic subacromial decompression: analysis of one- to three-year results. Arthroscopy. 1987;3(3):173–81.

This was one of the first outcome papers of arthroscopic subacromial decompression and its use in chronic impingement. It was an analysis of the 1–3 year results in 50 consecutive cases. Eighty percent had advanced stage II impingement without rotator cuff tear and 20 % had full-thickness tears of the rotator cuff. Patients were evaluated pre and postoperatively on the University of California, Los Angeles (UCLA) Shoulder Rating Scale, which includes an assessment of pain, function, range of motion, strength, and patient satisfaction. Eighty-eight percent of the cases were rated "satisfactory" (excellent or good), and 12 % were rated "unsatisfactory" (fair or poor). At the time the author concluded that the procedure was technically demanding.

Norlin R. Arthroscopic subacromial decompression versus open acromioplasty. Arthroscopy. 1989;5(4):321–3.

This early study is often cited. This randomised trial of only 20 patients divided patients into arthroscopic subacromial decompression or an open acromioplasty for treatment of refractory impingement. The arthroscopic group showed a more rapid recovery and better range of motion in the follow-up period. The time for surgery was shorter in the arthroscopic group and it was concluded that this was a superior technique.

Ellman H, Kay SP. Arthroscopic subacromial decompression for chronic impingement. Two- to five-year results. J Bone Joint Surg Br. 1991;73(3):395–8.

Another commonly quoted early paper on the outcome of arthroscopic subacromial decompression. This procedure was performed on 65 patients with impingement symptoms and no full thickness tear. (Patients with a partial tear were included). They were evaluated at 2–5 years after the procedure. On the UCLA shoulder rating scale, 89 % of the cases in this study achieved a satisfactory result and this compared favourably with results reported following open acromioplasty with decreased morbidity and good medium term results.

Brox JI, Staff PH, Ljunggren AE, Brevik JI. Arthroscopic surgery compared with supervised exercises in patients with rotator cuff disease (stage II impingement syndrome). BMJ. 1993;307(6909):899–903.

The aim of this randomized clinical study was to compare the effectiveness of arthroscopic decompression with a supervised exercise program and placebo soft laser treatment in 125 patients with resistant stage II impingement. Blinded evaluation using a Neer shoulder score was performed by one clinician at 6 months. No differences were found between the three groups in duration of sick leave and daily intake of analgesics. After 6 months there was no significant difference in improvement in Neer scores between surgery and supervised exercises. The condition improved significantly compared with placebo in both groups given the active treatments. The conclusion reached was that surgery or a supervised exercise regimen significantly, and equally, improved rotator cuff disease compared with placebo.

Haahr JP, Andersen JH. Exercises may be as efficient as subacromial decompression in patients with subacromial stage II impingement: 4-8-years' follow-up in a prospective, randomized study. Scand J Rheumatol. 2006;35(3):224–8.

This a randomized controlled trial (RCT) of 90 patients treated with subacromial decompression or graded physiotherapy and exercises for stage II impingement symptoms. Patients were followed up for 4–8 years. Outcomes were reported absence from work, self reported function, working capability and employment status. Eighty-eight percent responded to the questionnaire. Cases undergoing surgery tended to have more time off work during the first year, but the difference was not significant. Self-reported outcomes after 4–8 years did not differ between treatment groups. They concluded that the results of surgery were equal to conservative treatment.

Coghlan JA, Buchbinder R, Green S, Johnston RV, Bell SN. Surgery for rotator cuff disease. Cochrane Database Syst Rev. 2008;(1):CD005619.

This was one of a series of Cochrane reviews on treatments around the shoulder. The purpose was to determine the effectiveness and safety of surgery for rotator cuff disease. It was a systematic review of the literature and only studies described as randomised or quasi-randomised clinical trials (RCTs), studying participants with rotator cuff disease and surgical interventions compared to placebo, no treatment, or any other treatment were included. Fourteen RCT were identified with 829 patients but trials included a range of diagnosis. The trials that compared open or arthroscopic decompression with an exercise programme, physiotherapy or graded exercise showed no differences in outcome. In the six trials that compared arthroscopic with open subacromial decompression there were no significant differences at any time period although there was a tendency towards a quicker recovery in the arthroscopic group. Based on the trials (all susceptible to Bias) no firm conclusions could be drawn with regards the effectiveness of these procedures for rotator cuff disease. There appeared to be no difference between the arthroscopic or open decompression and active non-operative management.

Magaji SA, Singh HP, Pandey RK. Arthroscopic subacromial decompression is effective in selected patients with shoulder impingement syndrome. J Bone Joint Surg Br. 2012;94(8): 1086–9.

This study analysed 83 patients who had symptoms for more than 6 months due to subacromial impingement and undergoing arthroscopic decompression. While continuing with physiotherapy they waited a further 6 months for surgery. The patients were divided into groups on the basis of clinical and radiological criteria. The criteria were: temporary benefit from steroid injection, mid arc pain, a consistently positive Hawkins sign and radiological evidence of impingement. Group A fulfilled all four criteria, group B three criteria and group C two criteria. The Oxford shoulder score was recorded at 3 and 12 months postoperatively. At 1 year patients in all groups showed improvement in scores, but patients in group A had a higher mean score (p=0.01). At 1 year patients in groups A and B did better than those in group C (p=0.01). The authors concluded that arthroscopic subacromial decompression (SAD) is a beneficial intervention in selected patients. The four criteria could help identify patients in whom it is likely to be most effective.

Chahal J, Mall N, MacDonald PB, Van Thiel G, Cole BJ, Romeo AA, et al. The role of subacromial decompression in patients undergoing arthroscopic repair of full-thickness tears of the rotator cuff: a systematic review and meta-analysis. Arthroscopy. 2012;28(5):720–7.

This was a systematic review of the literature to determine the efficacy of arthroscopic repair of full-thickness rotator cuff tears with and without subacromial decompression. The literature was reviewed for eligible randomised controlled studies. Four studies with 373 patients were included in the analysis. A meta-analysis of shoulder-specific outcome measures (American Shoulder and Elbow Surgeons [ASES] or Constant scores) or the rate of reoperation between patients treated with subacromial decompression and those treated without it showed no statistically significant differences. The authors concluded that on the basis of the available literature there is no difference in the outcome of rotator cuff repair with or without subacromial decompression.

Rotator Cuff Tears and Repairs

Rotator Cuff Tears and Their Natural History

Clement ND, Nie YX, McBirnie JM. Management of degenerative rotator cuff tears: a review and treatment strategy. Sports Med Arthrosc Rehabil Ther Technol. 2012;4(1):48.

This is an article discussing all aspects of rotator cuff tear and a comprehensive literature review. It goes on to discuss the epidemiology and incidence of rotator cuff tear in the asymptomatic population (54 % of patients aged 60 will have a partial tear or full thickness tear on magnetic resonance imaging (MRI) scanning and approximately 30 % will have ultrasound changes). The article describes the evidence for diagnosis along with the clinical signs. The natural history of the tear is discussed along with suggestions for the management and repair techniques. Whilst there is a good literature review it is apparent that the principles used in the decision making are based on limited evidence.

Tashjian RZ. Epidemiology, natural history, and indications for treatment of rotator cuff tears. Clin Sports Med. 2012; 31(4):589–604.

This is a review of the epidemiology, natural history and indications for the treatment of rotator cuff disorders. The salient features in this review are:

Aetiology is multifactorial (age, trauma, genetics, smoking).
Tear incidence increases with age (more than 50 % in their 80's have a tear).
Substantial full thickness tears are likely to progress/ enlarge with time.
Pain or worsening pain usually suggests progression.
Larger full thickness tears that are symptomatic have a high rate of tear progression.
Smaller tears have a lesser rate of progression.

Yamaguchi K, Tetro AM, Blam O, Evanoff BA, Teefey SA, Middleton WD. Natural history of asymptomatic rotator cuff tears: a longitudinal analysis of asymptomatic tears detected sonographically. J Shoulder Elbow Surg. 2001;10(3):199–203.

This study examines longitudinally the natural history of asymptomatic rotator cuff tears over a 5-year period with the aim of assessing the risk for development of symptoms and tear progression. A review of consecutive bilateral sonograms done from 1989 to 1994 revealed 58 potential patients with unilateral symptoms who had contralateral asymptomatic rotator cuff tears. Primary and repeat sonograms were reassessed for tear size and location by two independent experienced radiologists blinded to the clinical data results.

Fifty-one percent of the previously asymptomatic patients became symptomatic over a mean of 2.8 years. Development of symptoms was associated with a significant increase in pain and decrease in function. The authors concluded that there appears to be a risk for tear size progression over time.

Melis B, DeFranco MJ, Chuinard C, Walch G. Natural history of fatty infiltration and atrophy of the supraspinatus muscle in rotator cuff tears. Clin Orthop Relat Res. 2010;468(6): 1498–505.

The aim of this study was to determined the speed of appearance and progression of fatty infiltration and correlate this with muscle atrophy. One thousand six hundred and eighty-eight patients with rotator cuff tears were retrospectively reviewed and the number of tendons torn, aetiology of the tear, time between onset of shoulder symptoms and diagnosis of rotator cuff tear recorded. Moderate supraspinatus fatty infiltration (on computed tomography [CT] or MRI) appeared an average of 3 years after onset of symptoms and severe fatty infiltration at an average of 5 years after the onset of symptoms. A positive tangent sign appeared at an average of 4.5 years after the onset of symptoms. The authors suggested that rotator cuff repair should be performed before the appearance of fatty infiltration (Stage 2) and atrophy.

Yamaguchi K, Ditsios K, Middleton WD, Hildebolt CF, Galatz LM, Teefey SA. The demographic and morphological features of rotator cuff disease. A comparison of asymptomatic and symptomatic shoulders. J Bone Joint Surg Am. 2006; 88(8):1699–704.

Five hundred and eighty-eight consecutive patients in whom a standardized ultrasound study had been performed for the assessment of unilateral shoulder pain were evaluated with regard to the presence and size of rotator cuff tears in each shoulder. Demographic factors that were analyzed included age, gender, side, and cuff thickness and correlated with the presence of pain. Thirty-six percent had an intact rotator cuff bilaterally, 34 % had a unilateral rotator cuff tear (either partial or full thickness), and 30 % had a bilateral tear.

The presence of rotator cuff disease was highly correlated with age. The average age was 48.7 years for patients with no rotator cuff tear, 58.7 years for those with a unilateral tear, and 67.8 years for those with a bilateral tear. In patients with a bilateral rotator cuff tear in whom one tear was symptomatic and the other tear was asymptomatic, the symptomatic tear was significantly larger. Patients who presented with a full-thickness symptomatic tear had a 35.5 % prevalence of a full-thickness tear on the contralateral side.

Arthroscopic vs Mini Open Rotator Cuff Repair

Walton JR, Murrell GA. A two-year clinical outcomes study of 400 patients, comparing open surgery and arthroscopy for rotator cuff repair. Bone Joint Res. 2012;1(9):210–7.

This study compared the clinical outcome of the two techniques over a 2 year or longer follow-up period. Two hundred open repairs were compared with 200 arthroscopic repairs performed by a single surgeon. Pain measurements were similar although the arthroscopic group reported less night pain at 6 months. The arthroscopic group demonstrated an earlier return of strength, achieving near maximal recovery by 6 months postoperatively whereas the open rotator cuff repair (RCR) patients took longer to reach the same recovery level. The arthroscopic group had a shorter operating time and a lower re-tear rate. The authors concluded that the arthroscopic repair involved less extreme pain than open RCR, earlier functional recovery, a shorter operative time and better repair integrity.

van der Zwaal P, Thomassen BJ, Nieuwenhuijse MJ, Lindenburg R, Swen JW, van Arkel ER. Clinical outcome in all-arthroscopic versus mini-open rotator cuff repair in small to medium-sized tears: a randomized controlled trial in 100 patients with 1-year follow-up. Arthroscopy. 2013;29(2):266–73.

This study evaluated the 1 year outcome of the two techniques in small to medium sized full thickness rotator cuff tears. One hundred patients were randomized at the time of surgery. Patients were evaluated before and 6, 12, 26, and 52 weeks after surgery using the Disabilities of the Arm, Shoulder, and Hand (DASH) score, the Constant score. A visual analog scale (VAS)-pain/impairment score, and measurement of active forward flexion/external rotation were used as secondary outcomes. Ultrasound was used at 1 year to assess cuff integrity. Overall, mean primary and secondary postoperative outcome scores did not statistically significantly differ between the treatment groups. At 6 weeks DASH score, VAS-pain and -impairment, and active forward flexion were significantly more improved in the arthroscopic group. Re-tear rates were similar in the two groups. The authors concluded that the outcomes measured do not differ in the two groups at 1 year but those treated arthroscopically may benefit at an earlier stage.

Cho CH, Song KS, Jung GH, Lee YK, Shin HK. Early postoperative outcomes between arthroscopic and mini-open repair for rotator cuff tears. Orthopedics. 2012;35(9):e1347–52.

This study randomized 60 patients with tears smaller than 3 cm into arthroscopic or mini open surgery. The early postoperative outcomes were then compared. Pain level, range of motion and complications were compared between the two groups from immediately postoperatively to 6 months postoperatively. At day 1 and 2 there was significantly less pain in the arthroscopic group although at 6 months there was no difference between the two groups. No significant difference existed in postoperative range of motion, duration of rehabilitation, shoulder stiffness, or complications between the two groups. Arthroscopic and mini-open repair appear to have similar clinical outcomes in the early postoperative period.

Lindley K, Jones GL. Outcomes of arthroscopic versus open rotator cuff repair: a systematic review of the literature. Am J Orthop (Belle Mead NJ). 2010;39(12):592–600.

This was a systematic review of ten studies comparing arthroscopic and mini-open full thickness rotator cuff tear repairs. There were no statistically significant differences between groups when ASES, UCLA and pain scores were compared within each study in terms of these data points. The incidence of re-tears was also the same. There may be decreased short-term pain in patients who undergo arthroscopic repairs.

Double Row vs Single Row Techniques for Rotator Cuff Repair

Sheibani-Rad S, Giveans MR, Arnoczky SP, Bedi A. Arthroscopic single-row versus double-row rotator cuff repair: a meta-analysis of the randomized clinical trials. Arthroscopy. 2013;29(2):343–8.

There has been controversy for a number of years with regard to the best techniques for rotator cuff repair and in particular the role of double row and single row repair. This was a meta-analysis of prospective randomized level 1 studies. The functional outcome scores included the American Shoulder and Elbow Surgeons (ASES) shoulder scale, the Constant shoulder score, and the University of California, Los Angeles (UCLA) shoulder rating scale were analysed. Five studies were identified. The authors found no significant differences in the clinical outcomes between the two types of repair in all outcomes measured.

Lapner PL, Sabri E, Rakhra K, McRae S, Leiter J, Bell K, Macdonald P. A multicenter randomized controlled trial comparing single-row with double-row fixation in arthroscopic rotator cuff repair. J Bone Joint Surg Am. 2012;94(14):1249–57.

A multicenter, randomized double blind controlled study of the two techniques in 90 patients comparing functional outcomes. The main outcome score was the Western Ontario rotator cuff index (WORC) at 24 months. The Constant score, ASES score and strength were used as secondary outcomes. At the end of the study period anatomical outcomes were assessed with MRI or ultrasound. The patient demographics were the same in each group and preoperative WORC scores did not differ. The WORC score did not differ at any time period up to 24 months between the two groups. The Constant score, ASES score, and strength did not differ significantly between groups at any time point. There was a tendency towards better healing rates with small tears and a double row technique.

Carbonel I, Martinez AA, Calvo A, Ripalda J, Herrera A. Single-row versus double-row arthroscopic repair in the treatment of rotator cuff tears: a prospective randomized clinical study. Int Orthop. 2012;36(9):1877–83.

One hundred and sixty patients with a full thickness tear of the rotator cuff were randomized into the two techniques. Results were evaluated by use of the University of California, Los Angeles (UCLA), American Shoulder and Elbow Surgeons (ASES) and Constant score, the Shoulder Strength Index (SSI) and range of motion. MRI was performed at 2 years. There was a 100 % follow-up rate. This study showed that at 2 years there was a significant difference in the clinical outcome in favour of the double row technique and this was even more pronounced in tears over 30 mm. There were no differences in the healing rates observed.

DeHaan AM, Axelrad TW, Kaye E, Silvestri L, Puskas B, Foster TE. Does double-row rotator cuff repair improve functional outcome of patients compared with single-row technique? A systematic review. Am J Sports Med. 2012;40(5): 1176–85.

This was a systematic analysis of the available literature of level I or II studies to compare double row techniques with single row to test the hypothesis that double-row fixation, although biomechanically superior, has no clinical benefit with respect to re-tear rate or improved functional outcome. Seven studies were identified that fulfilled the authors' criteria. There was no difference in the functional (ASES, Constant and UCLA) outcome scores. There was a trend towards a higher re-tear rate for the single row repair of 43 % compared with the double row technique of 27 % although this did not reach significance.

Anterior Shoulder Instability

Predicting Recurrent Instability

Hoelen MA, Burgers AM, Rozing PM. Prognosis of primary anterior shoulder dislocation in young adults. Arch Orthop Trauma Surg. 1990;110(1):51–4.

One hundred and ninety-six primary traumatic dislocations were identified from a single hospital over a 5 year period and followed up for an average of 4 years. Eighty-seven percent were available for the study. The most important factor involved in the prediction of recurrent dislocation was the age at initial presentation. The highest recurrence rate was found in patients of 30 years and younger (64 %). A fracture of the greater tuberosity improved the prognosis significantly.

Hovelius L, Lind B, Thorling J. Primary dislocation of the shoulder. Factors affecting the two-year prognosis. Clin Orthop Relat Res. 1983;(176):181–5.

This was a multicenter trial from Sweden. Two hundred and fifty-five patients with a primary shoulder dislocation were followed up for 2 years. In patients 22 years of age or younger, there was a 47 % recurrence rate. In the 23–29 year age group it was 28 % and this reduced to 13 % in the 30–40 year age group. The greatest risk for recurrence was in patients 17–19 years of age, 53 % of whom had at least one recurrence. Sex, type of trauma or physical activities seemed to have no relationship with recurrence rates.

Hovelius L, Olofsson A, Sandström B, Augustini BG, Krantz L, Fredin H, et al. Non-operative treatment of primary anterior shoulder dislocation in patients forty years of age and younger. A prospective twenty-five-year follow-up. J Bone Joint Surg Am. 2008;90(5):945–52.

This paper presents the outcome after 25 years of 255 patients with a primary shoulder dislocation who were managed with or without immobilization and rehabilitation. All 227 living patients (229 shoulders) completed the follow-up questionnaire, and 214 patients completed the Disabilities of the Arm, Shoulder and Hand (DASH) questionnaire. Forty-three percent had not redislocated, and 7 % redislocated once. 14.4 % of shoulders became stable with time. Eight percent continued with recurrent instability. Twenty-seven percent had undergone surgery for the treatment of recurrent instability. Only 2 of 24 shoulders with a fracture of the greater tuberosity at the time of the primary dislocation redislocated (p < 0.001). In conclusion after 25 years, half of the primary anterior shoulder dislocations that had been treated non-operatively in patients with an age of 12–25 years had not recurred or had become stable over time.

Robinson CM, Howes J, Murdoch H, Will E, Graham C. Functional outcome and risk of recurrent instability after primary traumatic anterior shoulder dislocation in young patients. J Bone Joint Surg Am. 2006;88(11):2326–36.

This was a prospective cohort study of 252 patients (age 15–35) who sustained a primary traumatic dislocation and were treated with immobilization and rehabilitation. There was regular clinical follow-up to assess whether recurrent instability had developed. Functional assessments were made and were compared for two subgroups: those who had not had instability develop and those who had received operative stabilization to treat recurrent instability. Instability developed in 55.7 % of the shoulders within the first 2 years after the primary dislocation and increased to 66.8 % by the fifth year. Younger male patients were most at risk. Of those that developed instability 87 % developed this within 2 years.

Early Surgery vs Conservative Management of First Time Dislocations

Smith GC, Chesser TJ, Packham IN, Crowther MA. First time traumatic anterior shoulder dislocation: a review of current management. Injury. 2013;44(4):406–8.

This is a review of current literature and the management of the first time traumatic dislocation of the shoulder. Currently in the UK 90 % of cases are treated non-operatively initially although there is an increasing trend towards early stabilization. The typical length of immobilization after the dislocation is 3–6 weeks although again the trend is towards less time or no immobilization with mixed evidence for and against. The risk of recurrent instability ranges from 25 to 95 % after non-operative management reflecting a range of populations and follow-up periods. It is estimated that if all those under the age of 25 with a first time dislocation undergo surgery then 30 % will undergo unnecessary operations. On review of the literature the authors conclude that there is little benefit in immobilization, the evidence for bracing is limited, recurrence rates can be reduced by early arthroscopic stabilization.

Jakobsen BW, Johannsen HV, Suder P, Søjbjerg JO. Primary repair versus conservative treatment of first-time traumatic anterior dislocation of the shoulder: a randomized study with 10-year follow-up. Arthroscopy. 2007;23(2):118–23.

This study took 76 patients after a first time dislocation and randomized them into conservative treatment (sling for 1 week with subsequent rehabilitation) or into a surgical group and subsequent similar rehabilitation. After a minimum of a 2 year follow-up 56 % in the conservative group had recurrence of their dislocation as compared with 3 % in the surgically treated group. Of those that had not dislocated 39 % in the conservative and 7 % in the operative group had anterior apprehension. At 10 years 72 % of the surgical group rated their shoulder good or excellent in contrast to the conservative group in which 75 % had unsatisfactory results because of recurrent instability, pain or stiffness. The authors concluded that open repair produces superior results compared with conservative treatment in acute first time dislocations

Robinson CM, Jenkins PJ, White TO, Ker A, Will E. Primary arthroscopic stabilization for a first-time anterior dislocation of the shoulder. A randomized, double-blind trial. J Bone Joint Surg Am. 2008;90(4):708–21.

The aim of this study was to assess the efficacy of a primary arthroscopic Bankart repair. Eighty-eight adults under the age of 35 with a first time anterior dislocation of the shoulder were randomized to arthroscopic lavage alone or arthroscopic lavage with an arthroscopic Bankart repair. The patients were followed up for 2 years and assessed with 3 scores, range of movement, patient satisfaction and complications. In the group that received a Bankart repair the risk of dislocation over the 2 years was reduced by 76 % and instability by 82 % compared with lavage alone. Patient satisfaction was higher and the functional scores were also significantly better. The conclusion was that early arthroscopic repair confers benefit distinct from the benefit of the therapeutic arthroscopy.

Kirkley A, Werstine R, Ratjek A, Griffin S. Prospective randomized clinical trial comparing the effectiveness of immediate arthroscopic stabilization versus immobilization and rehabilitation in first traumatic anterior dislocations of the shoulder: long-term evaluation. Arthroscopy. 2005;21(1): 55–63.

A prospective randomized clinical trial comparing the effectiveness of immediate arthroscopic stabilization versus immobilization and rehabilitation after a first traumatic anterior dislocation of the shoulder. Forty patients younger than 30 years with a first traumatic anterior shoulder dislocation, were randomized into immediate arthroscopic stabilization (plus rehabilitation) or immobilization with subsequent rehabilitation. At an average of 75 months follow-up there was a significant difference in recurrent dislocation rates but little difference in the functional scores. It is suggested that immediate stabilization is the treatment of choice in the subset of patients who are less than 30 and high level athletes.

Kirkley A, Griffin S, Richards C, Miniaci A, Mohtadi N. Prospective randomized clinical trial comparing the effectiveness of immediate arthroscopic stabilization versus immobilization and rehabilitation in first traumatic anterior dislocations of the shoulder. Arthroscopy. 1999;15(5):507–14.

Forty patients below the age of 30 with a first time dislocation were randomized into immobilization for 3 weeks and subsequent rehabilitation or arthroscopic stabilization within

4 weeks with subsequent identical rehabilitation. A blinded research assistant performed all follow-up evaluations. At 24 months, there was a statistically significant difference in the rate of redislocation (47 % compared with 15.9 % in favour of the surgically treated group). At an average 32 months follow-up, a significant reduction in redislocation and improvement in disease-specific quality of life was apparent in the arthroscopically stabilized group.

Owens BD, DeBerardino TM, Nelson BJ, Thurman J, Cameron KL, Taylor DC, et al. Long-term follow-up of acute arthroscopic Bankart repair for initial anterior shoulder dislocations in young athletes. Am J Sports Med. 2009; 37(4):669–73.

An evaluation of a cohort of young patients who had undergone acute arthroscopic repair of Bankart lesions for a first time dislocation to assess the long-term outcome. The mean follow-up was 11.7 years with a range from 9 to 14. Eighty-two percent of the originally identified cohort was available for review. Of the nine lost to follow-up there were two recurrences. Overall there was a redislocation rate of 14.3 %. 21.4 % had reported subluxations. At final follow-up the subjective scores were good (Western Ontario Shoulder instability score or WOSI, ASES, Short Form-36 [SF-36], Rowe, Simple Shoulder Test and Tegner). The authors conclude that in this group of patients that acute arthroscopic Bankart repair results in excellent subjective function and return to sport with an acceptable rate of recurrence and reoperation.

Arthroscopic Compared with Open Stabilization

Bottoni CR, Smith EL, Berkowitz MJ, Towle RB, Moore JH. Arthroscopic versus open shoulder stabilization for recurrent anterior instability: a prospective randomized clinical trial. Am J Sports Med. 2006;34(11):1730–7.

This was a prospective randomized study comparing arthroscopic anterior stabilization with open stabilization performed by one surgeon in a consecutive series of 64 patients. Post-operative evaluation included the range of motion, stability and a range of subjective assessments. This took place at a mean of 32 months. Failure was defined as a further dislocation, subluxation or symptoms that prevented return to work. The mean operative time was significantly shorter for the arthroscopic repairs (59 vs 149 min). There were 3 clinical failures (2 open stabilizations, 1 arthroscopic stabilization) by the established criteria. Subjective evaluations were equal in both groups. The clinical outcomes after arthroscopic and open stabilization are comparable.

Archetti Netto N, Tamaoki MJ, Lenza M, dos Santos JB, Matsumoto MH, Faloppa F, et al. Treatment of Bankart lesions in traumatic anterior instability of the shoulder: a randomized controlled trial comparing arthroscopy and open techniques. Arthroscopy. 2012;28(7):900–8.

In this study 50 patients (aged less than 40 years) with recurrent instability and the presence of an isolated Bankart lesion were randomly assigned to arthroscopic or open stabilization with metallic anchors. The primary outcomes included the Disabilities of the Arm, Shoulder and Hand (DASH) questionnaire and functional outcomes. Mean follow-up was just over 3 years with an 82 % follow-up rate. There was no difference in UCLA scores, Rowe scores, complications or failures. There was a tendency towards better DASH scores in the arthroscopic group although this did not seem clinically relevant. Both techniques are effective treatments.

Harris JD, Gupta AK, Mall NA, Abrams GD, McCormick FM, Cole BJ, et al. Long-term outcomes after Bankart shoulder stabilization. Arthroscopy. 2013;29(5):920–33.

The aim of this study was to analyse the results of the long-term outcome of those that had undergone an arthroscopic or open Bankart repair for post-traumatic recurrent instability without significant glenoid bone loss. This involved a systematic review of the literature of level I-IV evidence with a minimum of 5 year follow-up. Twenty-six studies (1,781 patients) were analysed. The mean length of clinical follow-up was 11 years. There was no significant difference in recurrence of instability with arthroscopic (11 %) versus open (8 %) techniques. There was no significant difference in instability recurrence with arthroscopic suture anchor versus open Bankart repair (8.5 % vs 8 %). There was no difference in the two groups in functional scores, rates or osteoarthritis Both techniques therefore result in similar long-term clinical outcomes, with no significant difference in the rate of recurrent instability, clinical outcome scores, or rate of return to sport. However, generally the study quality was poor, with most studies having Level III or IV Evidence.

Superior Labral Tear from Anterior to Posterior (Slap) Lesions

Snyder SJ, Karzel RP, Del Pizzo W, Ferkel RD, Friedman MJ. SLAP lesions of the shoulder. Arthroscopy. 1990;6(4):274–9.

This was the first paper to identify and classify SLAP lesions on the basis of a retrospective review of more than 700 shoulder arthroscopies and based on 37 patients with these lesions. The most common clinical complaints were pain, greater with overhead activity, and a painful catching or popping in the shoulder.

The authors described four types of lesion. Type I (fraying or degeneration of the superior labrum), Type II (detachment of the superior labrum and biceps anchor), Type III (bucket handle tear of the superior labrum with the remaining superior anchor attached) and type IV (bucket handle tears of the labrum with extension into the long head of biceps [LHB]).

Meserve BB, Cleland JA, Boucher TR. A meta-analysis examining clinical test utility for assessing superior labral anterior posterior lesions. Am J Sports Med. 2009;37(11):2252–8.

The reported accuracy of clinical tests for the presence of SLAP lesions is variable. The purpose of this meta-analysis was to determine which clinical tests are superior to others for diagnosing the presence or absence of these lesions. Six of 198 identified studies satisfied the eligibility criteria. Active compression, anterior slide, crank, and Speed tests were analysed. The accuracy of the anterior slide test was significantly inferior to that of the active compression, crank, and Speed tests. There was no significant difference in test accuracy found among active compression, crank, and Speed tests.

Brockmeier SF, Voos JE, Williams RJ 3rd, Altchek DW, Cordasco FA, Allen AA, et al. Outcomes after arthroscopic repair of type-II SLAP lesions. J Bone Joint Surg Am. 2009; 91(7):1595–603.

This was one of the first prospective studies on the results of arthroscopic anchor repairs of SLAP lesions. Forty-seven patients with a type II SLAP lesion were prospectively evaluated before and 2 years after surgery. The American Shoulder and Elbow Surgeons (ASES) score and L'Insalata outcome scores and physical examination were used. At an average of 2.7 years, the median ASES and L'Insalata scores had significantly improved. Eighty-seven percent rated the outcome as good or excellent. Those with a traumatic aetiology had significantly better patient reported outcome than those with an atraumatic history although there was no difference in outcome scores. Overall, 74 % of the 34 athletes were able to return to their preinjury level of competition. Ninety-two percent of the 12 athletes who reported a discrete traumatic event were able to return to their previous level of competition.

Sayde WM, Cohen SB, Ciccotti MG, Dodson CC. Return to play after Type II superior labral anterior-posterior lesion repairs in athletes: a systematic review. Clin Orthop Relat Res. 2012;470(6):1595–600.

The purpose of this systematic review was to assess patient satisfaction and return to sports in throwing and other athletes. A total of 506 patients with Type II SLAP tears were reviewed from 14 studies with a 2 years or more follow-up; of these, 327 had SLAP lesions repaired by anchor, 169 by tacks, and 10 by staples. Of the 506 patients, 198 were overhead athletes with a pooled subset of 81 identified baseball players. From the pooled results 83 % had "good-to-excellent" patient satisfaction and 73 % returned to their previous level of sports whereas only 63 % of overhead athletes returned to their previous level. Anchor repair was slightly better than tack repair

Osteoarthritis of the Shoulder

Hemiarthroplasty vs Total Shoulder Replacement for OA of the Shoulder

Sandow MJ, David H, Bentall SJ. Hemiarthroplasty vs total shoulder replacement for rotator cuff intact osteoarthritis: how do they fare after a decade? J Shoulder Elbow Surg. 2013;22(7):877–85.

This study compared the outcome of hemiarthroplasty (HA) and total shoulder replacement (TSR) in osteoarthritis (OA) with a minimum of a 10 year follow-up. Thirty-three patients were intraoperatively randomized to HA or TSR after glenoid exposure (13 HA and 20 TSR). At 6 months and 1 year, the TSR patients had less pain than the HA patients, becoming more apparent at 2 years. There were no differences between the groups at 10 years with respect to pain, function, and daily activities. No patients in the HA group rated their shoulders as pain-free at 10 years; 42 % of the surviving TSR patients rated their shoulders as pain-free at 10 years. Sixty-nine percent of the hemiarthroplasties and 90 % of the total shoulders remained in situ at death or at the 10-year review. TSR seems to have advantages over HA with respect to pain and function at 2 years, and there has not been a reversal of the outcomes on longer follow-up.

Singh JA, Sperling J, Buchbinder R, McMaken K. Surgery for shoulder osteoarthritis: a Cochrane systematic review. J Rheumatol. 2011;38(4):598–605.

A Cochrane Systematic Review of clinical trials of adults with shoulder OA, comparing surgical techniques (total shoulder arthroplasty, hemiarthroplasty, implant types, and fixation) to placebo, sham surgery, nonsurgical modalities, and no treatment to determine the benefits and harm of surgery. There were no controlled trials of surgery versus placebo or nonsurgical interventions. Seven studies with 238 patients were included. Two studies compared total shoulder arthroplasty (TSA) to hemiarthroplasty (n = 88).

Hemiarthroplasty showed significantly worse ASES scores and a trend towards a higher revision rate in hemiarthroplasty compared with TSR. Only one study provided data on pain scores and showed no difference between these two groups or outcomes on the SF-36 or adverse events. The authors concluded that TSR is associated with better shoulder function, with no other demonstrable clinical benefits compared to hemiarthroplasty.

Sperling JW, Cofield RH, Schleck CD, Harmsen WS. Total shoulder arthroplasty versus hemiarthroplasty for rheumatoid arthritis of the shoulder: results of 303 consecutive cases. J Shoulder Elbow Surg. 2007;16(6):683–90.

Three hundred and three consecutive arthroplasties were reviewed in 247 patients with rheumatoid arthritis. There were 195 total shoulder arthroplasties and 108 hemiarthroplasties. One hundred and eighty-seven total shoulder arthroplasties and 95 hemiarthroplasties were available for a minimum 2 year follow-up. All 303 shoulders were included in the survival analysis. Both groups showed a significant long term pain relief, improvement in active abduction, and external rotation in both groups. There was not a significant difference in improvement in pain and motion comparing hemiarthroplasty and TSA for patients with a thin or torn rotator cuff. Among patients with an intact rotator cuff, improvement in pain and abduction were significantly greater with TSA, and the risk for revision lower. Glenoid erosion was present in 98 % of the hemiarthroplasties. Glenoid lucency was present in 72 % of the total shoulder arthroplasties. Among patients with an intact rotator cuff, TSA appears to be the preferred procedure for pain relief, improvement in abduction, and lower risk of revision surgery

Radnay CS, Setter KJ, Chambers L, Levine WN, Bigliani LU, Ahmad CS. Total shoulder replacement compared with humeral head replacement for the treatment of primary glenohumeral osteoarthritis: a systematic review. J Shoulder Elbow Surg. 2007;16(4):396–402.

The objective of this review was to analyze the effect of TSR compared with hemiarthroplasty on rates of pain relief, range of motion, patient satisfaction, and revision surgery in patients with primary OA. This involved a systematic review of the literature from 1966 to 2004. Pain data was converted to a 100-point score. Outcome assessment data were pooled when possible. The authors identified 23 studies, with a total of 1,952 patients and mean follow-up of 43.4 months. Compared with humeral head replacement (HHR), TSR provided significantly greater pain relief, forward elevation, external rotation and patient satisfaction. 6.5 % of all TSRs required revision surgery compared with 10.2 % for HHR. Only 1.7 % of all-polyethylene glenoid components required revision. The authors concluded that on the basis of this review that TSR has significantly better pain relief, range of motion, and satisfaction compared with HHR.

Pfahler M, Jena F, Neyton L, Sirveaux F, Molé D. Hemiarthroplasty versus total shoulder prosthesis: results of cemented glenoid components. J Shoulder Elbow Surg. 2006; 15(2):154–63.

This was a retrospective study that compared the results of 705 total shoulder arthroplasties (TSAs) with 469 hemiarthroplasties (HAs). All operations were performed with the same prosthesis (Aequalis). Patient demographics were the same in each group. The length of follow-up averaged 43 months (range, 24–110 months) in both groups. The postoperative functional outcome and subjective assessment demonstrated the superiority of TSA over HSA independent of age or rotator cuff status (Constant score, 65.7 vs 56.3 points). However X-ray analysis revealed radiolucent lines around the glenoid in 68 % of cases. Outcome was adversely affected by their presence.

Lo IK, Litchfield RB, Griffin S, Faber K, Patterson SD, Kirkley A. Quality-of-life outcome following hemiarthroplasty or total shoulder arthroplasty in patients with osteoarthritis. A prospective, randomized trial. J Bone Joint Surg Am. 2005; 87(10):2178–85.

The purpose of this study was to compare the quality-of-life outcome following hemiarthroplasty or total shoulder arthroplasty in patients with osteoarthritis of the shoulder. Forty-two patients were randomized to receive a hemiarthroplasty or a total shoulder arthroplasty. Patients were evaluated at 6 weeks and periodically to 24 months. Significant improvements in disease-specific quality of life were seen 2 years after both the total shoulder arthroplasties and the hemiarthroplasties. There were no significant differences in quality of life or functional scores between the two groups. The authors concluded that both total shoulder arthroplasty and hemiarthroplasty improve disease-specific and general quality-of-life measurements. Whilst there are no significant differences between the treatment groups there are only small numbers in the study.

Bryant D, Litchfield R, Sandow M, Gartsman GM, Guyatt G, Kirkley A. A comparison of pain, strength, range of motion, and functional outcomes after hemiarthroplasty and total shoulder arthroplasty in patients with osteoarthritis of the shoulder. A systematic review and meta-analysis. J Bone Joint Surg Am. 2005;87(9):1947–56.

A systematic review of the literature (1966–2004) to evaluate the function and range of motion in patients who have had either a hemiarthroplasty or a total shoulder replacement for OA of the shoulder. Four randomized clinical trials were found to be eligible. Analysis focused on the 2-year outcome. The studies revealed a total of 112 patients (50 managed with hemiarthroplasty and 62 managed with total shoulder arthroplasty). A significant moderate effect was detected in the function domain of the UCLA in favour of total shoulder arthroplasty. A significant difference in the pain score was found in favour of the total shoulder arthroplasty group. TSA showed a significant difference in forward elevation. The authors concluded that a minimum of 2 years of follow-up, total shoulder arthroplasty provided better functional outcome than hemiarthroplasty. It was not clear that these results are maintained over time.

Sperling JW, Cofield RH, Rowland CM. Minimum fifteen-year follow-up of Neer hemiarthroplasty and total shoulder arthroplasty in patients aged fifty years or younger. J Shoulder Elbow Surg. 2004;13(6):604–13.

This was a retrospective analysis of 78 Neer hemiarthroplasties and 36 Neer total shoulder arthroplasties performed in patients aged 50 years or less. Sixty-two hemiarthroplasties and 29 total shoulder arthroplasties had complete preoperative evaluation, operative records, and a minimum 15-year follow-up or follow-up until revision. Both procedures provided a significant long-term relief from pain and improvement of movement. There was not a significant difference between total shoulder arthroplasty and hemiarthroplasty with regard to pain relief, abduction, or external rotation. Glenoid erosion was present in 72 % of the hemiarthroplasties. Seventy-six percent of the glenoids showed periprosthetic lucency. The estimated survival rate for hemiarthroplasty was 82 % at 10 years and 75 % at 20 years. The estimated survival rate for total shoulder arthroplasty was 97 % at 10 years and 84 % at 20 years. There was an increased tendency for revision of hemiarthroplasty due to glenoid pain.

Orfaly RM, Rockwood CA Jr, Esenyel CZ, Wirth MA. A prospective functional outcome study of shoulder arthroplasty for osteoarthritis with an intact rotator cuff. J Shoulder Elbow Surg. 2003;12(3):214–21.

This prospective study compared the outcomes from 37 TSA procedures with 28 hemiarthroplasties, followed up for a mean of 4.3 years and comparing pain relief and functional outcome. The results suggested a modest superiority of TSA over hemiarthroplasty in the medium term. Because both TSA and hemiarthroplasty provide considerable and nearly comparable improvement, the authors considered that the long-term risks of glenoid wear and loosening need to be clearly defined before a definitive conclusion could be reached regarding the differential indications for these two procedures.

Edwards TB, Kadakia NR, Boulahia A, Kempf JF, Boileau P, Némoz C, et al. A comparison of hemiarthroplasty and total

shoulder arthroplasty in the treatment of primary glenohumeral osteoarthritis: results of a multicenter study. J Shoulder Elbow Surg. 2003;12(3):207–13.

Six hundred and one total shoulder arthroplasties and 89 hemiarthroplasties were performed for primary osteoarthritis of the shoulder. Patients were evaluated with a clinical examination, Constant score, and radiographic evaluation. The minimum follow-up was 2 years. Total shoulder arthroplasty provided better scores for pain, mobility, and activity than hemiarthroplasty. Fifty-six percent of total shoulder arthroplasties had a radiolucent line around the glenoid component. The authors concluded that total shoulder arthroplasty provides results superior to those of hemiarthroplasty in primary osteoarthritis

Singh JA, Sperling JW, Cofield RH. Revision surgery following total shoulder arthroplasty: analysis of 2588 shoulders over three decades (1976 to 2008). J Bone Joint Surg Br. 2011;93(11):1513–7.

A total of 2,207 patients underwent 2,588 TSAs at the Mayo clinic. Their mean age was 65.0 years (19–91) and 1,163 (53 %) were women. In 63 % the primary diagnosis was osteoarthritis. Overall there was an 8.2 % revision rate. At 5, 10 and 20 years, survival rates were 94.2, 90.2 and 81.4 % respectively. Men had a higher hazard ratio of revision of 1.72 and also those with rotator cuff disease (4.71).

Rotator Cuff Arthropathy and Reverse Shoulder Replacement

Young SW, Zhu M, Walker CG, Poon PC. Comparison of functional outcomes of reverse shoulder arthroplasty with those of hemiarthroplasty in the treatment of cuff-tear arthropathy: a matched-pair analysis. J Bone Joint Surg Am. 2013;95(10):910–5.

The aim of this level III study was to compare the early functional results of hemiarthroplasty with those of reverse shoulder arthroplasty in the management of cuff-tear arthropathy. One hundred and two primary hemiarthroplasties for rotator cuff-tear arthropathy were compared with those of 102 reverse shoulder arthroplasties performed for the same diagnosis. Patients were matched for age sex, comorbidities. OSS (Oxford shoulder scores) were collected 6 months postoperatively. The mean OSS at 6 months was 31.1 in the hemiarthroplasty group and 37.5 in the reverse shoulder arthroplasty group. No difference in mortality rate was seen between the two groups. The authors concluded on the basis of this that reverse shoulder arthroplasty resulted in a functional outcome that was superior to that of hemiarthroplasty but accepted longer term follow-up was required.

Smith CD, Guyver P, Bunker TD. Indications for reverse shoulder replacement: a systematic review. J Bone Joint Surg Br. 2012;94(5):577–83.

Nam D, Kepler CK, Neviaser AS, Jones KJ, Wright TM, Craig EV, et al. Reverse total shoulder arthroplasty: current concepts, results, and component wear analysis. J Bone Joint Surg Am. 2010;92 Suppl 2:23–35.

These two reviews are thorough literature reviews and current concepts of the reverse shoulder prosthesis, describing indications, outcomes and complications of the procedure.

Favard L, Levigne C, Nerot C, Gerber C, De Wilde L, Mole D. Reverse prostheses in arthropathies with cuff tear: are survivorship and function maintained over time? Clin Orthop Relat Res. 2011;469(9):2469–75.

This was a retrospective review of 527 reverse shoulder arthroplasties performed in 506 patients between 1985 and 2003. Clinical and radiographic assessment was performed in 464 patients with a minimum follow-up of 2 years and 148 patients with a minimum follow-up of 5 years (mean, 7.5 years; range, 5–17 years). Cumulative survival curves were established with end points being prosthesis revision and Constant-Murley score of less than 30 points. There were 107 complications in 18 % of the 489 patients. Survivorship free of revision was 89 % at 10 years. Survivorship to a Constant score of less than 30 was 72 % at 10 years. Progressive radiographic changes after 5 years and an increasing frequency of large notches with long-term follow-up were observed. This demonstrates despite a relatively low revision rate there is deterioration in scores and radiographic changes over 10 years. Caution shoulder be exhibited in recommending this for young patients.

Naveed MA, Kitson J, Bunker TD. The Delta III reverse shoulder replacement for cuff tear arthropathy: a single-centre study of 50 consecutive procedures. J Bone Joint Surg Br. 2011;93(1):57–61.

This single surgeon study evaluated the mid-term clinical and radiological results of this arthroplasty in a consecutive series of 50 shoulders in 43 patients with a painful pseudoparalysis from cuff arthropathy. A follow-up of 98 % was achieved, with a mean duration of 39 months (8–81). The mean age of the patients at the time of surgery was 81 years (59–95). The mean American Shoulder and Elbow score and OSS were significantly improved (19–65 for the ASES, 44–23 on the OSS). The mean maximum elevation improved from 55° pre-operatively to 105° at final follow-up. There were seven complications during the whole series, although only four patients required further surgery.

Nolan BM, Ankerson E, Wiater JM. Reverse total shoulder arthroplasty improves function in cuff tear arthropathy. Clin Orthop Relat Res. 2011;469(9):2476–82.

In this retrospective review 67 patients who underwent 71 primary reverse total shoulder arthroplasties (RTSAs) for cuff tear arthropathy were evaluated with the Constant and ASES score at an average of 24 (average, 24 months; range, 12–58 months). Complications were recorded. The average age was 74 years (range, 54–92 years). All scores improved significantly and forward flexion improved from 61° to 121° on average. External rotation was not improved. Forty-nine percent showed radiographic notching and the overall complication rate was 23 %. There were no reoperations. The long term results are still not known.

Wall B, Nové-Josserand L, O'Connor DP, Edwards TB, Walch G. Reverse total shoulder arthroplasty: a review of results according to etiology. J Bone Joint Surg Am. 2007;89(7):1476–85.

Two hundred and forty consecutive reverse total shoulder arthroplasties were performed in 232 patients with an average age of 72.7 years. Patients were grouped according to etiology, and the clinical and radiographic outcomes for each group were measured and compared. Although substantial clinical and functional improvement was observed in all etiology groups, patients with primary rotator cuff tear arthropathy, primary osteoarthritis with a rotator cuff tear, and a massive rotator cuff tear had better outcomes, on average, than patients who had post-traumatic arthritis and those managed with revision arthroplasty. Dislocation and infection were the most common complications.

Calcific Tendonitis

ESWT for Calcific Tendinitis

Huisstede BM, Gebremariam L, van der Sande R, Hay EM, Koes BW. Evidence for effectiveness of Extracorporal Shock-Wave Therapy (ESWT) to treat calcific and non-calcific rotator cuff tendinosis—a systematic review. Man Ther. 2011; 16(5):419–33.

This was a systematic review of studies and randomised controlled trials into the use of extracorporeal shock-wave therapy (ESWT) as an alternative treatment for calcific and non-calcific rotator cuff tendinosis. Seventeen RCTs (11 for calcific tendonitis) were included. Strong evidence was found for effectiveness in favour of high-ESWT versus low-ESWT in short-term in calcific tendonitis. No evidence was found for the effectiveness of ESWT to treat non-calcific rotator cuff (RC) tendinosis.

Moderate evidence was found in favour of high-ESWT versus placebo in short-, mid- and long-term and versus low-ESWT in mid- and long-term outcomes. High-ESWT was more effective (moderate evidence). This review shows that only high-ESWT is effective for treating calcific RC-tendinosis.

Hsu CJ, Wang DY, Tseng KF, Fong YC, Hsu HC, Jim YF. Extracorporeal shock wave therapy for calcifying tendinitis of the shoulder. J Shoulder Elbow Surg. 2008;17(1):55–9.

This was a prospective study in 66 consecutive patients using extracorporeal shock wave therapy (ESWT) for calcific tendinitis. All patients were randomly divided into two groups: treatment and control. The 33 patients in the treatment group received two courses of ESWT. The control group underwent sham treatment with a dummy probe. Patients were evaluated with Constant scores, pain scales and post procedure radiographs. The ESWT results were good to excellent in 87.9 % of shoulders (29/33) and fair in 12.1 % (4/33), and the control results were fair in 69.2 % (9/13) and poor in 30.1 % (4/13). The calcium deposit was completely eliminated in 21 %, decreased in volume in 36 % and unchanged in 45. In the control group 15 % had partial resorption and 85 % remained unchanged. In contrast, elimination was partial in 15.3 % and unchanged in 84.7 %.

Albert JD, Meadeb J, Guggenbuhl P, Marin F, Benkalfate T, Thomazeau H, et al. High-energy extracorporeal shock-wave therapy for calcifying tendinitis of the rotator cuff: a randomised trial. J Bone Joint Surg Br. 2007;89(3):335–41.

This prospective study randomised 80 patients with refractory calcific tendonitis into two groups delivering 2,500 extracorporeal shock waves at either high- or low-energy under fluoroscopic guidance. All calcific deposits measured 10 mm or more. Patients were re-evaluated at a mean of 110 (41–255) days after treatment. The increase in the Constant score was significantly greater in the high energy group. The improvement from the baseline level was significant in the high-energy group and was not significant in the low-energy group. Total or subtotal resorption of the calcification occurred in 15 % in the high-energy group and in 5 % in the low-energy group. The authors concluded that high-energy shock-wave therapy significantly improves symptoms in refractory calcifying tendinitis of the shoulder after 3 months of follow-up. The calcific deposit remains unchanged in size in the majority of patients.

Cacchio A, Paoloni M, Barile A, Don R, de Paulis F, Calvisi V. Effectiveness of radial shock-wave therapy for calcific tendinitis of the shoulder: single-blind, randomized clinical study. Phys Ther. 2006;86(5):672–82.

This single-blind, randomized, controlled study evaluated the effectiveness of radial shockwave therapy (RSWT) for the management of calcific tendinitis of the shoulder. The study included 90 patients with radiologically confirmed calcific tendonitis. After randomisation into control or treatment groups, pain and functional level and radiological outcome were evaluated before and after treatment and at a 6-month follow-up. The treatment group had improvement in all the parameters analysed. The calcification disappeared in 87 % and partially in 13 %. Only 8.8 % of the patients in the control group displayed partially reduced calcification. The results suggest that the use of RSWT for the management of calcific tendinitis of the shoulder is safe and effective, leading to a significant reduction in pain and improvement of shoulder function after 4 weeks, without adverse effects.

Barbotage for Calcific Tendinopathy

Comfort TH, Arafiles RP. Barbotage of the shoulder with image-intensified fluoroscopic control of needle placement for calcific tendinitis. Clin Orthop Relat Res. 1978;(135): 171–8.

One of the first studies of needle lavage or barbotage in calcific tendonitis and reported on the outcome in only nine patients. Followed up for 9 years. The deposit was localised with image intensifier and the deposit irrigated and aspirated.

X-rays taken on follow-up show complete disappearance of the lesion in eight of the cases. One patient had early recurrence of symptoms out of the three who had postbarbotage cortisone injection. Barbotage is simple, effective, with virtually no complications. Failures of the method were apparently due to difficulty in locating the deposit with the needle.

Yoo JC, Koh KH, Park WH, Park JC, Kim SM, Yoon YC. The outcome of ultrasound-guided needle decompression and steroid injection in calcific tendinitis. J Shoulder Elbow Surg. 2010;19(4):596–600.

Thirty-five shoulders in 30 consecutive patients with painful calcific tendinitis were treated by ultrasound-guided needle decompression and subacromial corticosteroid injection. Patients were prospectively evaluated using American Shoulder and Elbow Surgeons (ASES) and Constant scores at 1, 3, and 6 months after the intervention. Size and morphology of the calcific deposits were compared with those in baseline radiographs at each visit. At 6 months after the index procedure 71.4 % showed significant improvements in the ASES and Constant scores. 28.6 % showed no symptom relief at the last follow-up. In those shoulders that showed an improvement in pain there was a significant reduction in the size of the calcific deposit but this did not occur in those with no pain relief. Needle decompression with subacromial steroid injection is effective in 71.4 % of calcific tendinitis within 6 months.

Surgery for Calcific Tendinitis

Ark JW, Flock TJ, Flatow EL, Bigliani LU. Arthroscopic treatment of calcific tendinitis of the shoulder. Arthroscopy. 1992;8(2):183–8.

This study evaluated the outcome of arthroscopic treatment of chronic resistant calcific tendinitis of the shoulder in 23 patients. The average age was 49 years (range 33–60) and average follow-up was 26 months (range 12–47).

Subacromial bursectomy was performed in all patients. Based on follow-up radiographs, 13 patients had partial calcium removal while 9 had complete removal of calcium. Fifty percent regained full motion and complete pain relief, 41 % patients had full motion and occasional episodes of pain, and 9 % remained with persistent pain. The authors concluded that arthroscopic calcium removal and subacromial bursectomy are reasonable alternatives in the treatment of chronic calcific tendinitis resistant to conservative treatment.

Balke M, Bielefeld R, Schmidt C, Dedy N, Liem D. Calcifying tendinitis of the shoulder: midterm results after arthroscopic treatment. Am J Sports Med. 2012;40(3):657–61.

This was a level 4 retrospective study of the mid term results of removal of the calcific deposit in 70 shoulders of 62 patients with a mean age of 54 years. Subacromial decompression in addition was performed in 44 patients. After a mean follow-up of 6 years (range, 2–13 years), patients were clinically investigated, and function was statistically evaluated using Constant and American Shoulder and Elbow Surgeons (ASES) scores. There were no differences in the overall ASES and constant scores between those that received decompression and those that did not. Ultrasound examination at last follow-up (48 shoulders) showed a partial supraspinatus tendon tear in 11 operated and 3 contralateral shoulders. The authors concluded that although the mid term results of arthroscopic treatment are good the rate of partial tearing may be increased after calcium removal. The numbers in the study were small.

Jerosch J, Strauss JM, Schmiel S. Arthroscopic treatment of calcific tendinitis of the shoulder. J Shoulder Elbow Surg. 1998;7(1):30–7.

This study evaluated 48 patients arthroscopically treated for calcific tendinitis. All patients were treated by removal of the calcific deposit whenever possible and resection of the coracoacromial ligament. Patients having a narrowed subacromial space or radiographic evidence of a spur also underwent an acromioplasty. The Constant score was used for postoperative assessment. Surgery significantly improved the Constant score. Those patients with postoperative elimination or reduction of the calcific deposits had significantly better outcomes than those who had no radiographic change. Acromioplasty did not improve the results. The authors concluded that the aim of surgery should be to remove the calcific deposit.

Marder RA, Heiden EA, Kim S. Calcific tendonitis of the shoulder: is subacromial decompression in combination with removal of the calcific deposit beneficial? J Shoulder Elbow Surg. 2011;20(6):955–60.

The aim of this study was to compare patients treated with decompression and debridement of the calcific deposit with those patients that had debridement of the deposit alone for calcific tendonitis. Fifty consecutive patients with calcific tendonitis refractory to non-operative measures were surgically treated by debridement as an isolated procedure (25 patients) or by debridement and concomitant subacromial decompression (25 patients). The two groups were retrospectively compared and the main outcome measure was pain and movement. Mean follow-up was 5 years with a minimum of 2 years. The group that had debridement alone showed a significantly shorter time to return to activity (11 vs 18 weeks) At the final evaluation there was no difference in the functional scores. It was concluded that debridement alone was a better surgical option.

Porcellini G, Paladini P, Campi F, Paganelli M. Arthroscopic treatment of calcifying tendinitis of the shoulder: clinical and ultrasonographic follow-up findings at two to five years. J Shoulder Elbow Surg. 2004;13(5):503–8.

Ninety-five shoulders with calcifying tendinitis of the rotator cuff were treated arthroscopically by the same surgeon and assigned to the same rehabilitation program with a mean follow-up of 36 months. Preoperative and postoperative clinical functional assessment was performed separately by three surgeons using the Constant score. At 24 months, improved Constant scores were inversely related to the number and size of residual calcifications in all patients. Ultrasound examination showed no cuff tears. As outcome seemed to relate strongly only to the presence of residual calcium deposits in the tendon, their complete removal is recommended.

Tillander BM, Norlin RO. Change of calcifications after arthroscopic subacromial decompression. J Shoulder Elbow Surg. 1998;7(3):213–7.

Fifty patients were reviewed after arthroscopic subacromial decompression. Twenty-five had calcific deposits in the rotator cuff visible on X-ray evaluation. Each patient with calcification was matched with a patient without calcification who had a similar state of the rotator cuff, date of surgery, age, and sex. The calcific deposits were left untouched in all cases. No significant difference was found in the postoperative outcome between the patients in the two groups measured by the Constant score. Postoperative X-ray evaluations revealed a disappearance or decrease in size of the calcific deposits in 19 (79 %) of the patients. These results provide new information on the course of calcifying tendinitis, which may indicate that we can leave calcific deposits untouched within the rotator cuff when performing arthroscopic subacromial decompression.

Conservative Treatment for Calcific Tendinitis

Cho NS, Lee BG, Rhee YG. Radiologic course of the calcific deposits in calcific tendinitis of the shoulder: does the initial radiologic aspect affect the final results? J Shoulder Elbow Surg. 2010;19(2):267–72.

The study enrolled 87 consecutive patients (92 shoulders) who were diagnosed with calcific tendinitis and underwent conservative treatment. The mean age at the time of first visit was 53.2 years. The mean follow-up period was 16.1 months. At the final follow-up, there was a significant increase in the Constant and UCLA scores. There were 7 excellent (8 %), 59 good (64 %), and 26 poor (28 %) results. Twelve percent revealed complete resolution of calcific deposits; 50 % decreased in size; 20 % had no change in size; 18 % increased in size. Significant clinical improvement can be expected with conservative treatment over 16 months with 72 % of excellent or good results regardless of the location, radiologic type and size, and initial symptoms of calcific deposits.

Frozen Shoulder

Robinson CM, Seah KT, Chee YH, Hindle P, Murray IR. Frozen shoulder. J Bone Joint Surg Br. 2012;94(1):1–9.

An excellent review of frozen shoulder discussing the epidemiology, pathoanatomy and histological/biochemical changes. There is a thorough literature review discussing the natural history and different treatments available. A treatment algorithm is suggested.

Hand GC, Athanasou NA, Matthews T, Carr AJ. The pathology of frozen shoulder. J Bone Joint Surg Br. 2007; 89(7):928–32.

In this study 22 patients treated for refractory frozen shoulder by arthroscopic release had biopsies taken and histological and immunocytochemical analysis was performed to identify the types of cell present at a mean time from onset of 15 months (3–36).

The tissue was characterised by the presence of fibroblasts, proliferating fibroblasts and chronic inflammatory cells. The infiltrate of chronic inflammatory cells was predominantly made up of mast cells, with T cells, B cells and macrophages also present. The pathology of frozen shoulder includes a chronic inflammatory response with fibroblastic proliferation which may be immunomodulated.

Vastamäki H, Kettunen J, Vastamäki M. The natural history of idiopathic frozen shoulder: a 2- to 27-year follow-up study. Clin Orthop Relat Res. 2012;470(4):1133–43.

This was a retrospective review of 83 patients treated with frozen shoulder. The mean age at onset of symptoms was 53 years. Fifty-one of the 83 patients (52 shoulders) were treated with observation or benign neglect (untreated group), 32 had received some kind of non-operative treatment before the first consultation with the senior author (non-operative group). Twenty patients underwent manipulation. Duration of the disease, pain levels, range of motion (ROM), and Constant scores were recorded. The average duration of the condition was 15 months (range, 4–36 months) in the untreated group, and 20 months (range, 6–60 months) in the non-operative group. At the final follow-up the ROM had improved to the contralateral level in 94 % in the untreated group, and 91 % in the other groups. Fifty-one percent of patients in the untreated group, 44 % in the non-operative group, and 30 % in the manipulation group were totally pain free. The Constant scores were the same in all groups and reaching the normal age- and gender-related scores. The authors concluded that 94 % of patients with spontaneous frozen shoulder recovered to normal levels of function and motion without treatment.

Griggs SM, Ahn A, Green A. Idiopathic adhesive capsulitis. A prospective functional outcome study of non-operative treatment. J Bone Joint Surg Am. 2000;82-A(10):1398–407.

Seventy-five consecutive patients were treated with use of specific shoulder stretching exercises. Patients were evaluated prospectively with regard pain, range of motion, and function. Mean follow-up duration was 22 months (12–40). Ninety percent of the patients reported a satisfactory outcome. Ten percent were not satisfied, 7 % underwent manipulation and/or arthroscopic capsular release. Despite significant improvements in pain and range of motion in those conservatively managed, and high rate of patient satisfaction, there were still significant differences in the pain and motion of the affected shoulder when compared with those of the unaffected, contralateral shoulder. At the final outcome evaluation, the DASH scores demonstrated limitations when compared with known population norms, whereas the profiles of the SF-36 were comparable with those of age and gender-matched control populations. Patients with a greater severity of pain with activity at the initial evaluation had significantly lower DASH and Simple Shoulder Test scores at final evaluation.

Shaffer B, Tibone JE, Kerlan RK. Frozen shoulder. A long-term follow-up. J Bone Joint Surg Am. 1992;74(5):738–46.

This was a cohort of 62 patients with idiopathic frozen shoulder treated non-operatively and followed up at 26 months and at just under 12 years of follow-up (average 7 years). Fifty percent of these patients still had either mild pain or stiffness of the shoulder, or both. The range of motion averaged 161° of forward flexion, 157° of forward elevation, 149° of abduction, 65° of external rotation, and internal rotation to the level of the fifth thoracic spinous process. Sixty percent still demonstrated some restriction of motion as compared with study-generated control values.

Chambler AF, Carr AJ. The role of surgery in frozen shoulder. J Bone Joint Surg Br. 2003;85(6):789–95.

This review examines the evidence to support interventional procedures in treating frozen shoulder. Several series report good results with either open or arthroscopic releases however they often have small numbers and often without a control group. There is limited evidence that surgery truly changes the natural history of the condition.

Rookmoneea M, Dennis L, Brealey S, Rangan A, White B, McDaid C, et al. The effectiveness of interventions in the management of patients with primary frozen shoulder. J Bone Joint Surg Br. 2010;92(9):1267–72.

There is no consensus on how best to manage patients with frozen shoulder. The authors conducted a review of the evidence of the effectiveness of interventions used to manage primary frozen shoulder. In total, 758 titles and abstracts were identified and screened, which resulted in the inclusion of 11 systematic reviews. Although these met most of the quality criteria, there was insufficient evidence to draw firm conclusions about the effectiveness of treatments commonly used to manage a frozen shoulder, mostly due to poor methodology. More rigorous trials are required.

Vastamäki H, Vastamäki M. Motion and pain relief remain 23 years after manipulation under anesthesia for frozen shoulder. Clin Orthop Relat Res. 2013;471(4):1245–50.

The aim of this study was to evaluate the long-term effects of manipulation. They investigated 15 patients (16 shoulders; 12 in women) at 3 months, 7 years, and 19–30 years after manipulation under anesthesia (MUA) for frozen shoulder. The mean age at MUA was 48.5 years. Four patients had diabetes. At 7 years, improvement had occurred in forward flexion to 155°, abduction to 175°, external rotation to 51°, and internal rotation to the T7 level.

During the next 16 years, ROM deteriorated by 8–23° but still equaled that contralateral shoulder. The mean Constant score was 70 (range, 34–88). It was concluded that in this group of patients treatment of idiopathic frozen shoulder by MUA led to improvement in shoulder motion and function that was maintained at a mean 23 years after the procedure.

Thomas WJ, Jenkins EF, Owen JM, Sangster MJ, Kirubanandan R, Beynon C, et al. Treatment of frozen shoulder by manipulation under anaesthetic and injection: does the timing of treatment affect the outcome? J Bone Joint Surg Br. 2011;93(10):1377–81.

This was a retrospective review of a prospectively collected, single-surgeon, consecutive series of 246 patients with a primary frozen shoulder treated by MUA within 4 weeks of presentation. The mean duration of presenting symptoms was 28 weeks (6–156), and time to initial post-operative assessment was 26 days (5–126). The Oxford shoulder score (OSS) significantly improved by a mean of 16 points with a mean at this time of 43 (7–48). Linear regression analysis showed that there was no correlation between the duration of symptoms and the OSS at initial or long term follow-up. At a mean of 42 months there was a sustained improvement with a mean OSS of 44 (16–48). A good outcome can be expected which is independent of the duration of the presenting symptoms, and this improvement is maintained in the long term.

Quraishi NA, Johnston P, Bayer J, Crowe M, Chakrabarti AJ. Thawing the frozen shoulder. A randomised trial comparing manipulation under anaesthesia with hydrodilatation. J Bone Joint Surg Br. 2007;89(9):1197–200.

This study prospectively evaluated the outcome of manipulation under anaesthesia and hydrodilatation as treatments for adhesive capsulitis. There were 36 patients and a total of 38 shoulders. They were randomized into one of the two treatment groups. The mean age of the patients was 55.2 years (44–70) and the mean duration of symptoms was 33.7 weeks (12–76). The patient demographics were the same in both groups. At the final follow-up, 94 % of patients (17 of 18) were satisfied or very satisfied after hydrodilatation compared with 81 % (13 of 16) of those receiving a manipulation. The authors concluded that most of their patients were treated successfully, but those undergoing hydrodilatation did better than those who were manipulated.

Le Lievre HM, Murrell GA. Long-term outcomes after arthroscopic capsular release for idiopathic adhesive capsulitis. J Bone Joint Surg Am. 2012;94(13):1208–16.

This study included patients who had had a circumferential arthroscopic release by a single surgeon. Patient-reported pain scores, shoulder functional scores and shoulder range of motion were assessed preoperatively and at 1, 6, 12, 24, and 52 weeks and at a mean of 7 years after surgery. At a mean follow-up of 7 years (5–13), 43 patients (49 shoulders) had significant improvement in pain, patient-reported shoulder function, stiffness, and difficulty in completing activities compared with the findings at the initial presentation and the 1-year follow-up evaluation. Shoulder motion improved and was comparable with that of the contralateral shoulder. There were no complications. The authors concluded that in contrast to results reported for non-operative treatment, shoulder range of motion at 7 years was equivalent to that in the contralateral shoulder.

Hip

Martin L. Grover and Timothy Kane

Abstract The past half century has seen tremendous advances in treatment of hip arthritis. The outcomes of hip arthroplasty has become clearer, with long term outcome studies presented in this chapter, as have the basic sciences of tribology and wear which are also covered here. The problems of the failed hip replacement, dislocation, infection and revision surgery are dealt with. The past two decades have also seen an increased interest and understanding of the young adult hip, with impingement pathologies and hip arthroscopy which are covered with key references here.

Keywords Hip replacement • Surgical approaches to the hip joint • Uncemented total hip replacement • Cemented total hip replacement • Tribology and basic science • Revision arthroplasty • Infected hip arthroplasty • Dislocation • Avascular necrosis • Arthroscopy • Impingement • Labral pathology

M.L. Grover, MB, FRCS (✉)
T. Kane, MBBS, BSc, FRCS (T&O)
Department of Orthopaedics,
Queen Alexandra Hospital, Portsmouth,
Hampshire P06 3LY, UK
e-mail: mlgrover@doctors.org.uk; kanetimothy@yahoo.com

G. Bowyer, A. Cole (eds.), *Selected References in Trauma and Orthopaedics*, DOI 10.1007/978-1-4471-4676-6_3, © Springer-Verlag London 2014

Hip Replacement (General)

DeLee JG, Charnley J. Radiological demarcation of cemented sockets in total hip replacement. Clin Orthop Relat Res. 1976;(121):20–32.

This paper looked at the frequency of radiological demarcation of the cement-bone junction in the acetabulum in 141 Charnley low-friction arthroplasties at an average of 10 years. Sixty-nine percent showed demarcation of various degrees and 9.2 % had progressive migration of the socket. The vast majority of cases with demarcation were symptomless. In most cases where demarcation was accompanied by migration the operation notes suggested a technical explanation and in three cases low-grade sepsis was responsible.

Gruen TA, McNeice GM, Amstutz HC. "Modes of failure" of cemented stem-type femoral components: a radiographic analysis of loosening. Clin Orthop Relat Res. 1979;(141):17–27.

This was a retrospective radiographic zonal analysis of 389 total hip replacements. It indicated a 19.5 % incidence (76 hips) of radiological evidences of mechanical looseness, i.e., fractured acrylic cement and/or a radiolucent gap at the stem-cement or cement-bone interfaces. It found progressive loosening in 56 of the 76 hips and these were categorized into mechanical modes of failure. The four modes of failure characterizing stem-type component progressive loosening mechanisms consisted of stem pistoning within the acrylic (3.3 %), cement-embedded stem pistoning with the femur (5.1 %), medial midstem pivot (2.5 %), calcar pivot (0.7 %) and bending (fatigue) cantilever (3.3 %).

Note: The original description of radiographic zones provides a universal classification system to map failing cemented femoral components.

Brooker AF, Bowerman JW, Robinson RA, Riley LH Jr. Ectopic ossification following total hip replacement. Incidence and a method of classification. J Bone Joint Surg Am. 1973; 55(8):1629–32.

This paper led to the adoption of the Brooker classification for ectopic bone formation after total hip replacement.

Crowe JF, Mani VJ, Ranawat CS. Total hip replacement in congenital dislocation and dysplasia of the hip. J Bone Joint Surg Am. 1979;61(1):15–23.

This paper looked at the results of 31 total hip replacements (THRs) in 24 patients with either severe congenital dysplasia or dislocation. At an average follow-up of 4 years, 11 were excellent, 16 good, 1 fair in one, and 1 poor. The operative technique included superolateral bone grafts to increase the acetabular coverage in 6 hips. Twenty-seven hips required smaller and straighter femoral components than normal. The incidence of major complications was 19 %.

Sanchez-Sotelo J, Berry DJ, Trousdale RT, Cabanela ME. Surgical treatment of developmental dysplasia of the hip in adults: II. Arthroplasty options. J Am Acad Orthop Surg. 2002;10(5):334–44.

Total hip arthroplasty is the procedure of choice for most patients with symptomatic end-stage coxarthrosis secondary to hip dysplasia. The anatomic abnormalities associated with the dysplastic hip increase the complexity of hip arthroplasty. When pelvic bone stock allows, it is desirable to reconstruct the socket at or near the normal anatomic acetabular location. To obtain sufficient bony coverage of the acetabular component, the socket can be medialized or elevated, or a lateral bone graft can be applied. Femoral shortening is sometimes required, through metaphyseal resection with a greater trochanteric osteotomy and advancement or by a shortening subtrochanteric osteotomy. Uncemented acetabular components allow biologic fixation with potentially improved results compared with cemented cups, especially in young patients. The location of the acetabular reconstruction and the desired leg length influence the type of femoral reconstruction. Cemented and uncemented implants can be used in femoral reconstruction, depending on the clinical situation. The results of total hip arthroplasty demonstrate a high rate of pain relief and functional improvement. The long-term durability of cemented total hip arthroplasty reconstruction in these patients is inferior to that in the general population. The results of uncemented implants are promising, but only limited early and midterm data are available.

Sanchez-Sotelo J, Trousdale RT, Berry DJ, Cabanela ME. Surgical treatment of developmental dysplasia of the hip in adults: I. Nonarthroplasty options. J Am Acad Orthop Surg. 2002;10(5):321–33.

Hip dysplasia is a developmental disorder that results in anatomic abnormalities leading to increased contact pressure in the joint and, eventually, coxarthrosis. However, many patients with hip dysplasia become symptomatic before the development of severe degenerative changes because of abnormal hip biomechanics, mild hip instability, impingement, or associated labral pathology. Several non-arthroplasty treatment options are available. Because the primary deformity is mostly acetabular, for many patients, a reconstructive osteotomy that restores more nearly normal pelvic anatomy is preferable. The Bernese periacetabular osteotomy is presently favoured because it provides good correction while creating little secondary pelvic deformity or destabilizing the pelvis. Proximal femoral osteotomy is occasionally needed as a complement to pelvic osteotomy and may also be indicated as an isolated procedure when most deformity is located on the femoral side (coxa valga subluxans). Arthroscopy can be beneficial when symptoms seem to be related only to labral tears or loose bodies in the absence of severe structural abnormalities about the hip. Fusion and resection arthroplasty are rarely indicated.

Barrack RL, Mulroy RD Jr, Harris WH. Improved cementing techniques and femoral component loosening in young patients with hip arthroplasty. A 12-year radiographic review. J Bone Joint Surg Br. 1992;74(3):385–9.

This paper reviewed 50 'second-generation' cemented hip arthroplasties in 44 patients aged 50 years or less. The femoral stems were all collared and rectangular in cross-section with rounded corners. The cement was delivered by a gun into a medullary canal occluded distally with a cement plug. At an average of 12 years follow-up no femoral component was revised for aseptic loosening, and only one stem was definitely loose by radiographic criteria. By contrast, 11 patients had undergone revision for symptomatic aseptic loosening of the acetabular component and 11 more had radiographic signs of acetabular loosening.

Approaches to the Hip Joint

These papers provide details of the surgical approaches. Preservation of the neurovascular supply to the anterior fibres of gluteus maximus, regardless of the approach to the hip joint, is important if good function is to be maintained.

Dall D. Exposure of the hip by anterior osteotomy of the greater trochanter: a modified antero-lateral approach. J Bone Joint Surg Br. 1986;68(3):382–6.

Hardinge K. The direct lateral approach to the hip. J Bone Joint Surg Br. 1982;64(1):17–9.

Learmonth ID, Allan PE. The omega lateral approach to the hip. J Bone Joint Surg Br. 1996;78(4):559–61.

Gibson A. Posterior exposure of the hip joint. J Bone Joint Surg Br. 1950;32-B(2):183–6.

Moore AT. The Moore self-locking Vitallium prosthesis in fresh femoral neck fractures: a new low posterior approach (the southern exposure). In: AAOS Instructional Course Lectures, vol 16. St Louis: CV Mosby, Co.; 1959. p. 309–21.

McFarland B, Osborne G. Approach to the hip: a suggested improvement on Kocher's method. J Bone Joint Surg Br. 1954;36-B(3): 364–7.

English TA. The trochanteric approach to the hip for prosthetic replacement. J Bone Joint Surg Am. 1975;57(8):1128–33.

Ganz R, Gill TJ, Gautier E, Ganz K, Krügel N, Berlemann U. Surgical dislocation of the adult hip: a technique with full access to the femoral head and acetabulum without the risk of avascular necrosis. J Bone Joint Surg Br. 2001;83(8):1119–24.

Uncemented Total Hip Replacement

Dumbleton J, Manley MT. Hydroxyapatite-coated prostheses in total hip and knee arthroplasty. J Bone Joint Surg Am. 2004;86-A(11):2526–40.

Hydroxyapatite (HA) coated implants have demonstrated extensive bone apposition in animal models. The osseous interface develops even in the presence of gaps of 1 mm and relative motion of up to 500 μm. Development of implant-bone interfacial strength is due to the biological effects of released calcium and phosphate ions, although surface roughness leads to increased interface strength in the absence of interface gaps. The clinical results at 15 years after THR have demonstrated that HA-coated femoral stems perform as well as, and possibly better than, other types of cementless devices, with the added benefit of providing a seal against wear debris. Hydroxyapatite-coated acetabular components must have a mechanical interlock with bone in order to take advantage of the coating effects. Clinical analyses of these types of designs at 7 years have indicated good survivorship. The performance of HA-coated implant depends on coating properties (thickness, porosity, HA content, and crystallinity), implant roughness, and overall design. The most reliable predictor of the performance of a device is success in long-term clinical studies.

Cemented Total Hip Replacement

Schulte KR, Callaghan JJ, Kelley SS, Johnston RC. The outcome of Charnley total hip arthroplasty with cement after a minimum twenty-year follow-up. The results of one surgeon. J Bone Joint Surg Am. 1993;75(7):961–75.

Three hundred and thirty cemented Charnley THRs were performed with 262 patients between 1970 and 1972. At a minimum of 20 years after the index operation, 83 patients (98 THRs) were still living and the outcome of 322 (98 %) of the 330 arthroplasties was known at the latest follow-up evaluation. Of the 98 hips in the living patients, 85 % caused no pain, 14 % caused mild pain, and 1 % caused moderate pain. Fifty-three percent were in patients who did not use walking aids, and only 7 % were in patients who used support for walking because of the hip. At the minimum 20-year follow-up, 10 % of the 322 hips that had been followed had been revised: 2 % because of loosening with infection; 7 %, because of aseptic loosening; 1 %, because of dislocation.

Comment: This impressive single surgeon series sets out the results which can be achieved for cemented arthroplasty.

Wroblewski BM, Taylor GW, Siney P. Charnley low-friction arthroplasty: 19- to 25-year results. Orthopedics. 1992;15(4): 421–4.

This review from Wrightington of 57 Charnley THRs with a 19–25 year follow-up shows that clinical results remain excellent; clinical results bear no relation to the radiologic appearances of the bone-cement interface on the acetabular side; and the long-term problem is socket wear. The need for regular follow-up and study of factors affecting socket wear is emphasized.

Ling RS, Charity J, Lee AJ, Whitehouse SL, Timperley AJ, Gie GA. The long-term results of the original Exeter polished cemented femoral component: a follow-up report. J Arthroplasty. 2009;24(4):511–7.

This paper presents a long-term follow-up report of the results of the original Exeter polished cemented stems inserted between November 1970 and the end of 1975 by surgeons of widely differing experience using crude cementing techniques. From the original series of 433 hips, there were, at the end of 2003, 26 living patients with 33 hips. Of the latter, there were 25 hips in 20 patients with their original femoral components still in situ. With the end point reoperation for aseptic stem loosening, the survivorship is 93.5 %. The reoperation rate for aseptic femoral component loosening is 3.23 % into the 33rd year of follow-up.

Lewthwaite SC, Squires B, Gie GA, Timperley AJ, Ling RS. The Exeter Universal hip in patients 50 years or younger at 10–17 years' follow-up. Clin Orthop Relat Res. 2008;466(2): 324–31.

This paper reports the performance of the Exeter Universal hip in younger patients. It reviews the survivorship and the clinical and radiographic outcomes of this hip in 107 patients (130 hips) 50 years old or younger at the time of surgery. The mean age at surgery was 42 years. The minimum follow-up was 10 years. 12 hips had been revised, of which 9 had aseptic loosening of the acetabular component and one cup was revised for focal lysis and pain. One hip was revised for recurrent dislocation and one joint underwent revision for infection. X-rays demonstrated 14 (12.8 %) of the remaining acetabular prostheses were loose but no femoral components were loose. Survivorship of both stem and cup from all causes was 92.6 % at an average of 12.5 years. Survivorship of the stem from all causes was 99 % and no stem was revised for aseptic loosening. The Exeter Universal stem performed well, even in the young, high-demand patient.

Middleton RG, Howie DW, Costi K, Sharpe P. Effects of design changes on cemented tapered femoral stem fixation. Clin Orthop Relat Res. 1998;(355):47–56.

The effects of matte finish and modularity on loosening of tapered stems using the same cementing technique were studied prospectively. In 80 patients, 82 cemented Exeter primary stems were implanted at total hip revision by one surgeon using the same surgical and cementing technique throughout the series. The polished stems behaved differently than the matte surfaced stems behaved. Polished stems subsided in the cement mantle an average of 1 mm at 2 years after implantation, but without subsequent loosening of stems up to 12 years after implantation. Matte surfaced stems with metal centralizers had a higher loosening rate, and loss of fixation at the prosthesis to cement interface was identified as an early sign of loosening of these stems. At a mean 6-year follow-up, there were no revisions or radiographic evidence of loosening of the polished modular stems. It is concluded that matte finish results in increased loosening of tapered stems but the introduction of modularity did not.

Tribology and Basic Science

Bartz RL, Nobel PC, Kadakia NR, Tullos HS. The effect of femoral component head size on posterior dislocation of the artificial hip joint. J Bone Joint Surg Am. 2000;82(9):1300–7.

In addition to technical and patient-associated factors, prosthetic features have also been shown to influence stability of the artificial hip joint. This cadaveric study showed significant associations between the femoral head size and the degree of flexion at dislocation 10°, 20° and 30° of adduction. Increasing the femoral head size from 22 to 28 mm increased the range of flexion by an average of 5.6° prior to impingement and by an average of 7.6° prior to posterior dislocation; however, increasing the head size from 28 to 32 mm did not lead to more significant improvement in the range of joint motion. The site of impingement prior to dislocation varied with the size of the femoral head. With a 22-mm head, impingement occurred between the neck of the femoral prosthesis and the acetabular liner, whereas with a 32-mm head, impingement most frequently occurred between the osseous femur and the pelvis.

Schreurs BW, Buma P, Huiskes R, Slagter JL, Slooff TJ. Morsellized allografts for fixation of the hip prosthesis femoral component. A mechanical and histological study in the goat. Acta Orthop Scand. 1994;65(3):267–75.

To simulate femoral intramedullary bone stock loss in revision surgery of failed total hip arthroplasties, a method was developed using impacted trabecular bone grafts. In 14 goats a cemented total hip arthroplasty was performed, fixating the stem within a circumferential construction of bone allografts. After 6 or 12 weeks, 4 goats were used for mechanical tests and 3 for histology. The stability of the stems was determined in a loading experiment with roentgen-stereophotogrammetric analysis. One aseptic loosening was seen with gross movements. Histologically, revascularization and remodeling of the grafts were evident. Bone apposition and bone resorption of the grafts resulted in a mixture of graft and new bone. There was more new bone formation in the 12-week group, but the process was not yet completed. The use of impacted trabecular bone grafts in cases of severe intramedullary bone stock loss seems to be a promising revision technique.

Comment: The success of impaction bone grafting in revision hip surgery is now well established. This was one of the earlier basic science studies which set the scene for its widespread introduction. The importance of graft size and preparation is emphasised.

Charles MN, Bourne RB, Davey JR, Greenwald AS, Morrey BF, Rorabeck CH. Soft-tissue balancing of the hip: the role of femoral offset restoration. Instr Course Lect. 2005;54:131–41.

Inadequate soft-tissue balancing is a major yet often underemphasized cause of failure for primary and revision total hip arthroplasty. Accordingly, contemporary cemented and cementless hip prostheses have been designed with consideration of this issue, and this has substantially increased the long-term survival of total hip replacements. This paper offers a full description and anatomical study of the role of offset in soft tissue balancing at total hip arthroplasty. Detailed description of pre operative planning and intraoperative tests are provided. The dangers of simply increasing leg length to address inadequate soft tissue tension is discussed.

Gandhe A, Grover M. Head size, does it matter? Curr Orthop. 2008;22(3):155–164.

This paper looks at differing diameter of head size from a tribological point of view as well as clinical. Charnley set the debate in motion in his paper on Low Friction Arthroplasty with the emphasis on finding the ideal head size to reduce friction and therefore, it was thought, wear. As our understanding of tribology improved and with the development of more wear-resistant materials, the emphasis has shifted towards finding the ideal size to improve joint stability. The ability to use large diameter heads has provided an opportunity to expand the indications for total hip arthroplasty to include trauma and younger patients.

Comment: Although increasing the head size has been shown to reduce dislocation rates it has only a minimal effect on range of movement beyond 36 mm. The consequences of reducing the thickness of the acetabular bearing material gives rise to cause for concern.

Howcroft D, Head M, Steele N. Bearing surfaces in the young patient: out with the old and in with the new? Curr Orthop. 2008;22(3):177–84.

This review article looks at the alternatives for bearing surfaces in total hip arthroplasty. Metal on ultra high molecular weight polyethylene (UHMWPE) remains the gold standard but predictably fails by way of osteolysis secondary to polyethylene wear, particularly in the active patient. This has prompted a resurgence in the development and use of the previously tried but forgotten ceramic and metal articulations, as well as the advent of the new highly-crosslinked polyethylene.

Dumbleton JH, Manley MT, Edidin AA. A literature review of the association between wear rate and osteolysis in total hip arthroplasty. J Arthroplasty. 2002;17(5):649–61.

This literature review looks at wear and osteolysis measurement. The incidence of osteolysis increases as the rate of wear increases. The literature indicates that osteolysis rarely is observed at a wear rate of <0.1 mm/year. The paper suggests that a practical wear rate threshold of 0.05 mm/year would eliminate osteolysis. This wear threshold suggests that the new cross-linked polyethylenes would reduce osteolysis, provided that in vivo wear rates mirror those observed in vitro.

Comment: This review is a precursor to the widespread introduction of a new generation of highly cross linked polyethylene. If its behaviour in vivo is the same as in vitro, it should be capable of producing wear rates well below 0.05 mm/year and as a consequence reducing or eliminating osteolysis in the average patient.

Weinrauch PC, Bell C, Wilson L, Goss B, Lutton C, Crawford RW. Shear properties of bilaminar polymethylmethacrylate cement mantles in revision hip joint arthroplasty. J Arthroplasty. 2007;22(3):394–403.

Although cement-within-cement revision arthroplasty minimizes the complications associated with removal of secure polymethylmethacrylate (PMMA), failure at the interfacial region between new and old cement mantles remains a theoretical concern. This article assesses the variability in shear properties of bilaminar cement mantles related to duration of postcure and the use of antibiotic cements. Bilaminar cement mantles were 15–20 % weaker than uniform mantles and demonstrated variability in shear strength related to duration of postcure of the freshly applied cement. The use of Antibiotic Simplex did not significantly influence interfacial cement adhesion. Interfacial adhesion by mechanisms other than mechanical interlock plays a significant role in the bond formed between new and old PMMA cements, with an important contribution by diffusion-based molecular interdigitation. In the presence of a secure cement-bone interface, the authors recommend cement-within-cement revision techniques in suitable patients.

Comment: This article also provides a very useful overview of the composition and mechanical properties of PMMA cement.

Kurtz S, Medel FJ, Manley M. Wear in highly crosslinked polyethylenes. Curr Orthop. 2008;22(6):392–9.

This is a review of the applications of cross linked polyethylene for use in the hip. Basic science of cross linking is presented together with clinical studies comparing differing types of highly cross-linked polyethylene (HXLPE). The issue of in vivo oxidation and increased brittleness are discussed. Because of its improved wear-resistance, crosslinked polyethylene is now regarded as a desirable technology for hip articulations. The paper provides an overview of the basic science concepts and terminology surrounding crosslinked polyethylene and the two main thermal processing techniques: annealing or remelting the polymer after irradiative crosslinking. The second part of the review is a critical assessment of the literature on femoral head penetration and wear in crosslinked polyethylenes measured in clinical studies.

Leslie IJ, Williams S, Isaac G, Ingham E, Fisher J. High cup angle and microseparation increase the wear of hip surface replacements. Clin Orthop Relat Res. 2009;467(9):2259–65.

In vitro testing of large bearing metal on metal surface replacements demonstrated that increased cup inclination angle and micro separation produced substantial increase in wear rates together with larger wear particles. The importance of correct head and cup position impart a critical influence on the wear rate of these bearings.

Livermore J, Ilstrup D, Morrey B. Effect of femoral head size on wear of the polyethylene acetabular component. J Bone Joint Surg Am. 1990;72(4):518–28.

This was an early review following development of a technique to determine accurately the wear of acetabular components. Critical analysis of the volumetric and linear wear of three head sizes was undertaken: 385 hips were followed for at least 9.5 years after replacement. The smallest volumetric and rate of linear wear were associated with use of a femoral head that had a diameter of 28-mm. The greatest amount and mean rate of linear wear occurred with 22-mm components, but these differences were not statistically significant. The greatest volumetric wear and mean rate of volumetric wear were seen with 32-mm components. A wider radiolucent line in acetabular Zone 1 was associated with use of the 32-mm head. The amounts of resorption of the proximal part of the femoral neck and of lysis of the proximal part of the femur both correlated positively with the extent of linear and volumetric wear; this suggests an association between the amount of debris from wear and these changes in the femoral neck and proximal part of the femur.

Comment: This remains an often quoted and frequently used paper although, with the advent of highly cross linked polyethylene some of the conclusions are being challenged.

Kärrholm J, Gill RH, Valstar ER. The history and future of radiostereometric analysis. Clin Orthop Relat Res. 2006;448:10–21.

Extensive review article on the science and application of Radio Stereometric Analysis (RSA) in Orthopaedics.

Comment: This should be considered the gold standard in any study measuring the rate of wear of polyethylene acetabular components.

Scheerlinck T, Casteleyn PP. The design features of cemented femoral hip implants. J Bone Joint Surg Br. 2006;88(11): 1409–18.

This is a review of the literature of two basic stem designs in cemented THR: loaded taper (force-closed) or composite beam (shape-closed) designs. Both design principles are capable of producing successful long-term results, providing that their specific requirements of stem metallurgy, shape and surface finish, preparation of the bone and handling of the cement are observed.

Comment: This article is an important reminder to the operating surgeon of the need to understand that the principles of fixation of an individual cemented stem rely on its design philosophy.

Revision Arthroplasty

Paprosky WG, Perona PG, Lawrence JM. Acetabular defect classification and surgical reconstruction in revision arthroplasty. A 6-year follow-up evaluation. J Arthroplasty. 1994;9(1):33–44.

This paper provides a comprehensive description of the most often used classification system for acetabular deficiencies, based on findings from 147 cemented acetabular components which were revised with cementless hemispheric press-fit components. The acetabular defects were typed from 1 to 3 and reconstructed with a bulk or support allograft. Size, orientation, and method of fixation of the allografts play an important role in the integrity of structural allografts, while adequate remaining host-bone must be present to ensure bone ingrowth.

Weeden SH, Schmidt RH. The use of tantalum porous metal implants for Paprosky 3A and 3B defects. J Arthroplasty. 2007;22(6 Suppl 2):151–5.

Implants made from highly porous tantalum metal provide a surface that is highly conducive to bone ingrowth. This short-term follow-up reviews 43 acetabular revisions treated with tantalum acetabular implants, used for severe acetabular defects (Paprosky type 3A and 3B defects). The overall success rate was 98 %.

Johanson NA, Driftmier KR, Cerynik DL, Stehman CC. Grading acetabular defects: the need for a universal and valid system. J Arthroplasty. 2010;25(3):425–31.

The systems for grading acetabular bone loss preoperatively in revision THR are reviewed in this paper. Only one of the systems in use had useful reliability and validity.

Mandziak DG, Howie DW, Neale SD, McGee MA. Cement-within-cement stem exchange using the collarless polished double taper stem. J Arthroplasty 2007;22(7): 1000–6.

This paper provides a clinical and radiographic study of 23 revisions prospectively monitored up to 12 years. There were no subsequent stem revisions and no radiographic evidence of loosening. Subsidence of the stem (a design feature) was similar to that in primary arthroplasty with this stem.

Quinlan JF, O'Shea K, Doyle F, Brady Oh. In-cement technique for revision hip arthroplasty. J Bone Joint Surg 2006; 88(6):730–3.

This paper showed consistently high function using cement-in-cement rather than total cement removal in 51 patients followed up for a mean of 29 months. There were no radiological signs of loosening and good hip scores.

Masterson EL, Masri BA, Duncan CP. Surgical approaches in revision hip replacement. J Am Acad Orthop Surg. 1998;6(2): 84–92.

This paper gives a most useful overview of the challenges faced by the revision hip surgeon and details several approaches and techniques to deal with component extraction and bone loss. It emphasizes the importance of surgical approach and the potential need for an extended exposure.

Toms AD, Barker RL, Jones RS, Kuiper JH. Impaction bone-grafting in revision joint replacement surgery. J Bone Joint Surg Am. 2004;86-A(9):2050–60.

This is a current concepts review and as such includes the history of impaction bone grafting (with useful references), technical aspects of the procedure, together with classification of bone defects in both hip and knee. It emphasizes that morcellised graft must be sufficiently compacted to allow immediate mechanical stability. The most common complications are femoral diaphyseal fracture and excessive implant migration.

Gie GA, Linder L, Ling RS, Simon JP, Slooff TJ, Timperley AJ. Impacted cancellous allografts and cement for revision total hip arthroplasty. J Bone Joint Surg Br. 1993;75(1):14–21.

This early series reported success with the cemented impaction grafting technique and the Exeter stem.

Halliday BR, English HW, Timperley AJ, Gie GA, Ling RS. Femoral impaction grafting with cement in revision total hip replacement. Evolution of the technique and results. J Bone Joint Surg Br. 2003;85(6):809–17.

This is a detailed account of biomechanical and biological studies of impaction bone grafting and cement. It presents the results using a tapered polished stem in 207 patients with more than 5-years follow-up. Twelve required further surgery for femoral fracture (10) or loosening (2); 2 had early postoperative infection.

As a consequence of this experience, the authors adopted increased usage of a longer femoral stem in these revision cases especially when the host bone around the tip of the standard stem would be poor, when there was major bone loss or a femoral fracture.

Infected Hip Arthroplasty

Toms AD, Davidson D, Masri BA, Duncan CP. The management of peri-prosthetic infection in total joint arthroplasty. J Bone Joint Surg Br. 2006;88(2):149–55.

A comprehensive review of the management of periprosthetic infection with emphasis on a two stage procedure with an articulated spacer used between stages. A classification for infection presentation is put forward together with guidelines for diagnosis. The quadruple approach of clinical evaluation, serology (erythrocyte sedimentation rate [ESR] and C-reactive protein [CRP]), diagnostic imaging and microbiology is proposed. The value of pre-operative aspiration and culture is emphasized. Treatment options and potential pitfalls are discussed in detail.

Willis-Owen CA, Konyves A, Martin DK. Factors affecting the incidence of infection in hip and knee replacement: an analysis of 5277 cases. J Bone Joint Surg Br. 2010;92(8): 1128–33.

A large series (>5,000) of hip and knee replacements reviewed in detail revealing an overall infection rate of just below 1 %. Male gender and prolonged operating time (tourniquet time in total knee replacement) were the most predictive of infection.

Biring GS, Kostamo T, Garbuz DS, Masri BA, Duncan CP. Two-stage revision arthroplasty of the hip for infection using an interim articulated Prostolac hip spacer: a 10- to 15-year follow-up study. J Bone Joint Surg Br. 2009;91(11):1431–7.

This is a 10–15 year follow-up study reporting outcomes with this two stage procedure in 99 patients. Success rate for eradicating infection was 89 %, rising to 96 % after additional surgery was performed for a small number. This series produces further evidence of the efficacy of a two stage revision procedure for infection using an antibiotic eluting hip spacer.

Morley JR, Blake SM, Hubble MJ, Timperley AJ, Gie GA, Howell JR. Preservation of the original femoral cement mantle during the management of infected cemented total hip replacement by two-stage revision. J Bone Joint Surg Br. 2012;94(3):322–7.

This paper reports a series of 15 patients with 2-stage revision but with retention of the original well-fixed cement mantle. Two patients had positive cultures at the second stage, managed with 6-weeks of antibiotics. One had recurrent infection managed with a further revision.

Comment: A series that challenged some previously held views about complete removal of all inert material during debridement of an infected hip replacement. A well fixed and intact femoral cement mantle can be safely left in situ at the first stage revision procedure.

Stockley I, Mockford BJ, Hoad–Reddick A, Norman P. The use of two-stage exchange arthroplasty with depot antibiotics in the absence of long-term antibiotic therapy in infected total hip replacement. J Bone Joint Surg Br. 2008;90(2):145–8.

A series of over 100 patients treated by a two stage exchange procedure for chronically infected total hip replacement. In these cases a prolonged interval course of antibiotic therapy was not used but an antibiotic loaded spacer was used between stages. The authors report an 87.7 % success rate.

Comment: This and subsequent papers challenge the need to use prolonged courses of intravenous (IV) antibiotics provided thorough debridement and the use of antibiotic impregnated spacers are used for the first stage.

Oussedik SI, Dodd MB, Haddad FS. Outcomes of revision total hip replacement for infection after grading according to a standard protocol. J Bone Joint Surg Br. 2010;92(9): 1222–6.

A series of 50 patients with infected total hip replacements, assessed according to a standardised protocol, is presented. The 11 treated with single-stage revision had no recurrence of infection; the 9 treated with 2-stage revision had 2 recurrences which were both successfully treated with further 2-stage revision. The outcome scores were better for those treated with single-stage revision. Single stage exchange is successful in eradicating infection but identification of patients suitable for the single stage should be done appropriately.

Fitzgerald RH Jr. Infected total hip arthroplasty: diagnosis and treatment. J Am Acad Orthop Surg. 1995;3(5):249–62.

A comprehensive clinical review detailing the classification, diagnosis and management of periprosthetic infection.

Comment: Although the prevalence of infecting organisms has changed over the past decade and single stage revision is gaining in popularity, this work provides a very useful overview of the salient aspects of joint infection.

Hanssen AD, Spangehl MJ. Treatment of the infected hip replacement. Clin Orthop Relat Res. 2004;(420):63–71.

This paper proposes that the essence of successful treatment requires complete debridement of the infected and foreign material and appropriate anti-microbial treatment. The authors prefer 2-stage delayed reconstruction.

Matthews PC, Berendt AR, McNally MA, Byren I. Diagnosis and management of prosthetic joint infection. BMJ. 2009;338:b1773.

This is a comprehensive clinical review from the Oxford Group highlighting the importance of co-ordinated multidisciplinary team approach requiring both sound surgical and microbiological principles in the management of these cases.

Comment: Well referenced article particularly with some online references which are useful.

Atkins BL, Athanasou N, Deeks JJ, Crook DW, Simpson H, Peto TE, et al. Prospective evaluation of criteria for microbiological diagnosis of prosthetic joint infection at revision arthroplasty. The Osiris Collaborative Study Group. J Clin Microbiol. 1998;36(10):2932–9.

A prospective study establishing the criteria for microbiological diagnosis of joint infection combining histological findings with cultures from multiple specimens. Three hundred and thirty-four patients were studied of whom 41 had infection, but only 65 % of these were culture positive. The group recommend taking five or six specimens, and if three or more have indistinguishable organisms this implies infection. Gram stain was not felt to be helpful.

Comment: The work highlights the importance of obtaining multiple specimens and details how and from where the tissue samples should be obtained.

Dislocation

Blom AW, Rogers M, Taylor AH, Pattison G, Whitehouse S, Bannister GC. Dislocation following total hip replacement: the Avon Orthopaedic Centre experience. Ann R Coll Surg Engl. 2008;90(8):658–62.

A large multi surgeon audit of dislocation after total hip replacement in a single unit with an 8–11 year follow-up. Dislocation rates were approximately 4 % for the posterior and Hardinge approach and 0 % for the Omega approach. Almost 59 % of dislocations after primary total hip replacement became recurrent. Revision hip surgery produced increased rates of dislocation of 8.1 % of which 70 % became recurrent. The large majority of dislocations occurred within 2 months of surgery.

Bourne RB, Mehin R. The dislocating hip: what to do, what to do. J Arthroplasty. 2004;19(4 Suppl 1):111–4.

The authors look at the aetiology and management of dislocation following primary total hip replacement. Sixty percent dislocated in the first 5 weeks, and closed reduction was successful in 67 %. If recurrence occurs, then revision surgery brings about stability in only 61 %. Many techniques have been used for the operative treatment of recurrent dislocation: the paper sums up with a useful algorithm for the surgical management of the unstable total hip replacement.

Rogers M, Blom AW, Barnett A, Karantana A, Bannister GC. Revision for recurrent dislocation of total hip replacement. Hip Int. 2009;19(2):109–13.

An interesting review of a cohort of 70 patients undergoing revision surgery for recurrent dislocation, the majority following primary rather than revision surgery. Stability was achieved in 75 % of patients dislocating after primary and 50 % after revision total hip replacement. The authors had a higher success rate stabilising posterior dislocations following the posterior approach than anterior dislocations following the transgluteal (Hardinge) approach. Cup augmentation conferred stability in about 90 %.

Williams JT Jr, Ragland PS, Clarke S. Constrained components for the unstable hip following total hip arthroplasty: a literature review. Int Orthop. 2007;31(3):273–7.

A review analysing eight publications between 1994 and 2005 reporting the use of various types of constrained acetabular liner. The most common modes of failure are discussed and the authors conclude that this method is an option for patients who have failed management of instability with other implants, patients with cognitive problems and those with deficient abductors. The mean rate of redislocation following revision with a constrained liner was 10 %. It is suggested that their use is particularly relevant to elderly or low demand individuals with well positioned primary implants.

Comment: Constrained liners are prone to mechanical failure either of the locking mechanism itself or fixation of the implants due to impingement.

Yun AG, Padgett D, Pellicci P, Dorr LD. Constrained acetabular liners: mechanisms of failure. J Arthroplasty. 2005;20(4): 536–41.

The modes of failure were identified in 29 dislocating hips managed with constrained liners: failure of fixation to the pelvis; liner dissociation; biomaterial failure; femoral head dislocation. The authors point out the vulnerability to mechanical overload and emphasise the need to avoid impingement.

Berend KR, Lombardi AV Jr, Mallory TH, Adams JB, Russell JH, Groseth KL. The long term outcome of 755 consecutive constrained acetabular components in total hip arthroplasty. J Arthroplasty. 2005;20(7 Suppl 3):93–102.

A large series with long term results encompassing constrained cup use in primary conversion and revision operations. Despite their use further dislocation was common (17.5 %, 28.9 % if used for recurrent dislocation). The authors highlight particular aspects of previous history which pose a significant risk of failure, which occurred in 42 % on a long-term basis.

Grigoris P, Grecula MJ, Amstutz HC. Tripolar hip replacement for recurrent prosthetic dislocation. Clin Orthop Relat Res. 1994;(304):148–55.

An early paper describing the use of the tripolar hip replacement for recurrent dislocation in eight patients. All were stable at a mean of 4-years follow-up.

Comment: This prosthesis is gaining wider use and acceptance and is used by some as an alternative to either a large head or a constrained cup.

Avascular Necrosis

Steinberg ME, Hayken GD, Steinberg DR. A quantitative system for staging avascular necrosis. J Bone Joint Surg Br. 1995;77(1):34–41.

With the advent of magnetic resonance imaging (MRI), existing staging systems suggested by, amongst others, Ficat needed updating. This paper evaluates 1,000 hips over a 12 year period using bone Scan and MRI. Seven stages of avascular necrosis, 0 to VI, are suggested based upon the type of radiological change demonstrated. The extent of such involvement is then measured allowing more accurate evaluation and better comparison with the different methods of management.

Mont MA, Zywiel MG, Marker DR, McGrath MS, Delanois RE. The natural history of untreated asymptomatic osteonecrosis of the femoral head: a systematic literature review. J Bone Joint Surg Am. 2010;92(12):2165–70.

Sixteen published papers were reviewed to determine which asymptomatic hips (usually second side under observation) progressed to symptomatic disease or collapse of the femoral head. Radiographic and demographic factors were evaluated to determine their influence on progression and prognosis. Small medial lesions had the best prognosis, as less than 10 % collapsed. Sickle cell disease had the highest progression, whereas systemic lupus erythematosus (SLE) had the most benign course.

Nam KW, Kim YL, Yoo JJ, Koo KH, Yoon KS, Kim HJ. Fate of untreated asymptomatic osteonecrosis of the femoral head. J Bone Joint Surg Am. 2008;90(3):477–84.

Follow-up of 105 asymptomatic hips to determine natural outcome of non-traumatic avascular necrosis (AVN), followed for >5 years or until pain developed. The study confirmed that the larger the necrotic lesion the more likely the hip was to become painful. Two-thirds required surgery within 5 years. However small lesions of less than 30 % of the femoral head could be treated conservatively, as the vast majority had no symptoms for more than 5 years. Onset of pain was within 5 years of diagnosis in 94 % of those who became symptomatic.

Mont MA, Jones LC, Hungerford DS. Nontraumatic osteonecrosis of the femoral head: ten years later. J Bone Joint Surg Am. 2006;88(5):1117–32.

An in depth view of published studies on osteonecrosis, detailed descriptions of pathology, diagnosis, treatment and outcomes. The key point of this and more recent studies is the emphasis on early diagnosis and intervention prior to collapse of the femoral head. The interaction between risk factors and genetic predisposition was felt to be important.

Comment: Arthroplasty produces better results than joint preserving procedures if the head has already collapsed.

Korompilias AV, Lykissas MG, Beris AE, Urbaniak JR, Soucacos PN. Vascularised fibular graft in the management of femoral head osteonecrosis: twenty years later. J Bone Joint Surg Br. 2009;91(3):287–93.

An aspect of current management review looking at the indications, technique and results of free vascularised fibular grafting for the treatment of osteonecrosis of the femoral head preserving the joint. This article provides comprehensive details of the operative technique and data from several studies investigating this technique is analysed. The graft supports the subchondral plate with callus, the intra-osseous pressure is reduced, the necrotic segment is replaced, viable cortical and cancellous graft is added with osseo-inductive and osseo-conductive potential.

Comment: Once again the importance of early diagnosis is highlighted and the results of the procedure are predictably good if performed for Steinberg's stage I and II disease.

Arthroscopy, Impingement and Labral Pathology

Espinoza N, Beck M, Rothenfluh DA, Ganz R, Leunig M. Treatment of femoro-acetabular impingement: preliminary results of labral refixation. J Bone Joint Surg Am. 2007;89 (Suppl 2 Pt 1):36–53.

This is a superb description of the surgical technique of dislocation of the hip in adults. It presents detailed anatomical studies of the blood supply to the femoral head. There is a retrospective review of 60 hips treated by arthrotomy and dislocation, trimming of the acetabular rim and femoral chondroplasty. One group had labral resection whereas the other had labral reattachment; there were beeter clinical scores and less X-ray evidence of arthritis in the group that underwent labral reattachment.

Comment: This article should be read and digested by all who operate on the hip joint. It is especially relevant to the trans-gluteal approaches but also points out a recognised, but little discussed fact, concerning the position of insertion of gluteus maximus into the fascia lata which changes with advancing age. Preservation of the neurovascular supply to the anterior fibres of gluteus maximus, regardless of the approach used to the hip joint, is important if good function is to be maintained.

Malviya A, Stafford GH, Villar RN. Is hip arthroscopy for femoroacetabular impingement only for athletes? Br J Sports Med. 2012;46(14):1016–8.

This study was compared the outcome of 122 hip arthroscopies for femoroacetabular impingement (FAI) in athletes and non-athletes. The study demonstrated a positive and sustained impact of arthroscopic surgery for FAI in both the athletic and non-athletic population.

Tönnis D. Normal values of the hip joint for the evaluation of X-rays in children and adults. Clin Orthop Relat Res. 1976;(119):39–47.

This paper sets out the most commonly used grading system for hip dysplasias and femoro-acetabular impingement syndromes. The shaft-neck and anteversion angles were difficult to interpret but the head-acetabular relationship was important.

Tönnis D, Heinecke A. Acetabular and femoral anteversion: relationship with osteoarthritis of the hip. J Bone Joint Surg Am. 1999;81(12):1747–70.

A deep acetabulum, coxa vara and deformity secondary to slip (either overt or subclinical) should be considered precursors to osteoarthritis of the hip.

Reynolds D, Lucas J, Klaue K. Retroversion of the acetabulum. A cause of hip pain. J Bone Joint Surg. 1999;81(2):281–8.

One of the first articles to define retroversion of the acetabulum as a cause of premature osteoarthritis, particularly useful in its description of the radiological (cross over) signs associated with this condition.

Ganz R, Klaue K, Vinh TS, Mast JW. A new peri-acetabular osteotomy for the treatment of hip dysplasias. Technique and preliminary results. Clin Orthop Relat Res. 1988;(232): 26–36.

The Bernese osteotomy is described in detail in this paper. The joint is exposed through a Smith-Peterson approach then osteotomies around the acetabulum allow it to be rotated and re-orientated. The osteotomies are secured with two screws. No vascular impairment of the osteotomised fragment occurred but heterotopic ossification was a problem in 4, prior to the use of indomethacin prophylaxis.

Siebenrock KA, Schoeniger R, Ganz R. Anterior femoro-acetabular impingement due to acetabular retroversion. Treatment with periacetabular osteotomy. J Bone Joint Surg Am. 2003;85-A(2):278–86.

A case series study looking at the results of the Bernese (Ganz) peri-acetabular osteotomy performed on 29 hips for anterior impingement. The article describes in detail the diagnostic methods, distribution of labral lesions and pitfalls of this procedure. The results were good or excellent in 26 hips: 3 underwent further surgery for loss of reduction or persistent impingement.

Philippon MJ, Briggs KK, Yen YM, Kuppersmith DA. Outcomes following hip arthroscopy for femoroacetabular impingement with associated chondrolabral dysfunction: minimum two-year follow-up. J Bone Joint Surg Br. 2009; 91(1):16–23.

The paper carries useful reviews of existing work and emerging surgical techniques for FAI. One hundred and twenty-two patients were treated with hip arthroscopy: 23 had osteoplasty for a cam lesion, 3 had trimming of the acetabular rim for a pincer lesion and 86 had both procedures for mixed impingement. Outcomes following tight inclusion criteria for the study, predicted better outcome related to the preoperative modified Harris hip score with joint space narrowing of less than 2 mm and labral pathology being able to be repaired rather than debrided.

Beck M, Kalhor M, Leunig M, Ganz R. Hip morphology influences the pattern of damage to the acetabular cartilage: femoroacetabular impingement as a cause of early osteoarthritis of the hip. J Bone Joint Surg Br. 2005;87(7):1012–8.

A full review of the concepts of femoro-acetabular impingement is presented with clear distinction between cam and pincer impingement types. Over 300 hips were analysed at surgical dislocation for the treatment of intra-articular pathology and the pathological findings are presented. The influence and implication of labral and other intra-articular soft tissue damage is discussed.

Knee

Jayanth Paniker, Graeme R. Wilson, and Janardhan Rao

Abstract This chapter looks at the common problems of the arthritic knee, ligamentous dysfunction or meniscal tears. Publications concerning potential treatments for cartilage defects and deformity are reviewed and evidence presented concerning the range of knee arthroplasties: total, unicompartmental and patella-femoral resurfacing. Consideration is also given to the failed arthroplasty and the treatment options and subsequent outcomes from revision surgery. Reconstruction for ligamentous injuries is dealt with, as is knee dislocation. Up-to-date references on the perennial problem of anterior knee pain are included here.

J. Paniker, MBBS, MRCS, MSc(T&O), FRCS (T&O)
Department of Trauma and Orthopaedics,
Countess of Chester Hospital, Liverpool Road,
Chester, Cheshire, UK

G.R. Wilson, MBChB
Department of Accident and Emergency,
Royal Liverpool University Hospital,
Prescot Street, Liverpool, Merseyside L78XP, UK

J. Rao, BSc (Hons), MBChB, FRCS (Ed),
FRCS (Tr & Orth) (✉)
Department of Orthopaedics, Countess of Chester Hospital,
Liverpool Road, Chester, Cheshire CH1 2UL, UK
e-mail: janardhan.rao@coch.nhs.net

G. Bowyer, A. Cole (eds.), *Selected References in Trauma and Orthopaedics*, DOI 10.1007/978-1-4471-4676-6_4,
© Springer-Verlag London 2014

Keywords   Knee anatomy • Osteoarthritis • Knee arthro-plasty • Failed arthroplasty • Knee revision • Cartilage defects • Anterior cruciate ligament dysfunction • Anterior knee pain • Patellofemoral pain syndrome • Unicompartmental knee replacement • Valgus/varus knee deformity • Meniscal injuries • Knee dislocation • Knee ligament injuries • Common peroneal nerve injury

Anatomy

Arnoczky SP, Warren RF. Microvasculature of the human meniscus. Am J Sports Med. 1982;10(2):90–5.

This study changed our understanding of the meniscal anatomy and in turn affected our management of meniscal injuries. The medial and lateral menisci from 20 human cadavers were investigated by histology and tissue clearing. The menisci were found to be supplied by branches of the lateral, medial, and middle genicular arteries. The peripheral 10–25 % of the meniscus was found to be supplied by a peri-meniscal capillary plexus originating in the capsular and synovial tissues of the joint. The anterior and posterior horns of the menisci were found to have a good blood supply but the postero-lateral aspect of the lateral meniscus adjacent to the popliteal tendon was found to have a poor blood supply.

Warren LF, Marshall JL. The supporting structures and layers on the medial side of the knee: an anatomical analysis. J Bone Joint Surg Am. 1979;61(1):56–62.

This was the first paper to describe the layered approach to the medial structures of the knee. One hundred and fifty-four fresh cadaver specimens were dissected to define the layers. Layer 1 "the fascial layer", layer 2 "the superficial medial ligament" and layer 3 "the capsular layer". The study describes in great detail the consistent nature of these layers and the different components of each layer.

Terry GC, LaPrade RF. The posterolateral aspect of the knee. Anatomy and surgical approach. Am J Sports Med. 1996; 24(6):732–9.

Thirty cadaveric knees were dissected to obtain a detailed understanding of the anatomic structures of the posterolateral aspect of the knee, and a dependable surgical approach to evaluate injuries to these structures was developed. This was used on 71 consecutive patients who were operated on for posterolateral knee injuries. Three fascial incisions and one lateral midcapsular incision were used to provide surgical access. The following individual anatomic structures were identified: the layers of the iliotibial tract, long and short heads of the biceps femoris muscle, fibular collateral ligament, mid-third lateral capsular ligament, fabello-fibular ligament, posterior arcuate ligament, popliteus muscle complex, lateral coronary ligament, and posterior capsule. This study increased our understanding of the individual anatomic structures and the relationships between these components. The surgical approach described for the evaluation of these anatomic structures should aid the surgeon in properly assessing the injuries before surgical repair.

Osteoarthritis

Altman R, Asch E, Bloch D, Bole G, Borenstein D, Brandt K, et al. Development of criteria for the classification and reporting of osteoarthritis. Classification of osteoarthritis of the knee. Diagnostic and Therapeutic Criteria Committee of the American Rheumatism Association. Arthritis Rheum. 1986;29(8):1039–49.

This paper really is the cornerstone of knee osteoarthritis (OA). It contains the classification system devised by the Osteoarthritis Subcommittee of the Diagnostic and Therapeutic Criteria Committee. The objectives were to standardize the clinical definition of OA, in order to increase the accuracy of OA reporting, and increase the reliability of future OA research. They initially sub classified OA into 'Primary' and 'Secondary', with further subsets of each, using a combination of clinical, radiological, and laboratory data available.

Felson DT, Anderson JJ, Naimark A, Walker AM, Meenan RF. Obesity and knee osteoarthritis. The Framingham Study. Ann Intern Med. 1988;109(1):18–24.

This study tacked onto the back of the Framingham Study looking at the effect of obesity on cardiovascular health. The aim was to see if obesity preceded, and therefore was a cause of, OA. It was a 35 year prospective follow-up study where patients were seen 18 times (weighed on each occasion) and at the final consultation were questioned regarding symptoms of knee OA and had radiographs taken. The results proved that obesity preceded OA and could therefore be considered causative. Men consistently in the top weight quintile had a relative risk for developing OA of 1.51 compared to lighter men. Women in the top quintile had a relative risk of 2.07 and those in the second quintile had a relative risk of 1.44 when compared to lighter women.

Outerbridge RE. The etiology of chondromalacia patellae. J Bone Joint Surg Br. 1961;43-B(4):752–7.

The description of the macroscopic changes to the cartilage are described. Grade 1 – softening and swelling of the cartilage. Grade 2 – fragmentation and fissuring of ½ in. or less. Grade 3 is the same as grade 2 but more than ½ in. in diameter. Grade 4 is erosion of cartilage down to bone. This classification, originally used to describe chondromalacia patella, is now used to describe arthroscopic finding of the cartilage in most joints.

Kellgren JH, Lawrence JS. Radiological assessment of osteoarthrosis. Ann Rheum Dis. 1957;16(4):494–502.

The radiological classification of osteoarthritis that is used most commonly was formulated in this paper. In this study, 510 X-rays of multiple joints of 85 people in the age group 55–64 chosen at random were graded for osteo-arthrosis by two observers on four occasions to determine the extent of observer difference. Osteoarthrosis was divided into five grades 0–4 as reported briefly in a previous paper by the same authors. It showed moderate intra-observer reliability but poor interobserver reliability.

Moseley JB, O'Malley K, Petersen NJ, Menke TJ, Brody BA, Kuykendall DH, et al. A controlled trial of arthroscopic surgery for osteoarthritis of the knee. N Engl J Med. 2002; 347(2):81–8.

This key study changed the indications for arthroscopic procedures. In a randomised placebo controlled trial, 180 patients with osteoarthritis of the knee were randomly assigned to receive arthroscopic débridement, arthroscopic lavage, or placebo surgery. Patients in the placebo group received skin incisions and underwent a simulated débridement without insertion of the arthroscope. Patients and assessors of outcome were blinded to the treatment-group assignment. Of the total of 165 patients who completed the trial, there was no difference with regards to pain or function between either of the intervention groups and the placebo group. The Knee-Specific Pain Scale was similar in the placebo, lavage, and débridement groups, at 1 year and at 2 years. In this study the outcomes after arthroscopic lavage or arthroscopic débridement were no better than those after a placebo procedure for patients with osteoarthritis of the knee.

Knee Arthroplasty

Waters TS, Bentley G. Patellar resurfacing in total knee arthroplasty. A prospective, randomized study. J Bone Joint Surg Am. 2003;85-A(2):212–7.

In this prospective, randomized controlled trial patients (n=513) were randomized to either patellar resurfacing at Total Knee Replacement (TKR) or no patellar resurfacing. Mean follow-up was 5.3 years and 474 knees survived to follow-up. Thirty-five patients had bilateral TKRs, one with resurfacing and one without. At follow-up the prevalence of anterior knee pain (AKP) in the non-resurfacing group was

25.1 % compared to 5.3 % in the resurfacing group (statistically significant). Ten of 11 patients who went on to have a resurfacing due to AKP had complete relief of their AKP. Patients in the non-resurfacing group had significantly lower postoperative functional scores and patients who had bilateral TKRs were more likely to prefer the resurfaced side.

Burnett RS, Boone JL, McCarthy KP, Rosenzweig S, Barrack RL. A prospective randomized clinical trial of patellar resurfacing and nonresurfacing in bilateral TKA. Clin Orthop Relat Res. 2007;464:65–72.

This study looked at the long-term outcome differences of patella resurfacing versus non-resurfacing in patients undergoing bilateral total knee arthroplasty. Thirty-two patients (64 knees) were randomised to either resurfacing or non-resurfacing of the patella for the first total knee arthroplasty, and the second knee received the opposite treatment. All patients received the same cruciate-retaining total knee arthroplasty as a bilateral single-stage procedure. At a minimum follow-up of 10 years, the study found no differences with regard to range of motion, Knee Society Clinical Rating Score, satisfaction, revision rates, or anterior knee pain.

Tanzer M, Smith K, Burnett S. Posterior-stabilized versus cruciate-retaining total knee arthroplasty: balancing the gap. J Arthroplasty. 2002;17(7):813–9.

This was a prospective, double-blind, randomized controlled trial in which 40 knees were randomized to receive a cruciate retaining (CR) total knee replacement (TKR) (n=20), or a posterior stabilized (PS) TKR (n=20). Surgical technique was similar for both groups and all procedures were carried out by the senior author. At 2-year follow-up there was no significant difference between the two groups in terms of the Knee Society Clinical and Functional Scores, and no difference in radiological evaluation. All patients reported that they were happy with their TKR, and both groups reported significant increases between pre and postoperative functional scores.

Ackroyd CE, Newman JH, Evans R, Eldridge JD, Joslin CC. The Avon patellofemoral arthroplasty: five-year survivorship and functional results. J Bone Joint Surg Br. 2007; 89(3):310–5.

Mid-term results of 109 consecutive patellofemoral resurfacing arthroplasties in 85 patients were reported. The 5-year survival rate, with revision as the endpoint, was 95.8 %. There were no cases of loosening of the prosthesis. At 5 years the median Bristol pain score improved from 15 to 35, the median Melbourne score from 10 to 25, and the median Oxford score from 18 to 39. Successful results, judged on a Bristol pain score of at least 20 at 5 years, occurred in 80 % (66) of knees. The main complication was radiological progression of arthritis, which occurred in 25 patients (28 %).

Failed Arthroplasty/Knee Revision

Kurtz S, Ong K, Lau E, Mowat F, Halpern M. Projections of primary and revision hip and knee arthroplasty in the United States from 2005 to 2030. J Bone Joint Surg Am. 2007;89(4):780–5.

This study gave the projection figures for primary and revision total hip and knee arthroplasties that would be performed in the United States through 2030. The data was collected from the Nationwide Inpatient Sample (1990–2003) and United States Census Bureau. Projections performed using Poisson regression on historical procedure rates in combination with population projections from 2005 to 2030 estimated, that by 2030, the demand for primary total hip arthroplasties would grow by 174 % to 572,000 and primary total knee arthroplasties by 673 % to 3.48 million procedures. Total hip and total knee revisions are projected to grow by 137 and 601 %, respectively, between 2005 and 2030. The study aimed to provide information to assist in making future policy decisions related to the numbers of orthopaedic surgeons needed and the deployment of appropriate resources.

Kim J, Nelson CL, Lotke PA. Stiffness after total knee arthroplasty. Prevalence of the complication and outcomes of revision. J Bone Joint Surg Am. 2004;86-A(7):1479–84.

In this study, 1,000 consecutive primary total knee replacements were reviewed to determine the prevalence of stiffness, which was 1.3 %. There were no significant differences in age, gender, implant design, diagnosis, or the need for lateral release between the patients with and without stiffness. The results of 56 revisions performed because of stiffness were also evaluated. The mean Knee Society score had improved at the time of follow-up, in both the function score and the pain score. The mean flexion contracture decreased from 11.3 degrees to 3.2°, the mean flexion improved from 65.8° to 85.4°, and the mean arc of motion improved from 54.6° to 82.2°. The arc of motion improved in 93 % of the knees, and flexion increased in 80 %. Extension improved in 63 %, and it remained unchanged in 30 %. The study found that revision surgery was a satisfactory treatment option for stiffness however the benefits were modest.

Lewold S, Robertsson O, Knutson K, Lidgren L. Revision of unicompartmental knee arthroplasty: outcome in 1,135 cases from the Swedish Knee Arthroplasty study. Acta Orthop Scand. 1998;69(5):469–74.

In the prospective Swedish Knee Arthroplasty study, by the end of 1995, 1,135 of 14,772 primary unicompartmental knee arthroplasties (UKA) for localized, mainly medial arthrosis had been revised. The Marmor/Richards and St. Georg sledge/Endo-Link prostheses were used in 65 %. Mean age at revision was 72 years. Two hundred and thirty-two revisions were performed as an exchange UKA, 750 as a total knee arthroplasty (TKA) and 153 were revised by other modes. In medial UKA, the indication for revision was component loosening in 45 % and joint degeneration in 25 % and in lateral UKA, the corresponding figures were 31 and 35 %, respectively. After only 5 years, the risk of having a second revision was more than three times higher for failed UKAs revised to a new UKA (cumulative rerevision rate (CRRR 26 %) than for those revised to a TKA (CRRR 7 %).

Once failed UKA should be revised to a TKA, whatever the mode of failure. Not even joint degeneration of the unoperated compartment can be safely treated by adding contralateral components; CRRR after this procedure was 17 %, while it was 7 % when converted to a TKA.

Gill T, Schemitsch EH, Brick GW, Thornhill TS. Revision total knee arthroplasty after failed unicompartmental knee arthroplasty or high tibial osteotomy. Clin Orthop Relat Res. 1995;(321):10–8.

A retrospective matched-pair comparative analysis was done between 30 total knee arthroplasties following failed high tibial osteotomies and 30 total knee arthroplasties following failed unicompartmental knee arthroplasties. The groups were matched according to age, gender, type of prosthesis, primary disease, and length of follow-up. At a minimum follow-up of 2 years, the Knee Society Knee Score for the high tibial osteotomy group was significantly higher than that for the unicompartmental arthroplasty group. More osseous reconstructions were required in the unicompartmental revisions. Rates of component loosening were not significantly different between the groups. A failed unicompartmental knee arthroplasty and a failed high tibial osteotomy can be revised successfully to a total knee arthroplasty. The results confirm that revisions after unicondylar arthroplasty and high tibial osteotomy are technically demanding. In this series, the results of total knee arthroplasty following unicompartmental knee arthroplasty approached but did not equal those obtained after high tibial osteotomy.

Barrack RL, Engh G, Rorabeck C, Sawhney J, Woolfrey M. Patient satisfaction and outcome after septic versus aseptic revision total knee arthroplasty. J Arthroplasty. 2000;15(8):990–3.

A consecutive series of revision total knee arthroplasties performed at three university centres was prospectively studied. The same implant was used in all cases. The evaluation included a Knee Society clinical score (KSCS); SF-36; satisfaction survey; and radiographs preoperatively, at 6 and 12 months postoperatively, and annually thereafter. Follow-up averaging 36 months was obtained in 125 of 138 knees (91 %). Twenty-six of 28 infected knees were treated successfully with 2-stage exchange with an interval of 4–6 weeks using an anti-biotic-impregnated spacer block and intravenous antibiotics. The remaining 99 knees were revised for reasons other than infection. Preoperatively, patients with infection had a significantly decreased arc of motion and lower KSCS compared with patients without infection. Postoperatively, patients with infection continued to have a significantly decreased range of motion, markedly lower KSCS and a significantly lower function score. A significantly higher percentage of patients were unable to return to normal activities of daily living after septic versus aseptic revision total knee arthroplasty (24 % vs. 7 %). Despite the inferior functional result, patients expressed an equal degree of satisfaction with the results of their treatment in septic versus aseptic revision cases.

Leopold SS, Silverton CD, Barden RM, Rosenberg AG. Isolated revision of the patellar component in total knee arthroplasty. J Bone Joint Surg Am. 2003;85-A(1):41–7.

Forty knees with a Miller-Galante I prosthesis underwent isolated patellar revision (with or without lateral retinacular release). The Hospital for Special Surgery (HSS) knee scores were collected prospectively, and pre-operative and final follow-up radiographs were analyzed with respect to alignment, component position, and patellar tracking. At a mean follow-up of 62 months, 15 (38 %) of the 40 knees that had had an isolated revision of the patellar component failed a second time. Eight of them required additional operations at a mean of 49 months after the patellar revision. Seven knees that did not undergo reoperation but were deemed to be failures on the basis of the patients' symptoms, had an average HSS knee score of 72 points at the time of the final follow-up. Of the 25 knees that had not failed, the average HSS knee score at the time of the final follow-up was 87 points. Isolated patellar revision, with or without concurrent lateral retinacular release, was associated with a high rate of reoperation and a relatively low rate of success. In this study, elements of the implant design and component alignment contributed to the patellar component failure.

Cartilage Defects

Hangody L, Kish G, Kárpáti Z, Udvarhelyi I, Szigeti I, Bély M. Mosaicplasty for the treatment of articular cartilage defects: application in clinical practice. Orthopedics. 1998;21(7):751–6.

The operative technique and early results of mosaicplasty were described in this paper. A total of 227 patients with circumscript cartilage defects of weight-bearing surfaces of the knee were treated using this technique. The results in 57 patients who had >3 years follow-up were evaluated using Magnetic resonance imaging, computed tomography arthrographies, ultrasound, and arthroscopy. Using the modified Hospital for Special Surgery (HSS) knee scoring system, 91 % of the patients achieved a good or excellent result.

Peterson L, Brittberg M, Kiviranta I, Akerlund EL, Lindahl A. Autologous chondrocyte transplantation. Biomechanics and long-term durability. Am J Sports Med. 2002;30(1):2–12.

This paper evaluated the durability of autologous chondrocyte transplantation grafts in 61 patients treated for isolated cartilage defects on the femoral condyle or the patella and followed up for a mean of 7.4 years (range, 5–11). After 2 years, 50 of the 61 patients had good or excellent clinical results, and 51 of 61 had good or excellent results at 5–11 years later. Grafted areas from 11 of the patients were evaluated with an electromechanical indentation probe during a second-look arthroscopy procedure (mean follow-up, 54.3 months); stiffness measurements were 90 % or more of those of normal cartilage in eight patients. Eight of 12 biopsy samples taken from these patients showed hyaline characteristics. This study showed that autologous chondrocyte transplantation has reasonable long-term durability.

Bentley G, Biant LC, Vijayan S, Macmull S, Skinner JA, Carrington RW. Minimum ten-year results of a prospective randomised study of autologous chondrocyte implantation versus mosaicplasty for symptomatic articular cartilage lesions of the knee. J Bone Joint Surg Br. 2012;94(4):504–9.

Autologous chondrocyte implantation (ACI) and mosaicplasty are both accepted methods of treating symptomatic articular cartilage defects in the knee. This study presented a long-term randomised comparison of the two techniques in 100 patients at a minimum follow-up of 10 years. The mean age of the patients at the time of surgery was 31.3 years and the mean duration of symptoms pre-operatively was 7.2 years. The mean size of the lesion for the ACI group was 440.9 mm^2 and for the mosaicplasty group was 399.6 mm^2. Patients had a mean of 1.5 previous operations (0–4) to the articular cartilage defect. Patients were assessed using the modified Cincinnati knee score and the Stanmore-Bentley Functional Rating system. Ten of 58 (17 %) in the ACI group and 23 of 42 (55 %) in the mosaicplasty group ($p < 0.001$) had failed at 10 years. The functional outcome of those patients who underwent ACI compared with mosaicplasty was significantly better ($p = 0.02$).

This reiterated the early results from the same group which showed significant superiority of ACI over mosaicplasty for the repair of articular defects in the knee.

Vanlauwe J, Saris DB, Victor J, Almqvist KF, Bellemans J, Luyten FP, et al. Five-year outcome of characterized chondrocyte implantation versus microfracture for symptomatic cartilage defects of the knee: early treatment matters. Am J Sports Med. 2011;39(12):2566–74.

This paper published the 5 year results of a randomised controlled study of 112 people treated with either autologous chondrocyte implantation or microfracture. Fifty-one people were treated with autologous chondrocyte implantation (ACI) and 61 with microfracture. At 5 years, there was no significant difference in the average change from baseline of the Knee Injury and Osteoarthritis Outcome Score between the groups . There were seven failures in the ACI group and ten in the microfracture group. In patients with symptoms for less than 3 years, ACI obtained statistically significant and clinically relevant better results than microfracture. In patients with longer duration of symptoms there was no difference between the treatment groups.

Bartlett W, Skinner JA, Gooding CR, Carrington RW, Flanagan AM, Briggs TW, et al. Autologous chondrocyte implantation versus matrix-induced autologous chondrocyte implantation for osteochondral defects of the knee: a prospective, randomised study. J Bone Joint Surg Br. 2005;87(5):640–5.

This was the first prospective randomised study comparing autologous chondrocyte implantation with the use of porcine-derived type I/type III collagen as a cover (ACI-C) and matrix-induced autologous chondrocyte implantation (MACI) using a collagen bilayer seeded with chondrocytes. The study included 91 patients with chondral defects, of whom 44 received ACI-C and 47 MACI grafts. At 1 year both treatments resulted in improvement, with the mean modified Cincinnati knee score increasing by 17.6 in the ACI-C group and 19.6 in the MACI group (p=0.32). Arthroscopic assessments performed after 1 year showed a good to excellent International Cartilage Repair Society score in 79.2 % of ACI-C and 66.6 % of MACI grafts. Hyaline-like cartilage or hyaline-like cartilage with fibrocartilage was found in the biopsies of 43.9 % of the ACI-C and 36.4 % of the MACI grafts after 1 year. The study showed that the clinical, arthroscopic and histological outcomes are comparable for both ACI-C and MACI.

Saw K, Anz A, Merican S, Tay YG, Ragavanaidu K, Jee CS, McGuire DA. Articular cartilage regeneration with autologous peripheral blood progenitor cells and hyaluronic acid after arthroscopic subchondral drilling: a report of 5 cases with histology. Arthroscopy. 2011;27(4):493–506.

A look into the future of management of osteoarthritis. In this study five patients, with International Cartilage Repair Society grade III and IV lesions of the knee joint, underwent a second look arthroscopy and chondral core biopsy to evaluate the quality of articular cartilage regeneration after arthroscopic subchondral drilling followed by postoperative intraarticular injections of hyaluronic acid (HA) & autologous peripheral blood progenitor cells (PBPCs). Autologous PBPCs were harvested 1 week after surgery and injected intra-articularly into the operated knee. A total of five weekly intra-articular injections were given. Arthroscopy confirmed articular cartilage regeneration, and histologic sections showed features of hyaline cartilage. These five patients are part of a larger study, the results of which are yet to be published.

Anterior Cruciate Ligament Dysfunction

Kocabey Y, Tetik O, Isbell WM, Atay OA, Johnson DL. The value of clinical examination versus magnetic resonance imaging in the diagnosis of meniscal tears and anterior cruciate ligament rupture. Arthroscopy. 2004;20(7):696–700.

This was a prospective, longitudinal study in which 50 consecutive patients with knee injuries were assessed clinically by a sports fellow with 10 years of sports orthopaedic experience. Each patient then underwent magnetic resonance imaging (MRI) which was reported by a radiologist who had been given the relevant clinical information (as per real practice). Of the 50 patients, 26 had an Anterior Cruciate Ligament (ACL) tear. All 26 tears were diagnosed by both clinical examination and MRI, all 24 normal ACLs were detected on clinical examination but only 23 were detected by MRI, MRI had one false positive result. This paper showed that a competent orthopaedic surgeon can rely on their clinical evaluation of ACL status, and need not order MRI for all patients if they are confident in their diagnosis.

Kessler MA, Behrend H, Henz S, Stutz G, Rukavina A, Kuster MS. Function, osteoarthritis and activity after ACL-rupture: 11 years follow-up results of conservative versus reconstructive treatment. Knee Surg Sports Traumatol Arthrosc. 2008;16(5):442–8.

This was a retrospective cohort study looking at the long-term outcomes between operative (n=60) and conservative (n=49) management of an ACL rupture as an isolated injury. Patients were assigned to their group bases on consensus between them and the surgeon, no randomization took place. However, the surgeons who had done the initial operation were not part of this study, reducing bias. Mean follow-up was 11.1 years and included clinical evaluation and radiographic evaluation (only of the affected knee, therefore comparison to the uninjured knee was not possible). Patients were allowed to choose their own physiotherapist but followed a similar routine. At follow-up, patients from the ACL reconstruction group reported significantly higher International Knee Documentation Committee (IKDC) scores than the conservative group, and the reconstruction group performed significantly better on the KT 1000 testing compared to the healthy leg. Patients in the operative group were significantly less likely to require further surgery for meniscal tears. On radiographic examination, the conservative group were significantly less likely to develop osteoarthritis (24 % vs 45 %), however radiographs of the contralateral knee were unavailable. Return to sport was similar between the groups.

Pinczewski LA, Deehan DJ, Salmon LJ, Russell VJ, Clingeleffer A. A five-year comparison of patellar tendon versus four-strand hamstring tendon autograft for arthroscopic reconstruction of the anterior cruciate ligament. Am J Sports Med. 2002;30(4):523–36.

What began as a prospective randomized controlled trail comparing outcomes between the commonly used patellar tendon (PT) graft and the novel hamstring graft (HS) techniques for ACL reconstruction rapidly changed to a non-randomized study because patients were refusing randomization to the PT group because they, and their physical therapists, were seeing better results in the HS group (earlier discharge, earlier comfortable walking, and earlier return to work). The total number of patients reaching the inclusion criteria was 180 (n = 90 for each group) and patients were followed up clinically and radiographically for a minimum of 5 years. In the PT group there were three ruptured grafts, and in the HS group there were seven ruptured grafts (not significant), these were excluded from follow-up. There were no significant differences between groups in terms of functional outcomes and complications, but the PT group had a significantly greater chance of developing OA by radiographic interpretation, developing a fixed flexion deformity, developing anterior knee pain, and developing donor site pain.

Jameson SS, Dowen D, James P, Serrano-Pedraza I, Reed MR, Deehan D. Complications following anterior cruciate ligament reconstruction in the English NHS. Knee. 2012;19(1):14–9.

This paper presents, for the first time, the complication results from a national register of all ACL reconstructions (n = 13,941) done in the National Health Service. The register represents 2 years of prospective data collection concentrating on deep vein thrombosis (DVT), pulmonary embolism (PE), wound infection, readmission, and death. The results show that 0.75 % of patients developed a wound complciation (infection or haematoma), 0.25 % of patients required further surgery for wound complications, and 1.36 % of people were readmitted within 90 days (0.59 % with wound complications). Perhaps most importantly they found that there was an overall risk of 0.44 % of developing a venous thromboembolism (0.3 % DVT, 0.18 % PE, five patients had both a DVT and PE). Patients over 40 years old were significantly more likely to develop a DVT or PE.

Shelbourne KD, Nitz P. Accelerated rehabilitation after anterior cruciate ligament reconstruction. Am J Sports Med. 1990;18(3):292–9.

Few papers directly compare the outcomes of postoperative rehabilitation following ACL reconstruction. This paper presents retrospective research comparing two cohorts of ACL reconstruction patients. Group I (n = 350) underwent a traditional 'slow' rehabilitation with a splinted knee brace and agility work not beginning until 7 months post-operatively, and Group II (n = 450) underwent an 'accelerated' rehabilitation with no bracing, immediate range of motion work, and an earlier planned return to sport. The two cohorts did not run simultaneously and patients were not randomized to either group. The results showed that patients in Group II achieved an earlier return to full sporting activity, fewer problems with patellofemoral pain (and fewer operations to correct this), shorter time to full range of movement, and increased strength at an earlier time point. Importantly, all of this was achieved without compromising stability of the knee or putting the graft at risk. This paper shows that patients have a better outcome if they undergo an 'accelerated' rehabilitation.

Mohtadi NGH, Chan DS, Dainty KN, Whelan DB. Patellar tendon versus hamstring tendon autograft for anterior cruciate ligament rupture in adults. Cochrane Database Syst Rev. 2011;(9):CD005960.

This Cochrane review compared the outcomes of ACL reconstruction using patellar tendon (PT) versus hamstring tendon(s) (HT) autografts in ACL deficient patients. Nineteen randomized and quasi-randomized controlled trials providing outcome data (minimum 2 year follow-up) for 1,597 young to middle-aged adults were included. The review showed no statistically significant differences between the two graft choices for functional assessment (single leg hop test), return to activity, Tegner and Lysholm scores, and subjective measures of outcome. There were also no differences found between the two interventions for re-rupture or International Knee

Documentation Committee scores. PT reconstruction resulted in a more statically stable knee, though patients experienced more anterior knee problems and showed a statistically significant loss of knee extension and a trend towards loss of knee extension strength. HT reconstructions demonstrated a trend towards loss of knee flexion and a statistically significant loss of knee flexion strength. The review showed there was insufficient evidence to draw conclusions on differences between the two grafts for long-term functional outcome and the development of osteoarthritis.

Anterior Knee Pain (Patellofemoral Pain Syndrome)

Witvrouw E, Lysens R, Bellemans J, Cambier D, Vanderstraeten G. Intrinsic risk factors for the development of anterior knee pain in an athletic population. A two-year prospective study. Am J Sports Med. 2000;28(4):480–9.

A 2 year prospective follow-up study containing 282 male and female subjects enrolled on a physical education course. Readings were taken from each subject regarding anthropometric variables, motor performance (including muscle length and strength), joint laxity (general, not just knee), lower leg alignment, static and dynamic patellofemoral characteristics, and psychological characteristics. Twenty-four out of 282 subjects developed anterior knee pain (AKP) during the study. Four risk factors were significant in the development of AKP: shortened quadriceps muscle, altered vastus medialis obliquus muscle reflex response time, decreased explosive strength, and a hypermobile patella.

Witvrouw E, Werner S, Mikkelsen C, Van Tiggelen D, Vanden Berghe L, Cerulli G. Clinical classification of patellofemoral pain syndrome: guidelines for non-operative treatment. Knee Surg Sports Traumatol Arthrosc. 2005;13(2):122–30.

This paper refers to patellofemoral pain syndrome (PFPS) as a 'wastebasket' for numerous diagnoses in the knee, and

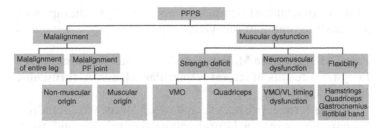

FIGURE 4.1   Classification system for PFPS (Adapted from Vanlauwe et al. (2011))

the authors quite sensibly suggest that before a management plan can be formulated it is important to understand *why* the patient is having pain and *where* the pain is originating from. They acknowledge that one management plan does not exist for treating PFPS, and perhaps this is because of the numerous pathologies occurring within or around the knee.

This paper is important because if a classification system is in place it enables orthopaedic surgeons and physiotherapists to create a management plan for each sub-diagnosis, and allows future research into PFPS to compare pathologies like-for-like (Fig. 4.1).

Clark DI, Downing N, Mitchell J, Coulson L, Syzpryt EP, Doherty M. Physiotherapy for anterior knee pain: a randomised controlled trial. Ann Rheum Dis. 2000;59(9):700–4.

An observer blind, prospective, randomized controlled trial containing 81 patients. Patients were randomized into four groups ('physiotherapy, taping and education', 'taping and education', 'physiotherapy and education', and 'education only') and followed up at 3 months and 12 months. All patients showed improvement in symptoms (using Western Ontario and McMasters Universities Osteoarthritis Index [WOMAC], visual analogue, and Hospital Anxiety and Depression [HAD] scores) at 3 and 12 months. Patients who received physiotherapy were significantly more likely to be discharged at 3 months. Patients who were discharged had significantly better results than those that were referred. Taping was shown not to influence outcome. This paper showed that physiotherapy was a successful treatment for AKP.

Panni AS, Tartarone M, Patricola A, Paxton EW, Fithian DC. Long-term results of lateral retinacular release. Arthroscopy. 2005;21(5):526–31.

A long term retrospective follow-up study. One hundred patients underwent a lateral retinacular release and were split into two groups based on pre-operative evaluation. Group I (n = 50) had anterior knee pain (AKP) with no patellar instability, and Group II (n = 50) had AKP with patellar instability. Mean follow-up at 97 months showed satisfactory results (good/excellent) in 70 % of Group I (compared to 71 % at 3 years) and 50 % of Group II (compared to 72 % at 3 years). These results are significantly different at 5 years, and the decrease in Group II is significant. The paper also showed that patients from Group I were significantly more likely to return to sports (80 % vs 60 %).

This paper is important because it shows that despite good initial results, results of lateral retinacular release diminish significantly with time if there was patellar instability to begin with, and that this same group of patients are significantly less likely to return to sports.

Fulkerson JP. Anteromedialization of the tibial tuberosity for patellofemoral malalignment. Clin Orthop Relat Res. 1983;(177):176–81.

Anteromedialization of the tibial tuberosity as a procedure to help in patellofemoral pain is described in this paper. The procedure was indicated only in patients who failed conservative management and had been identified to have isolated pathology of the patellofemoral joint with patella malalignment. The surgical technique is described in great detail. The paper also reports the results of eight patients who underwent the procedure with all patients achieving substantial relief of pre-operative pain and disability. Realignment of the patellofemoral mechanism and relief of patellofemoral contact stress can be achieved by this procedure, though careful patient selection is paramount to its success.

Unicompartmental Knee Replacement

Newman J, Pydisetty RV, Ackroyd C. Unicompartmental or total knee replacement: the 15-year results of a prospective randomised controlled trial. J Bone Joint Surg Br. 2009;91(1):52–7.

This paper represents the 15 year results of a previous 5 year study (Newman et al. 1998). Patients were reviewed at 8, 10, 12, and 15 years postoperatively, both clinically and radiologically. A number of patients from both groups were lost to follow-up due to death, frailty, and old age, however those that could filled in a questionnaire at home. During this time 4 unicompartmental knee replacements (UKRs) failed (3 revised) and 6 TKRs failed (4 revised), there was no significant difference between the groups. Full clinical evaluation was undertaken of surviving UKRs (n = 21) and TKRs (n = 19) and according to Bristol Knee Score 71.4 % of UKRs were graded excellent at 15 years, whilst only 52.6 % of TKRs were graded excellent.

Comment: The above paper shows that, for suitable candidates, UKR is an appropriate management option and provides results comparable with the TKR over the short and long term.

Weale AE, Newman JH. Unicompartmental arthroplasty and high tibial osteotomy for osteoarthrosis of the knee. A comparative study with a 12- to 17-year follow-up period. Clin Orthop Relat Res. 1994;(302):134–7.

Following the publication of an earlier review of this cohort of patients, which showed that results of unicompartmental arthroplasty were superior to high tibial osteotomy at 5–10 year follow-up, the authors aimed to see if this significant difference was still present long term, with a review between 12 and 17 years. Patients from both cohorts had died or been lost between the follow-ups, so only 21 osteotomies and 15 UKRs remained. Results showed a higher rate of revisions in the osteotomy group (17/49) compared to the UKR group (5/42), although no p-value was given. Overall knee scores were similar but when looking at pain alone, 80 % of the UKR group had none or mild pain, compared to 43 % of the osteotomy group, again no p-value was given. These results show that the superior results achieved with a UKR compared to a high tibial osteotomy are maintained long term.

Laurencin CT, Zelicof SB, Scott RD, Ewald FC. Unicompartmental versus total knee arthroplasty in the same patient. A comparative study. Clin Orthop Relat Res. 1991;(273):151–6.

This study followed up, for an average of 81 months, 23 patients who had a TKR in one knee and a UKR in the other knee on the same admission. Evaluation consisted of chart review, range of motion, and interview concentrating on patient preference with regards to pain, stability, feel, and ability to go up and down stairs. Thirteen patients had patella resurfacing and ten patients did not. More patients in the UKR group had none or mild pain (96 % vs 83 %), 44 % of patients preferred their UKR compared to 12 % who preferred the TKR (44 % had no preference), and the mean increase in range of movement in the UKR group was 17° (106° pre-op to 123° post-op) and in the TKR group it was 2° (108° pre-op to 110° post-op). Through statistical analysis it was determined that these results were not significantly different, although the trend is apparent.

Gleeson RE, Evans R, Ackroyd CE, Webb J, Newman JH. Fixed or mobile bearing unicompartmental knee replacement? A comparative cohort study. Knee. 2004;11(5):379–84.

This prospective study aimed to compare the short term outcomes between fixed and mobile bearings in a UKR. Most patients were randomized although some were put into a specific group depending on surgeon preference. Fifty-seven knees were in the 'fixed' group, compared to 47 in the 'mobile' group, minimum follow-up was 2.7 years with a mean of 4 years. Both bearings performed similarly in terms of Bristol Knee Score and Oxford Knee Score, but patients with a fixed bearing performed significantly better ($p = 0.013$) in terms of pain relief, and more patients in the fixed group had good or excellent outcomes compared to the mobile group (84 % vs 70 %). Both fixed and mobile groups had similar revision rates (3 vs 4) and 3 mobile bearings required reoperation to change the bearing thickness.

Berger RA, Meneghini RM, Jacobs JJ, Sheinkop MB, Della Valle CJ, Rosenberg AG, et al. Results of unicompartmental knee arthroplasty at a minimum of ten years of follow-up. J Bone Joint Surg Am. 2005;87(5):999–1006.

Sixty-two consecutive unicompartmental knee arthroplasties performed with cemented modular Miller-Galante implants in 51 patients were studied prospectively both clinically and radiographically. All patients had isolated unicompartmental disease without patellofemoral symptoms. In 38 patients (49 knees) with a minimum of 10 years of follow-up, a good/excellent result was recorded in 92 % and a fair result in 8 %. Two patients (two knees) with well-fixed components underwent revision to total knee arthroplasty because of progression of arthritis. At the time of the final follow-up, no component was loose radiographically and there was no evidence of periprosthetic osteolysis. Radiographic evidence of progression of loss of joint space was observed in 32 % of knees. Kaplan-Meier analysis revealed a survival rate of 98.0 % at 10 years and 95.7 % at 13 years, with revision or radiographic loosening as the end point. The survival rate was 100 % at 13 years with aseptic loosening as the end point.

This unicompartmental knee design has yielded excellent results, which were mirrored by similar good results in the UK National Joint Registry.

Pandit H, Jenkins C, Gill HS, Barker K, Dodd CA, Murray DW. Minimally invasive Oxford phase 3 unicompartmental knee replacement: results of 1000 cases. J Bone Joint Surg Br. 2011;93(2):198–204.

This prospective study describes the outcome of the first 1000 phase 3 Oxford medial unicompartmental knee replacements (UKRs) implanted using a minimally invasive surgical approach. The mean follow-up was 5.6 years (1–11) with 547 knees having a minimum follow-up of 5 years. At 5 years their mean Oxford knee score was 41.3 , the mean American Knee Society Objective Score 86.4, mean American Knee Society Functional Score 86.1, mean Tegner activity score 2.8. For the entire cohort, the mean maximum flexion was 130° at the time of final review. The incidence of implant-related re-operations was 2.9 %; of these 29 re-operations, two were revisions requiring revision knee replacement components, 17 were conversions to a primary total knee replacement, six were open reductions for dislocation of the bearing, three were secondary lateral UKRs and one was revision of a tibial component. The most common reason for further surgical intervention was progression of arthritis in the lateral compartment (0.9 %), followed by dislocation of the bearing (0.6 %) and revision for unexplained pain (0.6 %). If all implant-related re-operations are considered failures, the 10-year survival rate was 96 %. The survival rates are similar to those obtained with a standard open approach whereas the function is better.

Valgus/Varus Knee Deformity

Brouwer GM, van Tol AW, Bergink AP, Belo JN, Bernsen RM, Reijman M, et al. Association between valgus and varus alignment and the development and progression of radiographic osteoarthritis of the knee. Arthritis Rheum. 2007;56(4):1204–11.

This study used participants from the Rotterdam study to assess the relationship between malalignment and the development and progression of knee OA. Knee OA at baseline and at a mean follow-up 6.6 years was scored according to the Kellgren/Lawrence grading system. Alignment was measured by the femoro-tibial angle on radiographs at baseline. Multivariable logistic regression for repeated measurements was used to analyze the association. Of 2,664 knees, 1,012 (38 %) had normal alignment, 693 (26 %) varus alignment, and 959 (36 %) valgus alignment. Valgus alignment was associated with a borderline significant increase in development of knee OA (odds ratio [OR] 1.54), and varus alignment was associated with a twofold increased risk (OR 2.06). Stratification for body mass index showed that this increased risk was seen in overweight and obese individuals.

An increasing degree of varus alignment is associated with progression and development of knee OA particularly in overweight and obese persons.

Karachalios T, Sarangi PP, Newman JH. Severe varus and valgus deformities treated by total knee arthroplasty. J Bone Joint Surg Br. 1994;76(6):938–42.

This prospective case-controlled study compared the outcome of knee replacement in seriously deformed to those in slightly deformed knees. There were 51 knees with varus or valgus deformities greater than 20° matched for age, gender, disease, type of prosthesis and time of operation with a control group in which the alignment of the leg was within 5° of normal. The clinical outcome at a mean 5.5 years was similar in the two groups. Some deformity persisted in 14 patients in the first group, 13 of whom were initially in valgus. These patients had a significantly poorer mean clinical outcome. Lateral dislocation or subluxation of the patella was found in four knees, all of which had had valgus deformity of 30° or more.

Teeny SM, Krackow KA, Hungerford DS, Jones M. Primary total knee arthroplasty in patients with severe varus deformity. A comparative study. Clin Orthop Relat Res. 1991;(273):19–31.

Severe varus deformity in total knee arthroplasty (TKA) requires more attention to achieve bony alignment and ligament balancing. This paper evaluated the clinical and roentgenographic results in 27 knees (20 patients) with a minimum preoperative varus deformity of 20° in comparison with those of 40 knees (31 patients) with a deformity of less than 5° varus or valgus. The average knee evaluation score in the varus group was 89 points, and for the nondeformity group it was 92 points (p less than 0.02). There were no poor results in the varus deformity group and one poor result in the non-deformity group. Postoperative knee range of motion was 98° in the varus deformity group and 107° in the non-deformity group. The deformity was corrected to 3° varus in the deformity group and 0° varus in the non-deformity group. Cases with severe varus had longer operating times and mild residual varus deformity.

Ranawat AS, Ranawat CS, Elkus M, Rasquinha VJ, Rossi R, Babhulkar S. Total knee arthroplasty for severe valgus deformity. J Bone Joint Surg Am. 2005;87 Suppl 1(Pt 2):271–84.

This paper describes the inside-out soft-tissue release technique and its long-term results when performed in primary total knee arthroplasty in patients with a severe valgus knee deformity. Seventy-one patients (85 knees) had a valgus deformity of 10°, however only 35 patients (42 knees) had a minimum follow-up of 5 years.

The technique describes an inside-out soft-tissue release of the posterolateral aspect of the capsule with pie-crusting of the iliotibial band and resection of the proximal part of the tibia and distal part of the femur to provide a balanced, rectangular space. Cemented, posterior stabilized implants were used in all knees. The mean modified Knee Society clinical score improved from 30 to 93 points post-operatively, and the mean functional score improved from 34 to 81 points. There was no improvement in range of motion. The mean coronal alignment was corrected from 15° of valgus to 5° of valgus postoperatively. Three patients underwent revision surgery because of delayed infection, premature polyethylene wear, and patellar loosening in one patient each. The study shows that the inside-out release technique is reproducible and has good long-term results.

Sprenger TR, Doerzbacher JF. Tibial osteotomy for the treatment of varus gonarthrosis. Survival and failure analysis to twenty-two years. J Bone Joint Surg Am. 2003;85-A(3):469–74.

The long-term results of treatment of medial compartment gonarthrosis with a proximal tibial osteotomy were assessed in this study. Seventy-six valgus-producing high tibial osteotomies were performed in 66 patients with medial compartment gonarthrosis. The factors that were analyzed included postoperative valgus alignment, age, gender, and weight of the patient; preoperative Ahlbäck radiographic grade; adverse events; Workers' Compensation status; and public liability. Ten-year survival was 74, 70, and 65 % for conversion to arthroplasty, a Hospital for Special Surgery knee score of <70 points, and patient dissatisfaction, respectively. Radiographic valgus alignment between 8 and 16° at 1 year after the osteotomy had the most significant positive effect on survivorship for all end points (p<0.01). Complications occurred in 16 (21 %) of the 76 procedures. The study found that survival at 10 years was 90 %, when the valgus angle at 1 year was between 8 and 16°. The study recommended tibial osteotomy as an alternative to total knee arthroplasty, in patients less than 60 years old.

Hewett TE, Myer GD, Ford KR, Heidt RS, Jr., Colosimo AJ, McLean SG, et al. Biomechanical measures of neuromuscular control and valgus loading of the knee predict anterior cruciate ligament injury risk in female athletes: a prospective study. Am J Sports Med. 2005;33(4):492–501.

The study looked at whether female athletes in high-risk sports were at greater risk of ACL injury. Two hundred and five pre-screened female athletes in high-risk sports were prospectively measured for neuromuscular control using 3-dimensional kinematics (joint angles) and joint loads using kinetics (joint moments) during a jump-landing task. Nine athletes had a confirmed anterior cruciate ligament rupture. These 9 had significantly different knee posture and loading. Knee abduction angle (P<.05) at landing was 8° greater in anterior cruciate ligament-injured than in uninjured athletes. Anterior cruciate ligament-injured athletes had a 2.5 times greater knee abduction moment (P<.001) and 20 % higher ground reaction force (P<.05), whereas stance time was 16 % shorter; hence, increased motion, force, and moments occurred more quickly. Knee abduction moment predicted anterior cruciate ligament injury status with 73 % specificity and 78 % sensitivity; dynamic valgus measures showed a predictive r2 of 0.88. Knee motion and knee loading during a landing task are predictors of anterior cruciate ligament injury risk in female athletes.

Meniscal Injuries

Hede A, Larsen E, Sandberg H. Partial versus total meniscectomy. A prospective, randomised study with long-term follow-up. J Bone Joint Surg Br. 1992;74(1):118–21.

Two hundred patients with a meniscal lesion were randomly allocated to partial or total meniscectomy. The results were compared at 1 year and at a median of 7.8 years. At 1 year, 91 % who had partial and 80 % who had a total meniscectomy had an excellent functional outcome, though this dropped to 62 and 52 % respectively at the later follow-up. Patients with partial meniscectomy had higher Lysholm scores. Both groups showed equal progression of radiological evidence of joint narrowing. The incidence of mediolateral instability rose from 8 to 47 % and was more frequent after total than after partial meniscectomy. There was also more instability and greater rate of progression of joint narrowing in the lateral meniscectomy patients.

Hamberg P, Gillquist J, Lysholm J. A comparison between arthroscopic meniscectomy and modified open meniscectomy. A prospective randomised study with emphasis on postoperative rehabilitation. J Bone Joint Surg Br. 1984;66(2):189–92.

This prospective randomised study allocated 40 patients with a clinical diagnosis of a degenerative medial meniscal tear into four equal groups: arthroscopic partial meniscectomy, arthroscopic total meniscectomy, open partial meniscectomy and open total menscectomy. In the short term, there was no statistically significant difference between the groups with regards to lysholm knee score and muscle strength. The arthroscopic group had the best results with a significantly shorter surgical time, earlier return to work and better post-operative course.

Berthiaume MJ, Raynauld JP, Martel-Pelletier J, Labonté F, Beaudoin G, Bloch DA, et al. Meniscal tear and extrusion are strongly associated with progression of symptomatic knee osteoarthritis as assessed by quantitative magnetic resonance imaging. Ann Rheum Dis. 2005;64(4):556–63.

32 patients meeting American College of Rheumatology (ACR) criteria for symptomatic knee osteoarthritis were studied with knee MRI scans every 6 months for 2 years. The cartilage volumes of different knee regions were measured. Three indices of structural change in the medial and lateral menisci were evaluated: degeneration, tear, and extrusion. Twenty-four patients (75 %) had mild to moderate or severe meniscal damage. A highly significant difference in global cartilage volume loss was observed between severe medial meniscal tear and absence of tear (p = 0.002). An even greater difference was found between the medial meniscal changes and medial compartment cartilage volume loss (p < 0.0001). Similarly, a major difference was found between the presence of a medial meniscal extrusion and loss of medial compartment cartilage volume (p < 0.001). Meniscal tear and extrusion appear to be associated with progression of symptomatic knee osteoarthritis.

Morgan CD, Wojtys EM, Casscells CD, Casscells SW. Arthroscopic meniscal repair evaluated by second-look arthroscopy. Am J Sports Med. 1991;19(6):632–7; discussion 637–8.

Of 353 arthroscopic peripheral meniscal repairs performed using the "outside to inside" suturing technique with rasp preparation of the tear region, 74 repairs (50 medial and 24 lateral) were assessed by second-look arthroscopy and are the basis of this report. Results were graded as either healed, incompletely healed, or failed; these findings were correlated with clinical symptoms and associated ACL deficiency. Overall, asymptomatic healing occurred in 84 %, with 65 % healed and 19 % incompletely healed. The failure rate was 16 %. All failures were symptomatic while all healed and incompletely healed menisci were asymptomatic. Failure was associated with ACL deficiency in all cases. No failures occurred in either an ACL uninjured knee or an ACL reconstructed knee. Failure was also associated with tear location in the posterior horn of the medial meniscus. Eleven of 12 failures (92 %) involved posterior medial meniscal tears with only 1 failure located posterolaterally. Visual evidence of healing required a 4 month time interval.

Knee Dislocation

Schenck R. Classification of knee dislocations. Oper Tech Sports Med. 2003;11(3):193–8.

In this paper, Schenck introduces a describes an anatomic classification system for knee dislocations based on the number and type of ligaments ruptured (Table 4.1). This system is useful because it allows like cases to be studied, it makes it easier to direct management, and it allows simple communication between team members. It also gives an indication as to the severity of the injury, although this cannot be relied upon. Injuries to surrounding tissue should be given in the description, but not in the classification.

Green NE, Allen BL. Vascular injuries associated with dislocation of the knee. J Bone Joint Surg Am. 1977;59(2):236–9.

This case series of 245 knee dislocations (204 from previous literature and 41 new cases) was reviewed to determine the incidence of arterial injury and the results of its management. It was confirmed that anterior and posterior dislocations were both most common, and most commonly associated with popliteal artery injury. When both series were combined (n=245) it was found that 32 % of all dislocations were associated with arterial injury (with only 10 % of these recovering after reduction), patients with an anterior or posterior dislocation had a higher incidence of vascular damage of 39 and 44 % respectively. Again, combining the two series, an overall amputation rate of 86 % was found for those with vascular injury not operated on within 8 h,

TABLE 4.1 Anatomic classification of knee dislocation

KDI	One or both cruciate intact
KDII	Bicruciate rupture, collaterals intact
KDIII	Bicruciate rupture, one collateral rupture
	Subset KDIIIM or KDIIIL
KDIV	Bicruciate and both collaterals ruptured
KDV	Periarticular facture/dislocation
C	Add for arterial injury
N	Add for nerve injury

whereas for those operated on within 8 h, a limb survival rate of 89 % was noted.

Richter M, Bosch U, Wippermann B, Hofmann A, Krettek C. Comparison of surgical repair or reconstruction of the cruciate ligaments versus nonsurgical treatment in patients with traumatic knee dislocations. Am J Sports Med. 2002;30(5):718–27.

This retrospective study followed 89 patients with knee dislocations. Group I were managed surgically, with either repair or reconstruction (n = 63), and Group II were managed conservatively (n = 26). Mean follow-up at 8.2 years (range 2–25 years) showed statistically significantly better results for the surgical group compared to the non-surgical group in terms of Lysholm Score, Tegner Score, development of OA, Lachmann Test, and return to sport. Conclusions from this study say that it is beneficial to operate on the multiligament damaged traumatic knee dislocation.

Mariani PP, Santoriello P, Iannone S, Condello V, Adriani E. Comparison of surgical treatments for knee dislocation. Am J Knee Surg. 1999;12(4):214–21.

In this retrospective study, three surgical techniques were compared for the management of ruptured ACL and posterior cruciate ligament (PCL) in a knee dislocation. Group I (n = 11) had direct repair of both ligaments, Group II (n = 6) had reconstruction of the ACL with reattachment of the PCL, and Group III (n = 6) had reconstruction of both ligaments. At mean follow-up of 6.9 years, better results were achieved in Group III in terms of anteroposterior translation and IKDC evaluation.

Harner CD, Waltrip RL, Bennett CH, Francis KA, Cole B, Irrgang JJ. Surgical management of knee dislocations. J Bone Joint Surg Am. 2004;86-A(2):262–73.

In this retrospective study, patients were reviewed to determine whether acute operative management (<3 weeks from injury, n = 19) or delayed operative management (>3 weeks from injury, n = 12) produced the optimum results. Patients had a minimum follow-up of 24 months, and at this time patients in the acutely treated group performed significantly better on the Sports Activity Scale (89 vs 69), and performance on the Lysholm score (91 vs 80) and Knee Outcome Survey Activities of Daily Living (90 vs 84) approached significance but did not reach it.

Knee Ligament Injuries

Keller PM, Shelbourne KD, McCarroll JR, Rettig AC. Non-operatively treated isolated posterior cruciate ligament injuries. Am J Sports Med. 1993;21(1):132–6.

Forty patients with isolated Posterior Cruciate Ligament (PCL) injuries treated non-operatively were reviewed with a mean 6 year follow-up. Patients were reviewed using a modified Noyes questionnaire, clinical examination, isokinetic testing, and radiographic investigation. Questionnaire results showed that patients had pain (90 %), had problems walking (43 %), and had a limited activity level (65 %), and only 51 % of patient had achieved the recovery they were expecting. Longer time since injury was associated with worse knee score and worse radiographic appearence. Noyes score appeared to worsen with increased ligament laxity. Four patients required surgery. Quadriceps strength was unaffected. This study showed that patients with isolated tears of the PCL do not recover well if treated conservatively.

Ahn JH, Yoo JC, Wang JH. Posterior cruciate ligament reconstruction: double-loop hamstring tendon autograft versus Achilles tendon allograft—clinical results of a minimum 2-year follow-up. Arthroscopy. 2005;21(8):965–9.

This retrospective case-control study compared the results of patients who had undergone PCL reconstruction using a hamstring autograft (Group I, n = 18) with those who had an Achilles tendon allograft (Group II, n = 18). All patients had only PCL injury, or PCL injury with meniscal injury. At minimum 2 year follow-up, statistically significant improvements were observed in the cohort as a whole. Regarding IKDC scores, Group I achieved more 'normal' or 'nearly normal' knees (16 vs 14) but this difference was not significant. Regarding Lysholm Knee Score, patients in Group I had a significantly better improvement than patients in Group II (21.9 point increase vs 17.2 point increase respectively, $p < 0.01$). There was no significant difference between the groups with regard to posterior displacement measured using a Telos stress machine. Eight patients from Group I and 11 patients from Group II required removal of the post-tie screw, and 1 patient from Group II required surgery to increase range of movement.

Stannard JP, Brown SL, Farris RC, McGwin G Jr, Volgas DA. The posterolateral corner of the knee: repair versus reconstruction. Am J Sports Med. 2005;33(6):881–8.

This prospective study compared 57 tears of the posterolateral corner (PLC) which were either repaired (n = 35) if the tissue was deemed repairable, or reconstructed (n = 22) if not. At mean follow-up of 33 months, there was a significantly greater proportion of reconstructions that had been successful compared to repairs (91 % vs 67 %, $p = 0.03$). 12/13 failed repairs and 2/2 failed reconstructions underwent successful revision reconstruction. There was no difference in post operative range of motion. There were no significant differences between groups with regards to Lysholm scores, IKDC scores, SF-36 scores, and complication rates after revision operations had been performed. Following these results, the authors now only repair the PLC if there is a significant avulsion fracture allowing internal fixation with screws.

Reider B, Sathy MR, Talkington J, Blyznak N, Kollias S. Treatment of isolated medial collateral ligament injuries in athletes with early functional rehabilitation. A five-year follow-up study. Am J Sports Med. 1994;22(4):470–7.

This prospective, 5-year follow-up study reports on 34 athletes with grade III injuries to the medial collateral ligament (MCL) treated with early functional rehabilitation. The programme consisted of four goals and as soon as one was reached the next one was aimed for: (1) walks unassisted without a limp, (2) 90 % knee flexion, (3) full knee motion, and (4) complete a full running programme in one session with no pain/swelling and >90 % strength compared to contalateral leg. After the fourth goal was achieved, patients could return to sport. Mean Hospital for Special Surgery (HSS) score was 45.9/50. Most patients returned to full activity within 4 weeks, and all returned eventually, however it took between 2 and 4 months before most patients thought their knee was back to normal. Twenty-three patients still had at least one residual symptom in the knee at follow-up, consisting of mild pain, looseness, swelling, and crepitus. The authors claim that these results are comparable with earlier series of immobilisation, and surgical management, with minimal treatment related morbidity and an earlier return to sport.

Buzzi R, Aglietti P, Vena LM, Giron F. Lateral collateral ligament reconstruction using a semitendinosus graft. Knee Surg Sports Traumatol Arthrosc. 2004;12(1):36–42.

This retrospective case series analysed 13 lateral collateral ligament (LCL) injuries that had been reconstructed using a free semitendinosus graft. All patients had either ACL injury (n = 6) or PCL injury (n = 7) at the same time, all of these were reconstructed. At mean follow-up 60 months, the ACL group had 5 symptom free patients, and 1 patient complained of pain and swelling after mountain biking. IKDC scores were normal for 5, and nearly normal for 1 knee, and lateral joint opening was 0–2 mm for 5 knees, and 3–5 mm for 1 knee. In the PCL group, 4 patients were symptom free and 3 had mild to moderate pain and swelling after activity. IKDC scores were normal for 2 knees, and nearly normal for 5 knees, and lateral joint opening was 0–2 mm for 6 knees, and 3–5 mm for 1 knee. Eleven patients (85 %) returned to their pre-injury level of activity, and 2 (15 %) returned to one level lower.

Common Peroneal Nerve Injury

Ferraresi S, Garozzo D, Buffatti P. Common peroneal nerve injuries: results with one-stage nerve repair and tendon transfer. Neurosurg Rev. 2003;26(3):175–9.

This paper presented the results of 45 patients who suffered a common peroneal nerve (CPN) injury. The early patients (Group A, n = 6) were treated with nerve repair only, whereas the remainder (Group B, n = 39) were treated with nerve repair and transfer of the tibialis posterior muscle to regain foot dorsiflexion. The results for Group A were poor, with 5 patients having 'poor' results (M0 power) and 1 patient having a 'fair' result (M1-2). The results in Group B were far superior with 28 patients having 'good' results (M3+, considered acceptable for easy walking), 7 patients having a 'fair' result, and 4 patients having a 'poor' result. The authors concluded that nerve repair plus tibialis posterior transfer was the optimum management plan for patient with CPN injuries.

Garozzo D, Ferraresi S, Buffatti P. Surgical treatment of common peroneal nerve injuries: indications and results. A series of 62 cases. J Neurosurg Sci. 2004;48(3):105–12; discussion 112.

This series, used the same cohort as the study above, plus some extra patients (total n = 62), to assess the outcomes after CPN injury based on the mechanism of injury and the surgical timing. The results between Group A and Group B (as above) were similar to the above paper, with better results in the 'nerve repair and tendon transfer' patients, at 2 year follow-up. Causative mechanism did have an influence as to the outcome, with patients suffering 'sharp injuries and transections' having 100 % 'good' recovery and patients suffering knee dislocations having 74 % 'good' recovery. Other mechanisms had poorer outcomes: Crush Fractures (33 % 'good'), ankle sprain (0 % 'good'), and gunshots (0 % 'good'). The authors conclude, using their own experience and a review of the literature, that open wounds with complete nerve palsy should undergo surgical treatment as an emergency or within 1–2 days, closed injuries, with no spontaneous recovery within 4 months, should undergo surgical intervention, and any delay past this is associated with poor postoperative recovery. Both of these recommendations are regardless of mechanism of injury.

Kim DH, Murovic JA, Tiel RL, Kline DG. Management and outcomes in 318 operative common peroneal nerve lesions at the Louisiana State University Health Sciences Center. Neurosurgery. 2004;54(6):1421–8; discussion 1428–9.

Patients between 1967 and 1999 (n=318), were reviewed retrospectively with regards to injury mechanism, preoperative neurological status, lesion type, operative technique, and outcome. Results for mechanism of injury were: stretch/contusions without knee fracture/dislocation (44 %), tumours (13 %), lacerations (12 %), entrapments (9 %), stretch/contusions with knee fracture/dislocation (7 %), compressions (7 %), iatrogenic (4 %), and gunshot wounds (4 %). If intraoperative nerve action potentials (NAP) were found, neurolysis was performed, if no NAPs were found then either direct suture or graft repair was done. Of those without tumours (n=278), 107 (88 %) patients undergoing neurolysis had a good recovery, 16 (84 %) of patients undergoing end-to-end suture had a good recovery, but only 58 (42 %) of the patients undergoing graft repair had a good recovery. However, when graft length was considered, those with short grafts (<6 cm) did better than those with medium grafts (7–12 cm), and both did better than those with long grafts (13–24 cm) at 75 % good outcome vs 38 and 16 % respectively.

Niall DM, Nutton RW, Keating JF. Palsy of the common peroneal nerve after traumatic dislocation of the knee. J Bone Joint Surg Br. 2005;87(5):664–7.

In this case series of 55 patients with knee dislocation, 14 (25 %) had injury to the CPN, and all 14 had damage to PCL and posterolateral corner (PLC). Of the dislocations with damage to the PCL and PLC (n=34), 41 % had CPN injury. Complete CPN rupture was present in 4 patients, whilst 10 had contusions to the nerve. Those with contusions were treated conservatively, with the 3 patients with lesions <7 cm achieving full recovery within 16 months. Of the remaining 7 patients, 2 achieved no motor function and partial sensory function, 1 achieved movement (not considered useful) and partial sensory function, and 4 achieved functional movement (2 with full sensory recovery, 2 with partial sensory recovery). Of the 4 patients with CPN ruptures, 1 underwent ipsilateral cable grafting of the sural nerve and 2 patients had tendon transfers of tibialis posterior. The fourth patient was not described in detail but was recorded as having no recovery.

References

Newman JH, Ackroyd CE, Shah NA. Unicompartmental or total knee replacement? Five-year results of a prospective, randomised trial of 102 osteoarthritic knees with unicompartmental arthritis. J Bone Joint Surg Br. 1998;80(5):862–5.

Vanlauwe J, Saris DB, Victor J, Almqvist KF, Bellemans J, Luyten FP, et al. Five-year outcome of characterized chondrocyte implantation versus microfracture for symptomatic cartilage defects of the knee: early treatment matters. Am J Sports Med. 2011;39(12):2566–74.

Foot and Ankle

Gavin Bowyer

Abstract This chapter covers the key topics in elective adult foot and ankle orthopaedics. Degenerative change in the ankle and great toe joint, and Achilles tendon and tibialis posterior tendon dysfunction are common problems, as are the effects of diabetes and rheumatoid arthritis in the foot. These pathologies and treatment options are dealt with here with up-to-date references. The common deformity of hallux valgus and the less common, but challenging, cavovarus foot are also considered. References are presented which help to understand the pathology, treatment and outcomes.

Keywords Ankle arthritis • Tibialis posterior dysfunction • Pes cavus • Diabetic foot • Rheumatoid foot • Hallux valgus • Hallux rigidus • Achilles tendinopathy

G. Bowyer, MA, MChir, FRCS (Orth)
Department of Trauma and Orthopaedics,
University Hospital Southampton, NHS Trust,
Tremona Road, Southampton, Hampshire SO16 6YD, UK
e-mail: gwbowyer@aol.com

G. Bowyer, A. Cole (eds.), *Selected References in Trauma and Orthopaedics*, DOI 10.1007/978-1-4471-4676-6_5,
© Springer-Verlag London 2014

Ankle Arthritis

Haene R, Qamirani E, Story RA, Pinsker E, Daniels TR. Intermediate outcomes of fresh talar osteochondral allografts for treatment of large osteochondral lesions of the talus. J Bone Joint Surg Am. 2012;94(12):1105–10.

Large osteochondral defects of the talus present a treatment challenge. Fresh osteochondral allograft transplantation can be used for large lesions without the donor-site morbidity associated with other procedures such as autologous chondrocyte implantation or osteochondral autograft transfer. The average duration of follow-up in this paper was 4.1 years. The latest follow-up computed tomography (CT) evaluation identified failure of graft incorporation in 2 of 16 ankles. Osteolysis, subchondral cysts, and degenerative changes were found in 5, 8 and 7 ankles, respectively. Five ankles were considered failures, and two required a reoperation because of ongoing symptoms. Overall, ten patients had a good or excellent result; however, persistent symptoms remained in six of these patients. Only four were symptom-free.

Goldberg AJ, Macgregor A, Dawson J, Singh D, Cullen N, Sharp RJ, Cooke PH. The demand incidence of symptomatic ankle osteoarthritis presenting to foot & ankle surgeons in the United Kingdom. Foot (Edinb). 2012;22(3):163–6.

Ankle arthritis is a cause of major disability; however reports in the literature on the incidence of ankle osteoarthritis are rare. A survey and questionnaire of foot and ankle surgeons in UK was used to inform an estimate of the size of the problem. There are an estimated 29,000 cases of symptomatic ankle osteoarthritis being referred to specialists in the UK, representing a demand incidence of 47.7 per 100,000. About 3,000 definitive operations to treat end stage ankle osteoarthritis take place in the UK annually.

Hendrickx RP, Stufkens SA, de Bruijn EE, Sierevelt IN, van Dijk CN, Kerkhoffs GM. Medium- to long-term outcome of ankle arthrodesis. Foot Ankle Int. 2011;32(10):940–7.

This long term study looked for deterioration in outcome resulting from loss of ankle joint motion and adjacent joint arthritis. Isolated ankle arthrodesis cases were reviewed – there was follow-up data on 60 patients (66 ankles). There were 40 males and 26 females with a mean age at surgery of 47 years. In 60 ankles, fusion was obtained using a two-incision, three-screw technique. Fusion was achieved in 91 % after primary surgery. In six patients rearthrodesis was needed to obtain fusion. Ninety-one percent were satisfied with their clinical result. Infection occurred once. No other serious adverse events were encountered. In all contiguous joints significant progression of arthritis was appreciated, but the functional and clinical importance of these findings remains unclear.

DeGroot H 3rd, Uzunishvili S, Weir R, Al-omari A, Gomes B. Intra-articular injection of hyaluronic acid is not superior to saline solution injection for ankle arthritis: a randomized, double-blind, placebo-controlled study. J Bone Joint Surg Am. 2012;94(1):2–8.

Sixty-four patients with ankle osteoarthritis were randomly assigned to a single intra-articular injection of 2.5 mL of low-molecular-weight, non-cross-linked hyaluronic acid or a single intra-articular injection of 2.5 mL of normal saline solution. The American Orthopedic Foot & Ankle Society (AOFAS) clinical rating score in the hyaluronic acid group had improved from baseline by 4.9 and 4.9 points at 6 and 12 weeks post-injection, respectively, whereas the mean scores in the placebo group initially worsened by 0.4 point at 6 weeks and then improved by 5.4 points at 12 weeks. While the change at 12 weeks from baseline was substantial for both groups, the between-group differences were not significant.

Henricson A, Nilsson JÅ, Carlsson A. 10-year survival of total ankle arthroplasties: a report on 780 cases from the Swedish Ankle Register. Acta Orthop. 2011;82(6):655–9.

Records of uncemented 3-component total ankle replacements (TARs) were retrospectively reviewed. The overall survival rate fell from 0.81 (95 % CI: 0.79–0.83) at 5 years to 0.69 (95 % CI: 0.67–0.71) at 10 years. Excluding the STAR prosthesis, the survival rate for all the remaining designs was 0.78 at 10 years. Women below the age of 60 with osteoarthritis were at a higher risk of revision, but age did not influence the outcome in men or women with rheumatoid arthritis. Revisions due to technical mistakes at the index surgery and instability were undertaken earlier than revisions for other reasons. The results have slowly improved during the 18-year period investigated.

Gougoulias N, Khanna A, Maffulli N. How successful are current ankle replacements?: a systematic review of the literature. Clin Orthop Relat Res. 2010;468(1):199–208.

This is a systematic literature search of studies reporting on the outcome of total ankle arthroplasty. Thirteen Level IV studies of overall good quality reporting on 1,105 total ankle arthroplasties (234 Agility, 344 STAR, 153 Buechel-Pappas, 152 Hintegra, 98 Salto, 70 TNK, 54 Mobility) were included. Residual pain was common (range, 27–60 %), superficial wound complications occurred in 0–14.7 %, deep infections occurred in 0–4.6 % of ankles, and ankle function improved after total ankle arthroplasty. The overall failure rate was approximately 10 % at 5 years with a wide range (range, 0–32 %) between different centers. Superiority of an implant design over another cannot be supported by the available data.

Haddad SL, Coetzee JC, Estok R, Fahrbach K, Banel D, Nalysnyk L. Intermediate and long-term outcomes of total ankle arthroplasty and ankle arthrodesis. A systematic review of the literature. J Bone Joint Surg Am. 2007;89(9): 1899–905.

This systematic review identified 49 primary studies (10 arthroplasty, 39 arthrodesis, none directly comparative). The mean AOFAS Ankle-Hindfoot Scale score was 78.2 points for total ankle arthroplasty and 75.6 points for arthrodesis. Results were (arthroplasty vs arthrodesis): Excellent – 38 % vs 31 %; Good 30.5 % vs 37 %; Fair 5.5 % vs 13 %; Poor 24 % vs 13 %.

The 5-year implant survival rate was 78 % and the 10-year survival rate was 77 %. The revision rate following total ankle arthroplasty was 7 %, usually for loosening and/ or subsidence; the revision rate following arthrodesis was 9 % (usually for non-union). One percent of the patients who had undergone total ankle arthroplasty required a below-the-knee amputation compared with 5 % in the ankle arthrodesis group.

Comment: Data are sparse, and like is not compared with like – there were no comparative trials.

Tibialis Posterior Dysfunction

Aronow MS. Tendon transfer options in managing the adult flexible flatfoot. Foot Ankle Clin. 2012;17(2):205–26.

Tendon transfer is often used in surgery for posterior tibial tendon dysfunction. The flexor digitorum longus is most commonly transferred, although the flexor hallucis longus and peroneus brevis have also been described in the literature. This paper examines the advantages and disadvantages of the different tendons, the associated surgical techniques and the published results.

Nielsen MD, Dodson EE, Shadrick DL, Catanzariti AR, Mendicino RW, Malay DS. Non-operative care for the treatment of adult-acquired flatfoot deformity. J Foot Ankle Surg. 2011;50(3):311–4.

This retrospective cohort study focused on non-operative measures, including bracing, physical therapy, and non-steroidal anti-inflammatory drugs (NSAIDs) for adult-acquired flatfoot in 64 consecutive patients. Nonsurgical treatment was successful in 87.5 % over the 27-month observation period. Overall, 78 % of the patients were obese, but body mass index (BMI) was not statistically significantly associated with the outcome of treatment. Bracing tended to be successful but not when there was a split-tear of the tibialis posterior on magnetic resonance imaging

(MRI); a split-tear was associated with failure of non-operative treatment.

Parsons S, Naim S, Richards PJ, McBride D. Correction and prevention of deformity in type II tibialis posterior dysfunction. Clin Orthop Relat Res. 2010;468(4):1025–32.

This is a prospective study of 32 patients managed by split tibialis anterior transfer (to a navicular bone tunnel) and translational os calcis osteotomy for flexible pes planus deformity after failed conservative treatment. The average follow-up was 5.1 years. Twenty-nine of the 32 patients could perform a single heel rise test at 12 months. The mean postoperative American Orthopaedic Foot and Ankle Society hindfoot score was 89 [good].

Deland JT. Adult-acquired flatfoot deformity. J Am Acad Orthop Surg. 2008;16(7):399–406.

This is a review of posterior tibial tendon dysfunction/insufficiency, also known as adult-acquired flatfoot deformity. This encompasses a wide range of deformities, varying in location, severity, and rate of progression. The paper proposes prompt early, aggressive nonsurgical management. If this fails then surgical correction should be strongly considered to avoid worsening of the deformity. The goal of surgery is to achieve proper alignment and maintain as much flexibility as possible in the foot and ankle complex.

Bluman EM, Title CI, Myerson MS. Posterior tibial tendon rupture: a refined classification system. Foot Ankle Clin. 2007;12(2):233–49.

Since Johnson's and Strom's classification system in 1989 an increasingly complex array of deformities of the foot has been recognized in association with posterior tibial tendon rupture (PTTR). This paper looks at ankle and hindfoot valgus, forefoot supination, forefoot abduction, and medial column instability, then presents a refined classification for PTTR, with suggestions for potential treatments for each stage.

Knupp M, Hintermann B. The Cobb procedure for treatment of acquired flatfoot deformity associated with stage II insufficiency of the posterior tibial tendon. Foot Ankle Int. 2007;28(4):416–21.

The Cobb procedure involves the use of a split anterior tibial tendon (ATT) graft that is re-routed through the first cuneiform to the proximal stump of the posterior tibial tendon (PTT). In this study of 22 patients followed up for a mean of 2 years, the overall clinical results were excellent in 9 patients (41 %), good in 12 (54.5 %), fair in 1 (4.5 %), and poor in none. None of the patients had decreased power of the anterior tibial tendon compared to the contralateral foot. Nineteen patients (86 %) were able to wear shoes without shoe modifications.

Alvarez RG, Marini A, Schmitt C, Saltzman CL. Stage I and II posterior tibial tendon dysfunction treated by a structured non-operative management protocol: an orthosis and exercise program. Foot Ankle Int. 2006;27(1):2–8.

Forty-seven consecutive patients with stage I or II posterior tibial tendon dysfunction were treated non-operatively with articulated ankle foot orthosis or foot orthosis, high-repetition exercises, aggressive plantarflexion activities, and high-repetition home exercise program that including Achilles stretching. After a median of ten physical therapy visits over a median period of 4 months, 39 (83 %) of the 47 patients had successful subjective and functional outcomes, and 42 patients (89 %) were satisfied. Five patients (11 %) required surgery after failure of non-operative treatment.

Trnka HJ. Dysfunction of the tendon of tibialis posterior. J Bone Joint Surg Br. 2004;86(7):939–46.

Comment: A very well written review covering the aetiology and patho-anatomy, presentation, classification, treatment (operative and non-operative) in this condition and the acquired adult pes planus.

Wacker JT, Hennessy MS, Saxby TS. Calcaneal osteotomy and transfer of the tendon of flexor digitorum longus for stage-II dysfunction of tibialis posterior. Three- to five-year results. J Bone Joint Surg Br. 2002;84(1):54–8.

Prospective study of surgery in 51 patients with painful flexible flatfoot without fixed forefoot supination deformity (classical stage-II dysfunction of the PTT) treated by a medial displacement calcaneal osteotomy and transfer of the tendon of flexor digitorum longus. In 44 patients reviewed at 3–5 years, the mean AOFAS ankle/hindfoot rating scale improved from 48.8 before operation to 88.5 at follow-up. The operation failed in two patients who later had a calcaneocuboid fusion. The outcome in 43 patients was rated as good to excellent for pain and function, and in 36 good to excellent for alignment. There were no poor results.

Pes Cavus

Younger AS, Hansen ST Jr. Adult cavovarus foot. J Am Acad Orthop Surg. 2005;13(5):302–15.

Comment: A superb, detailed review which looks at the aetiology of cavovarus foot deformity (hereditary motor sensory neuropathy/Charcot-Marie-Tooth [HMSN/CMT], cerebral palsy [CP], Stroke, residual club foot, talar injury) and the resulting pathology (strong peroneus longus and tibialis posterior leading to hindfoot varus and pronated forefoot). This leads to lateral foot overload, ankle instability, peroneal tendonitis and stress fractures, with degeneration in the overloaded joints. Gait examination and the Coleman block test are key to assessing the foot. Surgery is aimed at rebalancing the tendons (tendon transfer and osteotomy) before joints and tendons become imbalanced; fixed bony deformity is addressed with osteotomy and fusion.

Burns J, Landorf KB, Ryan MM, Crosbie J, Ouvrier RA. Interventions for the prevention and treatment of pes cavus. Cochrane Database Syst Rev. 2007;(4):CD006154.

This systematic review assesses the effects of interventions for the prevention and treatment of pes cavus. Only one trial (custom-made foot orthoses) fully met the inclusion criteria. Two additional cross-over trials (off-the-shelf foot orthoses and footwear) were also included. In one randomised controlled trial, custom-made foot orthoses were significantly more beneficial than sham orthoses for treating chronic musculoskeletal foot pain associated with pes cavus.

Casasnovas C, Cano LM, Albertí A, Céspedes M, Rigo G. Charcot-Marie-tooth disease. Foot Ankle Spec. 2008;1(6):350–4.

Charcot-Marie-Tooth disease (CMT) or hereditary motor and sensory neuropathy constitutes a genetically heterogeneous group of diseases that affect the peripheral nervous system. CMT is characterized by degeneration or abnormal development of the peripheral nerve and is transmitted with different genetic patterns. Features include: an awkward high-stepping gait, tripping; distal muscular atrophy of all extremities; foot deformities, such as cavus foot. The classification of CMT is complex and updated as new genes and mutations are found. CMT should be suspected in any patient with cavus foot, particularly if other members of the family have been diagnosed with the disease. Treatment decisions must be individualized and based on a clear history, careful examination, and well-defined patient goals.

Leeuwesteijn AE, de Visser E, Louwerens JW. Flexible cavovarus feet in Charcot-Marie-Tooth disease treated with first ray proximal dorsiflexion osteotomy combined with soft tissue surgery: a short-term to mid-term outcome study. Foot Ankle Surg. 2010;16(3):142–7.

Surgical correction of cavovarus foot deformity consisted of dorsiflexion osteotomy at the base of the first metatarsal combined with tendon transfers. Secondary calcaneal osteotomy was performed in cases of persistent varus of the calcaneus. Seventy percent of the patients could walk barefoot after the operation and 77 % of the patients had less pain after surgery. Pressure callosities diminished in 81 %.

Foot function was considered better after surgery by 84 %. Ninety percent were satisfied with the correction of the deformity.

Ward CM, Dolan LA, Bennett DL, Morcuende JA, Cooper RR. Long-term results of reconstruction for treatment of a flexible cavovarus foot in Charcot-Marie-Tooth disease. J Bone Joint Surg Am. 2008;90(12):2631–42.

Cavovarus foot deformity is common in patients with Charcot-Marie-Tooth disease. Multiple surgical reconstructive procedures have been described, but few authors have reported long-term results. This study evaluated the long-term results of a reconstruction consisting of dorsiflexion osteotomy of the first metatarsal, transfer of the peroneus longus to the peroneus brevis, plantar fascia release, transfer of the extensor hallucis longus to the neck of the firstmetatarsal, and in selected cases, transfer of the tibialis anterior tendon to the lateral cuneiform. Results showed lower rates of degenerative changes and reoperations as compared with those reported at the time of long-term follow-up of patients treated with triple arthrodesis.

Diabetic Foot

Robinson AH, Pasapula C, Brodsky JW. Surgical aspects of the diabetic foot. J Bone Joint Surg Br. 2009;91(1):1–7.

A comprehensive review of the literature relating to the pathology and management of the diabetic foot is presented. This should provide a guide for the treatment of ulcers, Charcot neuro-arthropathy and fractures involving the foot and ankle in diabetic patients.

Lipsky BA, Berendt AR, Cornia PB, Pile JC, Peters EJ, Armstrong DG, et al. Executive summary: 2012 Infectious Diseases Society of America clinical practice guideline for the diagnosis and treatment of diabetic foot infections. Clin Infect Dis. 2012;54(12):1679–84.

Diabetic foot infections (DFIs) often begin in a wound, most often a neuropathic ulceration. It is important to distinguish infection from colonisation and to classify the extent of the infection, and vascular status of the limb. Most DFIs are polymicrobial. Most require some surgical intervention, ranging from minor (debridement – send tissue for culture) to major (resection, amputation). Empiric antibiotic therapy for acute infection can be narrowly targeted at G+ve cocci, but those at risk for infection with antibiotic-resistant organisms or with chronic, previously treated, or severe infections usually require broader spectrum regimens. Osteomyelitis occurs in many diabetic patients with a foot wound and can be difficult to diagnose (optimally defined by bone culture and histology) and treat (often requiring surgical debridement or resection, and/or prolonged antibiotic therapy). Wounds must also be properly dressed and off-loaded of pressure, and patients need regular follow-up. Multidisciplinary foot teams improve outcome.

Lowery NJ, Woods JB, Armstrong DG, Wukich DK. Surgical management of Charcot neuroarthropathy of the foot and ankle: a systematic review. Foot Ankle Int. 2012;33(2): 113–21.

Charcot neuroarthropathy (CN) of the foot and ankle is an extremely challenging clinical dilemma and surgical management can be highly complicated. The current literature on this topic comprises retrospective case series and expert opinions. Furthermore, surgery in patients with CN of the foot and ankle (the use of exostectomy, fusion, and Achilles tendon lengthening for CN) is guided by studies with low levels of evidence to support our current surgical practices.

Mueller MJ, Sinacore DR, Hastings MK, Strube MJ, Johnson JE. Effect of Achilles tendon lengthening on neuropathic plantar ulcers. A randomized clinical trial. J Bone Joint Surg Am. 2003;85-A(8):1436–45.

Limited ankle dorsiflexion has been implicated as a contributing factor to plantar ulceration of the forefoot in diabetes. This study compared outcomes for diabetics with a neuropathic plantar ulcer treated with a total-contact cast with and without Achilles tendon lengthening. Twenty-nine (88 %) of 33 ulcers in the total-contact cast group and all 30 ulcers (100 %) in the Achilles tendon lengthening group healed. Of those available for follow-up at 7 months, 59 % in the total-contact cast group and 15 % of the Achilles tendon lengthening group had an ulcer recurrence. Of those available for follow-up at 2 years, 81 % of the total-contact cast group and 38 % in the Achilles tendon lengthening group had ulcer recurrence.

Rheumatoid Foot

Scott DL, Pugner K, Kaarela K, Doyle DV, Woolf A, Holmes J, et al. The links between joint damage and disability in rheumatoid arthritis. Rheumatology (Oxford). 2000;39(2): 122–32.

This literature review found 23 reports on the progression of joint damage, 12 reports on the progression of disability and 25 reports dealing with their interrelationship. Joint damage progresses constantly over the first 20 years of rheumatoid arthritis (RA). It accounts for approximately 25 % of disability in established RA. The link between damage and disability is strongest in late (>8 years) RA. However, avoiding or reducing joint damage in both early and established/ late RA is likely to maintain function.

Bohay DR, Brage ME, Younger AS. Surgical treatment of the ankle and foot in patients with rheumatoid arthritis. Instr Course Lect. 2009;58:595–616.

Rheumatoid arthritis can be as devastating for the joints of the foot and ankle as for other joints of the lower and upper extremities. Early conservative treatment often is provided by a primary care provider or rheumatologist. Drug and injection therapies are used with footwear modifications, activity restrictions, and orthoses. Surgery often is the last treatment modality available to the patient; it has the potential to relieve pain and improve function.

van der Heide HJ, Louwerens JW. Reconstructing the rheumatoid forefoot. Foot Ankle Surg. 2010;16(3):117–21.

This single surgeon series involved repositioning of the metatarsophalangeal (MTP) subluxation or dislocation of the lesser rays in 54 feet (39 patients). In cases of severe deformity or degeneration of the 1st MTP joint, an arthrodesis was performed. When, in addition to repositioning the MTP joints, an arthrodesis of the hallux was performed, the mean AOFAS-forefoot score was 69.80 at a mean of 40 months postoperatively. In cases with no operation on the hallux, the AOFAS score was 42.2. When comparing the patients who were satisfied and those who were not, the most important factor was also fusion of the 1st MTP joint, without a fusion only 50 % was satisfied, with a fusion the satisfaction rate was 93 %.

Jaakkola JI, Mann RA. A review of rheumatoid arthritis affecting the foot and ankle. Foot Ankle Int. 2004;25(12): 866–74.

This article reviews the clinical presentation, evaluation, and treatment of rheumatoid arthritis affecting the foot and ankle. Rheumatoid arthritis is a systemic disease. Approximately 20 % of patients with rheumatoid arthritis present initially with foot and ankle symptoms, and most patients will eventually develop foot and ankle symptoms. Although early intervention includes conservative measures, operative treatment often is needed to adequately treat rheumatoid patients. Treatment of foot and ankle problems in patients with rheumatoid arthritis is directed to maintaining ambulatory capacity.

Bibbo C, Goldberg JW. Infectious and healing complications after elective orthopaedic foot and ankle surgery during tumor necrosis factor-alpha inhibition therapy. Foot Ankle Int. 2004;25(5):331–5.

Thirty-one patients with rheumatoid arthritis undergoing elective foot and ankle surgery over a 12-month period were prospectively followed for the development of complications in the postoperative period. All patients continued their anti-rheumatoid drugs in the peri-operative period. Patients were then stratified into two groups based on the use of immuno-modulation via TNF-alpha inhibition (group 1) versus patients who did not receive TNF-alpha inhibition therapy (group 2). At mean follow-up of 10.6 months (group 1) and 9.7 months (group 2), healing or infectious complications were similar in both groups. However, when total complications (healing+infection) were analyzed, group 1 (TNF-alpha inhibition, "higher risk") patients demonstrated a lower complication rate (p=0.033).

Comment: This is an important paper presenting evidence for management of these patients taking powerful immune-modulating drugs.

Hallux Valgus

Easley ME, Trnka HJ. Current concepts review: hallux valgus part II: operative treatment. Foot Ankle Int. 2007;28(6): 748–58.

Comment: A well written and extensively referenced review of the operative options, and their rationale.

Ferrari J, Higgins JP, Prior TD. Interventions for treating hallux valgus (abductovalgus) and bunions. Cochrane Database Syst Rev. 2004;(1):CD000964.

This systematic review found that the methodological quality of the 21 included trials was generally poor and trial sizes were small. Few studies considered conservative treatments. The duration of follow-up was short in most trials; few trials maintained follow-up for 3 years. The evidence from the trials included suggested that orthoses and night splints did not appear to be any more beneficial in improving outcomes than no treatment. Surgery (chevron osteotomy) was shown to be beneficial compared to orthoses or no treatment, but when compared to other osteotomies, no technique was shown to be superior to any other. It was notable that the numbers of participants in some trials remaining dissatisfied at follow-up were consistently high (25–33 %), even when the hallux valgus angle and pain had improved.

Comment: A further Cochrane review was carried out in 2009 but has been withdrawn – findings were similar to this one.

Myerson MS, Badekas A. Hypermobility of the first ray. Foot Ankle Clin. 2000;5(3):469–84.

Hypermobility of the first ray is one of the causative components in common foot problems (such as hallux valgus) with a large intermetatarsal angle and metatarsus primus varus. Clinically, hypermobility is evaluated by determining sagittal motion (the grasping test) and transverse motion (the clinical squeeze test). The authors' surgical treatment of choice is arthrodesis of the tarsometatarsal joint (as part of the hallux valgus correction), exostectomy, capsulorraphy, and distal soft tissue release to correct and stabilize the first metatarsal at the apex of the deformity.

The main complications associated with the Lapidus procedure and its modifications are non-union, malunion, and dorsal elevation of the first metatarsal. Although radiographic non-union is the most frequent complication, only 25 % of the patients with this condition have associated clinical findings; the results have been defined as good or excellent in two series.

Perera AM, Mason L, Stephens MM. The pathogenesis of hallux valgus. J Bone Joint Surg Am. 2011;93(17):1650–61.

This paper proposes that the first ray is an inherently unstable axial array that relies on a fine balance between its static (capsule, ligaments, and plantar fascia) and dynamic stabilizers (peroneus longus and small muscles of the foot) to maintain its alignment. In some feet, there is a genetic predisposition for a nonlinear osseous alignment or a laxity of the static stabilizers that disrupts this muscle balance. Poor footwear plays an important role in accelerating the process, but occupation and excessive walking and weight-bearing are unlikely to be notable factors. In any patient, a number of factors have come together to cause the hallux valgus.

Bai LB, Lee KB, Seo CY, Song EK, Yoon TR. Distal chevron osteotomy with distal soft tissue procedure for moderate to severe hallux valgus deformity. Foot Ankle Int. 2010;31(8): 683–8.

This study looked at 76 patients (86 feet) that underwent distal chevron osteotomy with a distal soft tissue procedure for symptomatic moderate to severe hallux valgus deformity. At a mean follow-up of 31 months, 94 % of the patients were very satisfied or satisfied. Average AOFAS score improved from 54.7 points preoperatively to 92.9 at final follow-up. Average hallux valgus angle changed from 36.2° preoperatively to 12.4° at final follow-up, and average first-second intermetatarsal angle changed from 17.1° to 7.3°. There were no cases of avascular necrosis of the metatarsal head.

Maffulli N, Longo UG, Marinozzi A, Denaro V. Hallux valgus: effectiveness and safety of minimally invasive surgery. A systematic review. Br Med Bull. 2011;97:149–67.

Minimally invasive techniques for hallux valgus correction include arthroscopy, percutaneous and minimum incision surgery. In the last few decades, several techniques have been increasingly used. Data are lacking to allow definitive conclusions on the use of these techniques for routine management of patients with hallux valgus. Given the limitations of the current case series, especially the extensive clinical heterogeneity, it is not possible to determine clear recommendations regarding the systematic use of minimally invasive surgery for hallux valgus correction, even though preliminary results are encouraging.

Fuhrmann RA, Zollinger-Kies H, Kundert HP. Mid-term results of Scarf osteotomy in hallux valgus. Int Orthop. 2010;34(7):981–9.

A retrospective study on 178 Scarf osteotomies with a mean follow-up of 44.9 months. At follow-up the mean AOFAS score had improved significantly, but only 55 % of the feet showed a perfect realignment of the first ray. Patients with a hallux valgus angle exceeding 30° and pre-existing degenerative changes at the 1st metatarsophalangeal joint (MTPJ) displayed inferior clinical results. Nearly 20 % of the patients suffered from pain at this joint; attributed to onset or worsening of arthritis at the joint. Radiographic criteria (hallux valgus, first intermetatarsal angle, hallux valgus interphalangeus, MTP 1 joint congruency, arthritic lesions at MTP 1) worsened with time.

Hallux Rigidus

Zammit GV, Menz HB, Munteanu SE, Landorf KB, Gilheany MF. Interventions for treating osteoarthritis of the big toe joint. Cochrane Database Syst Rev. 2010;(9):CD007809.

Osteoarthritis affecting the big toe joint of the foot (hallux limitus or rigidus) is a common and painful condition. Although several treatments have been proposed, few have been adequately evaluated. This Cochrane review identified only one trial worthy of inclusion; that involved physiotherapy for the affected joint, and that presented a high risk of bias.

Comment: As is so often the case, there is a paucity of quality evidence for interventions even in this common condition.

Coughlin MJ, Shurnas PS. Hallux rigidus: demographics, etiology, and radiographic assessment. Foot Ankle Int. 2003; 24(10):731–43.

This study evaluated the demographics, etiology, and radiographic findings associated with hallux rigidus. The condition was not associated with elevatus, first ray hypermobility, a long first metatarsal, Achilles or gastrocnemius tendon tightness, abnormal foot posture, symptomatic hallux valgus, adolescent onset, shoewear, or occupation. Hallux rigidus was associated with hallux valgus interphalangeus, bilateral involvement in those with a familial history, unilateral involvement in those with a history of trauma, and women. A flat or chevron-shaped metatarsophalangeal joint was more common in hallux rigidus patients. At the initial examination 81 % of patients had radiographic and clinical evidence of unilateral disease, but at the final follow-up 79 % of patients had radiographic and clinical evidence of bilateral disease (mean of 8.9 years later).

Coughlin MJ, Shurnas PS. Hallux rigidus. Grading and long-term results of operative treatment. J Bone Joint Surg Am. 2003;85-A(11):2072–88.

This paper evaluated the long-term results of the operative treatment of hallux rigidus and assessed a clinical and radiographic grading of hallux rigidus. Treatment consisted of arthrodesis (mean follow-up 6.7 years) or cheilectomy (mean follow-up 9.7 years). There was significant improvement in dorsiflexion and total motion following the cheilectomies and significant improvement in postoperative pain and AOFAS scores in both treatment groups. Ninety-seven percent had a good or excellent subjective result, and 92 % of the cheilectomy procedures were successful in terms of pain relief and function. Cheilectomy was used with predictable success to treat Grade-1 and 2 and selected Grade-3 cases. Arthrodesis should be performed in patients with Grade-4 hallux rigidus or Grade-3 hallux rigidus with <50 % of the metatarsal head cartilage remaining at the time of surgery.

Roukis TS. The need for surgical revision after isolated cheilectomy for hallux rigidus: a systematic review. J Foot Ankle Surg. 2010;49(5):465–70.

Isolated cheilectomy has been proposed for treatment of hallux rigidus due to the perceived safety, efficacy, and ability to revise with repeat cheilectomy, implant or interpositional arthroplasty, or arthrodesis. Twenty-three studies, describing 706 cheilectomies, met the inclusion criteria, with 62 (8.8 %) undergoing surgical revision in the form of arthrodesis, an arthroplasty (interpositional, silicone, resectional) or repeat cheilectomy. Only 12 studies specified the grade of hallux rigidus as: 19.9 % grade 1, 40.6 % grade II, 36.6 % grade III, and 2.9 %. Revision was commoner in higher grade arthritis.

Brewster M. Does total joint replacement or arthrodesis of the first metatarsophalangeal joint yield better functional results? A systematic review of the literature. J Foot Ankle Surg. 2010;49(6):546–52.

This systematic review of the literature compared the functional outcomes of arthrodesis and joint replacement in first metatarsophalangeal surgery. It found 10 studies eligible for inclusion: 5 featured arthrodesis and 5 featured total joint replacement. Overall, arthrodesis achieves better functional outcomes than total joint replacement.

Comment: This paper includes the comment that "The operative techniques and prostheses for joint replacements are however still in an early stage of development and advances still need to be achieved to produce a more successful and anatomical prosthesis that could be functionally superior to an arthrodesis". The published results in the literature consistently show early promising results and poorer mid term results across a range of prostheses – it is rare to find long term results for replacement arthroplasty.

Dawson-Bowling S, Adimonye A, Cohen A, Cottam H, Ritchie J, Fordyce M. MOJE ceramic metatarsophalangeal arthroplasty: disappointing clinical results at two to eight years. Foot Ankle Int. 2012;33(7):560–4.

This reports on the mid-term results of 31 cases with the MOJE, a ceramic press fit arthroplasty undertaken for painful hallux. There was radiological loosening in 16 and 1 component fracture. Eight implants were been revised. In patients who had not undergone subsequent fusion, 15 had less than 36° of movement, 9 had 36–45°, 4 were in the 46–60 range, and only 1 had more than 60°. There were no infections. Previous studies had suggested favourable initial outcomes with the MOJE but in this series the reoperation rate of 26 % at up to 8 years and loosening in 52 % was worrying.

Achilles Tendinopathy

Maffulli N, Sharma P, Luscombe KL. Achilles tendinopathy: aetiology and management. J R Soc Med. 2004;97(10):472–6.

Comment: This paper provides an authoritative, well-referenced review of this condition including the anatomy, pathological features, presentation and management. It is available as a free full-text paper online through PubMed.

Wiegerinck JI, Kerkhoffs GM, van Sterkenburg MN, Sierevelt IN, van Dijk CN. Treatment for insertional Achilles tendinopathy: a systematic review. Knee Surg Sports Traumatol Arthrosc. 2013;21(6):1345–55.

This systematic review of the literature was performed to identify surgical and non-surgical therapeutic studies for insertional Achilles tendinopathy. Fourteen trials met the inclusion criteria evaluating 452 procedures in 433 patients. Five surgical techniques were evaluated; all had a good patient satisfaction (mean 89 %).

It is not possible to draw conclusions regarding the best surgical treatment for insertional Achilles tendinopathy. Extracorporeal shock wave therapy (ESWT) seems effective in patients with non-calcified insertional Achilles tendinopathy. Although both eccentric exercises resulted in a decrease in visual analog scale (VAS) score, full range of motion eccentric exercises shows a low patient satisfaction compared to floor level exercises and other conservative treatment.

Deans VM, Miller A, Ramos J. A prospective series of patients with chronic Achilles tendinopathy treated with autologous-conditioned plasma injections combined with exercise and therapeutic ultrasonography. J Foot Ankle Surg. 2012;51(6):706–10.

This prospective case series examined 26 patients with painful Achilles tendinopathy for a minimum duration of 6 months, treated with intratendinous autologous-conditioned plasma injection followed by a standardized rehabilitation protocol. Results showed statistically significant improvements in terms of pain, other symptoms, activities of daily living, sports activities, and quality of life.

de Vos RJ, Weir A, van Schie HT, Bierma-Zeinstra SM, Verhaar JA, Weinans H, et al. Platelet-rich plasma injection for chronic Achilles tendinopathy: a randomized controlled trial. JAMA. 2010;303(2):144–9.

This stratified, block-randomized, double-blind, placebo-controlled trial looked at 54 patients aged 18–70 years with chronic tendinopathy 2–7 cm above the Achilles tendon insertion. Treatments were eccentric exercises (usual care) with either a platelet-rich plasma (PRP) injection (PRP group) or saline injection (placebo group).

The mean Victorian Institute of Sports Assessment-Achilles (VISA-A) score improved significantly after 24 weeks in the PRP group by 21.7 points and in the placebo group by 20.5 points; the PRP injection compared with a saline injection did not result in greater improvement in pain and activity.

Comment: This shows the value of an RCT compared to a case series reported in the paper by Deans et al., above.

Bell KJ, Fulcher ML, Rowlands DS, Kerse N. Impact of autologous blood injections in treatment of mid-portion Achilles tendinopathy: double blind randomised controlled trial. BMJ. 2013;346:f2310.

This RCT looked at the effectiveness of two peritendinous autologous blood injections in addition to a standardised eccentric calf strengthening programme in improving pain and function in patients with mid-portion Achilles tendinopathy. The administration of two unguided peritendinous autologous blood injections 1 month apart, in addition to a standardised eccentric training programme, provides no additional benefit in the treatment of mid-portion Achilles tendinopathy.

Kiewiet NJ, Holthusen SM, Bohay DR, Anderson JG. Gastrocnemius recession for chronic noninsertional achilles tendinopathy. Foot Ankle Int. 2013;34(4):481–5.

This small case series of 12 patients, underwent gastrocnemius recession for refractory Achilles tendinopathy. The mean pain score significantly decreased and the mean AOFAS ankle and hindfoot score was significantly improved when compared with previously published scores for patients who underwent Achilles debridement with flexor hallucis longus (FHL) transfer. The authors conclude that gastrocnemius recession for the treatment of refractory Achilles tendinopathy was a viable treatment option following the failure of non-operative management.

Al-Abbad H, Simon JV. The effectiveness of extracorporeal shock wave therapy on chronic Achilles tendinopathy: a systematic review. Foot Ankle Int. 2013;34(1):33–41.

Extracorporeal shock wave therapy (ESWT) is hypothesized to be an effective alternative intervention to surgery when other conservative therapies fail. This systematic review investigated the effectiveness of ESWT in the treatment of insertional and non-insertional Achilles tendinopathies.

Four of the included studies were RCTs, and two were pre-post study designs. Overall, the review showed satisfactory evidence for the effectiveness of low-energy ESWT in the treatment of chronic insertional and non-insertional Achilles tendinopathies at a minimum 3 months' follow-up before considering surgery if other conservative management fails. However, combining ESWT with eccentric loading appears to show superior results.

Schon LC, Shores JL, Faro FD, Vora AM, Camire LM, Guyton GP. Flexor hallucis longus tendon transfer in treatment of Achilles tendinosis. J Bone Joint Surg Am. 2013; 95(1):54–60.

This study of 56 older, sedentary patients with insertional or midsubstance Achilles tendinosis looked at surgical debridement of the Achilles tendon with flexor hallucis longus tendon transfer. The study found significant improvement in terms of Achilles tendon function, physical function, and pain intensity in this group of relatively inactive, older, overweight patients. When present, hallux weakness had minimal functional sequelae.

Kang S, Thordarson DB, Charlton TP. Insertional Achilles tendinitis and Haglund's deformity. Foot Ankle Int. 2012;33(6):487–91.

This retrospective radiographic review of patients with insertional Achilles tendinitis showed that Haglund's deformity (enlargement of the posterosuperior prominence of the calcaneus) was not indicative of insertional Achilles tendinitis and was present in asymptomatic patients. Also, a majority of the insertional Achilles tendinitis patients had calcification at the tendon insertion.

Pearce CJ, Carmichael J, Calder JD. Achilles tendinoscopy and plantaris tendon release and division in the treatment of non-insertional Achilles tendinopathy. Foot Ankle Surg. 2012;18(2):124–7.

This consecutive series of 11 patients with a minimum of 2 years follow-up found that Achilles tendinoscopy and division of the plantaris tendon are encouraging but further studies are required to compare it to other treatments. It is minimally invasive and low risk so should not affect the ability to perform a formal open procedure if unsuccessful.

Alfredson H. Midportion Achilles tendinosis and the plantaris tendon. Br J Sports Med. 2011;45(13):1023–5.

Seventy-three consecutive tendons with chronic painful mid-portion Achilles tendinosis, were treated with US + Doppler-guided scraping, via a medial incision. If there was a plantaris tendon located in close relation to the medial Achilles, it was extirpated. Preliminary clinical results of the combined procedure, were very promising. A thickened plantaris tendon located in close relation to the medial Achilles seemed common in patients with chronic painful midportion tendinosis. The authors conclude that role of the plantaris tendon in midportion Achilles tendinosis needs to be further evaluated.

Alfredson H. Ultrasound and Doppler-guided mini-surgery to treat midportion Achilles tendinosis: results of a large material and a randomised study comparing two scraping techniques. Br J Sports Med. 2011;45(5):407–10.

This paper evaluated the clinical results of ultrasound (US) and colour Doppler-guided mini-surgery (scraping) outside the ventral tendon in a randomised study, compare two different techniques for surgical scraping. After surgery (follow-up mean 11 months), the mean VAS was 3 in 111 tendons (89 %) from satisfied patients back in full Achilles tendon loading activity. In the randomised study, there were no significant differences in the results between open treatment with a scalpel and percutaneous treatment with a needle.

Silbernagel KG, Brorsson A, Lundberg M. The majority of patients with Achilles tendinopathy recover fully when treated with exercise alone: a 5-year follow-up. Am J Sports Med. 2011;39(3):607–13.

This case series of 34 patients 51 ± 8.2 years old, were evaluated 5 years after initiation of exercise treatment. Eighty percent fully recovered from the initial injury; of these, 65 % had no symptoms, and 15 % had a new occurrence of symptoms, 20 % had continued symptoms.

Increased fear of movement might have a negative effect on the effectiveness of exercise treatment; therefore, a pain-monitoring model should be used when patients are treated with exercise.

Rompe JD, Nafe B, Furia JP, Maffulli N. Eccentric loading, shock-wave treatment, or a wait-and-see policy for tendinopathy of the main body of tendo Achillis: a randomized controlled trial. Am J Sports Med. 2007;35(3):374–83.

This RCT compares the effectiveness of three management strategies-group for chronic non-insertional Achilles tendinopathy: eccentric loading; repetitive low-energy shock-wave therapy (SWT); and wait and see. In the 75 patients enrolled, at 4-month follow-up, eccentric loading and low-energy SWT showed comparable results. The wait-and-see strategy was ineffective.

van der Plas A, de Jonge S, de Vos RJ, van der Heide HJ, Verhaar JA, Weir A, et al. A 5-year follow-up study of Alfredson's heel-drop exercise programme in chronic midportion Achilles tendinopathy. Br J Sports Med. 2012; 46(3):214–8.

This RCT evaluated the 5-year outcome of patients with chronic midportion Achilles tendinopathy treated with the classical Alfredson's heel-drop (eccentric) exercise programme.

In 46 patients (58 tendons), the VISA-A score significantly increased from 49.2 at baseline to 83.6 after 5 years and from the 1- to 5-year follow-up from 75.0 to 83.4.

39.7 % of the patients were completely pain-free at follow-up and 48.3 % had received one or more alternative treatments. After the 3-month Alfredson's heel-drop exercise programme, almost half of the patients had received other therapies. Although improvement of symptoms can be expected at long term, mild pain may remain.

Jonsson P, Alfredson H, Sunding K, Fahlström M, Cook J. New regimen for eccentric calf-muscle training in patients with chronic insertional Achilles tendinopathy: results of a pilot study. Br J Sports Med. 2008;42(9):746–9.

This paper investigated a new model of painful eccentric training ("Alfredson Regime") for chronic painful insertional Achilles tendinopathy. Twenty-seven patients performed a painful eccentric training regimen without loading into dorsiflexion. This was done as 3×15 reps, twice a day, 7 days/week, for 12 weeks. In this short-term pilot study this regime showed promising clinical results in 67 % of the patients.

Fahlström M, Jonsson P, Lorentzon R, Alfredson H. Chronic Achilles tendon pain treated with eccentric calf-muscle training. Knee Surg Sports Traumatol Arthrosc. 2003; 11(5):327–33.

Seventy-eight consecutive patients with chronic painful Achilles tendinosis at the mid-portion and 30 consecutive patients with chronic insertional Achilles tendon pain were treated with eccentric calf-muscle training for 12 weeks. Most patients were recreational athletes. In 90 of the 101 Achilles tendons (89 %) with chronic painful mid-portion Achilles tendinosis, treatment was satisfactory and the patients were back on their pre-injury activity level after the 12-week training regimen. In these patients, the amount of pain during activity decreased significantly. On the contrary, in only ten of the tendons (32 %) with chronic insertional Achilles tendon pain was treatment satisfactory.

Ribbans WJ, Collins M. Pathology of the tendo Achillis: do our genes contribute? Bone Joint J. 2013;95-B(3):305–13.

This review summarises present knowledge of the influence of genetic patterns on the pathology of the Achilles tendon, with a focus on the possible biological mechanisms by which genetic factors are involved in the aetiology of tendon pathology.

Part II
Trauma

Spine Trauma

Guy Selmon

Abstract This chapter deals with injury to the cervical and lumbar spine, setting out mechanisms of injury, the consequences of trauma for the skeletal and neurological structures and its implication for the patient. The rationale behind treatment options is presented, as well as the outcomes. Importantly, there are references on the general management of the spinal injury patient, for the non-specialist who will not be expected to operate on these patients, but who can so markedly influence outcome if initial management is suboptimal.

Keywords Spine trauma • Thoracolumbar burst fractures • Cervical spine fractures

G. Selmon, MBBS, FRCS, FRCS (Tr and Orth)
Department of Trauma and Orthopaedics,
The Conquest Hospital, The Ridge,
St. Leonards on Sea, East Sussex, TN37 7RD, UK
e-mail: guyselmon@hotmail.com

G. Bowyer, A. Cole (eds.), *Selected References in Trauma and Orthopaedics*, DOI 10.1007/978-1-4471-4676-6_6,
© Springer-Verlag London 2014

Thoracolumbar Burst Fractures

Gnanenthiran SR, Adie S, Harris IA. Non-operative versus operative treatment for thoracolumbar burst fractures without neurological deficit: a meta-analysis. Clin Orthop Relat Res. 2012;470(2):567–77.

This meta-analysis compared pain and function in patients with thoracolumbar burst fractures, without neurological deficit, treated non-operatively and surgically. Four trials, including two randomized controlled trials (RCTs) with a total of 79 patients, were identified. Follow-up ranged from 24 to 118 months. No difference was identified between the groups in pain, function and return to work. Surgery was associated with higher complication rates and higher costs.

Boerger TO, Limb D, Dickson RA. Does 'canal clearance' affect neurological outcome after thoracolumbar burst fractures? J Bone Joint Surg Br. 2000;82(5):629–35.

This paper reviewed the world literature regarding the surgical treatment of patients with thoracolumbar burst fractures with neurological deficit. Sixty publications met minimal inclusion criteria with only three being prospective studies. There was no apparent advantage of surgical over non surgical treatment as regards neurological improvement. Surgery, in the belief it might improve neurological deficit, could not be justified. They believed that the neurological damage occurred at the time of injury.

Denis F. The three column spine and its significance in the classification of acute thoracolumbar spinal injuries. Spine (Phila Pa 1976). 1983;8(8):817–31.

This classic publication introduces the concept of the middle column. A retrospective review of 412 thoracolumbar injuries, the paper goes on to explain the division of spinal injuries into minor and major. Major injuries were classified into compression fractures, burst fractures, seat-belt-type injuries and fracture dislocations.

Yi L, Jingping B, Gele J, Baoleri X, Taixiang W. Operative versus non-operative treatment for thoracolumbar burst fractures without neurological deficit. Cochrane Database Syst Rev. 2006;(4):CD005079.

This Cochrane review aimed to identify RCTs which compared operative versus non-operative treatment for thoracolumbar burst fractures without neurological deficit. They identified one trial. This did not show a statistical difference in pain or function, return to work rates, radiographic findings or average length of hospital stay. There was no correlation with degree of kyphosis or percentage of correction lost and any clinical symptoms.

Cervical Spine Fractures

Nourbakhsh A, Shi R, Vannemreddy P, Nanda A. Operative versus non-operative management of acute odontoid Type II fractures: a meta-analysis. J Neurosurg Spine. 2009;11(6):651–8.

This meta-analysis aimed to establish the appropriateness of criteria described in the literature as indications for surgery for these specific fractures. They identified a statistically significant higher fusion rate for the surgically treated group compared to external immobilization (halo vest or collar) in patients over the age range of 45–55. This was not the case in patients younger than this. Operative treatment is recommended for older patients and patients with significant posterior displacement (greater than 4–6 mm).

Koivikko MP, Kiuru MJ, Koskinen SK, Myllynen P, Santavirta S, Kivisaari L. Factors associated with non-union in conservatively-treated type-II fractures of the odontoid process. J Bone Joint Surg Br. 2004;86(8):1146–51.

The results of nearly 70 patients with type 2 odontoid peg fractures treated in halo vests were reviewed. 46 % had united. Factors associated with non-union included a fracture gap of more than 1 mm, posterior displacement of more than 5 mm, a delay of more than 4 days in the start of treatment and posterior redisplacement of more than 2 mm.

Shoulder Trauma

Andrew Cole

Abstract This chapter covers fractures of the clavicle and injuries to the acromio-clavicular joint. The shoulder is dealt with, reviewing injury patterns, treatment options and outcomes for glenoid and proximal humeral injuries. Fractures of the humeral shaft are also reviewed with updates on the treatment options as well as consideration of the potential radial nerve injuries which may be associated with these fractures.

Keywords Fractures of the clavicle • Lateral clavicle fractures • Acromioclavicular joint dislocation • Diaphyseal humeral fractures • Radial nerve palsy • Proximal humeral fractures • Scapular and glenoid fractures

A. Cole, BSc (Hons), MBBS, FRCS (Tr and Orth)
Department of Trauma and Orthopaedics,
University Hospital Southampton, NHS Trust,
Southampton, Hampshire SO16 6YD, UK
e-mail: andrew.cole@uhs.nhs.uk, andycole34@btopenworld.com

G. Bowyer, A. Cole (eds.), *Selected References in Trauma and Orthopaedics*, DOI 10.1007/978-1-4471-4676-6_7,
© Springer-Verlag London 2014

Fractures of the Clavicle

McKee RC, Whelan DB, Schemitsch EH, McKee MD. Operative versus non-operative care of displaced midshaft clavicular fractures: a meta-analysis of randomized clinical trials. J Bone Joint Surg Am. 2012;94(8):675–84.

Recent studies have suggested an increasing role for operative intervention in midshaft clavicle fractures. This was a systematic review of randomized studies available comparing operative and non-operative management of these fractures. Six studies including 412 patients were reviewed. The non-union rate was higher in the non-operatively treated patients at 14.5 % compared with 1.5 % of those treated operatively. The rate of symptomatic mal-union was 8.5 % in the non-operative group compared to zero in the operatively treated group. The authors concluded that operative treatment provides a significantly lower non-union and symptomatic malunion rate with an earlier return to function. There is however little evidence that surgical intervention provides a better long term functional outcome.

Virtanen KJ, Malmivaara AO, Remes VM, Paavola MP. Operative and non-operative treatment of clavicle fractures in adults. Acta Orthop. 2012;83(1):65–73.

This was systematic review of the medical literature from 1966 to 2011. It identified six randomized controlled trials (RCTs) with 631 patients and seven controlled studies with 559 patients. Their conclusions were that surgery provides earlier functional improvement, although at 6 months there is little difference between the two groups. Delayed and non-union were more common in those groups treated non-operatively. Overall non-union rates in non-operatively managed patients ranged from 0–29 % and 0–4 % in those managed with surgery. The precise method of surgery seems to have little influence on the rates of union.

Zlowodzki M, Zelle BA, Cole PA, Jeray K, McKee MD; Evidence-Based Orthopaedic Trauma Working Group. Treatment of acute midshaft clavicle fractures: systematic review of 2144 fractures: on behalf of the Evidence-Based Orthopaedic Trauma Working Group. J Orthop Trauma. 2005;19(7):504–7.

This study was designed to systematically summarize and compare results of different treatment options. (non-operative, operative, extramedullary and intramedullary fixation) in the management of displaced midshaft clavicle fractures. The group reported a 4 % non-union rate in total. The non-union rate in the non-operatively treated group was 6 % for all fractures and 15 % for displaced fractures. When treated non-operatively, fracture displacement, fracture comminution, female gender, and age were associated with non-union. The review included three randomized controlled trials with methodological limitations, and also retrospective cohort studies and case series. There was only one study comparing different operative methods. Functional outcome measures were not analyzed.

Lateral Clavicle Fractures

Stegeman SA, Nacak H, Huvenaars KH, Stijnen T, Krijnen P, Schipper IB. Surgical treatment of Neer type-II fractures of the distal clavicle. Acta Orthop. 2013;84(2):184–90.

This meta-analysis reviewed the available surgical techniques in the management of the Neer type II lateral clavicular fractures. After searching the available literature, no comparative studies were found. Twenty-one studies (8 prospective and 13 retrospective cohort studies) were selected for the meta-analysis. The 21 studies selected included 350 patients with a distal clavicular fracture. Union was achieved in 98 % of the patients. Functional outcome was similar between the treatment modalities. Hook-plate fixation was associated with a 11-fold increased risk of major complications compared to intramedullary fixation and a 24-fold increased risk compared to suture anchoring.

The authors concluded that if surgical treatment of a distal clavicle fracture is considered, a fixation procedure with a low risk of complications and a high union rate such as plate fixation or intramedullary fixation should be used. The hook-plate fixation had an increased risk of implant-related complications.

Oh JH, Kim SH, Lee JH, Shin SH, Gong HS. Treatment of distal clavicle fracture: a systematic review of treatment modalities in 425 fractures. Arch Orthop Trauma Surg. 2011;131(4):525–33.

The authors of this paper reviewed articles from January 1990 to September 2009. They identified 425 cases from 21 studies. Sixty patients were treated non-operatively and 365 surgically. From 365 patients who were treated surgically. One hundred and five had a coracoclavicular stabilization, 162 had a hook plate, 42 intramedullary fixation, 16 interfragmentary fixation, and 40 K-wire plus tension band wiring.

Nonsurgical treatment resulted in a 33.3 % non-union rate. Surgical treatment resulted in a 1.6 % non-union rate, there was however a higher complication rate, (22.2 %). There did not appear to be a significantly different non-union rate between the surgical modalities, however, there was a higher complication rate in cases of hook plating and k wire tension band wiring.

The authors concluded that for nonsurgical treatment, the functional outcomes were generally acceptable despite the high non-union rate. If surgical treatment is considered, intramedullary screw fixation, coraco-clavicular stabilization and interfragmentary fixation would be preferred because of their lower complication rate.

Acromioclavicular Joint Dislocation

Weaver JK, Dunn HK. Treatment of acromioclavicular injuries, especially complete acromioclavicular separation. J Bone Joint Surg Am. 1972;54(6):1187–94.

Neviaser, in 1968, first introduced the concept of using the coracoacromial (CA) ligament for acromioclavicular (AC) joint repair. The ligament was detached from the coracoid and transferred to the distal end of the clavicle. The repair was then augmented with fixation across the AC joint.

This is the classic 1972 paper of the original description of the Weaver Dunn procedure for stabilization of the acromio-clavicular joint (ACJ) a modification of the method described by Nevaiser. This new procedure involved the release of the coracoacromial ligament from the acromion, resection of the distal end of the clavicle and transfer of the CA ligament to the lateral end of the clavicle, more closely replicating the coracoclavicular (CC) ligaments.

It was described for 12 acute dislocations and 3 chronic cases with an average follow-up of 35 months. Eleven cases were rated as good, 3 fair and 1 poor result (recurrence).

Phillips AM, Smart C, Groom AF. Acromioclavicular dislocation. Conservative or surgical therapy. Clin Orthop Relat Res. 1998;(353):10–7.

The purpose of this study was to perform an up to date literature review to clarify available information influencing decision making in severely displaced acromioclavicular dislocation. Twenty-four papers were retrieved with 1,172 patients. Eight hundred and thirty-three were treated surgically with a follow-up of 43.7 months. Non-operatively treated patients were followed up for 60.4 months. Overall, 88 % of surgically treated patients and 87 % of nonsurgically treated patients had a satisfactory outcome.

Surgical vs. nonsurgical complications most commonly encountered were the need for further surgery (59 % versus 6 %), infection (6 % versus 1 %), and deformity (3 % versus 37 %).

Surgery did not appear to result in a quicker return to activity. Pain was the same in both groups. Surgery did not appear to improve the range of motion or strength (both of which were slightly better in the non-operative group). The authors concluded that there does not seem to be any reason to recommend an operative procedure to a patient with a Rockwood type III injury based on the evidence available at that time.

Beitzel K, Cote MP, Apostolakos J, Solovyova O, Judson CH, Ziegler CG, et al. Current concepts in the treatment of acromioclavicular joint dislocations. Arthroscopy. 2013;29(2):387–97.

This is a systematic review of the literature. It attempts to compare operative vs non-operative management, early vs delayed treatment and the various types of reconstruction (anatomic vs non anatomic) in AC joint dislocations. In all, 20 studies were identified as fulfilling the selection criteria. These consisted of 14 comparing operative with non-operative treatment, 4 comparing early with delayed surgical intervention, and 2 comparing anatomic with nonanatomic surgical techniques. In all there were 162 techniques described for reconstruction of the AC joint!

The authors concluded that there is a lack of evidence to support treatment options for patients with AC joint dislocations. There is a general consensus for non-operative treatment of Rockwood type I and II injuries, initial nonsurgical treatment of type III injuries, and operative intervention for Rockwood type IV to VI injuries.

Further research is needed to determine if differences exist regarding early versus delayed surgical intervention and anatomic versus nonanatomic surgical techniques in the treatment of patients with AC joint dislocations.

Diaphyseal Humeral Fractures

Non-operative Management

Klenerman L. Fractures of the shaft of the humerus. J Bone Joint Surg Br. 1966;48(1):105–11.

This was one of the first papers to look at the amount of malunion that could be accepted after a fracture of the mid-shaft of the humerus. Because the glenohumeral joint has an exceptional range of motion in many planes, deformity is well tolerated after union. Klenerman showed in his paper that acceptable results could be achieved even after 20° of anterior bowing, 30° of varus angulation, 15° of malrotation, and 3 cm of shortening.

Sarmiento A, Kinman PB, Galvin EG, Schmitt RH, Phillips JG. Functional bracing of fractures of the shaft of the humerus. J Bone Joint Surg Am. 1977;59(5):596–601.

This was the first paper from Sarmiento and his team describing functional bracing of the humerus. They reported on 51 cases of shaft fractures treated with a functional brace, individually molded or prefabricated. It maintained good alignment of the fragments and permitted rapid union. They concluded that bracing appeared to provide a desirable physiological environment conducive to rapid healing. Non-unions were not encountered in nonpathological fractures. They also suggested that healing times were rapid and the morbidity attached to the method was minimum.

Sarmiento A, Zagorski JB, Zych GA, Latta LL, Capps CA. Functional bracing for the treatment of fractures of the humeral diaphysis. J Bone Joint Surg Am. 2000;82(4): 478–86.

In 2000 Sarmiento updated his original paper recording the outcomes of patients treated over a 12 year period between 1978 and 1990. Nine hundred and twenty-two patients with a fracture of the humeral diaphysis were treated with functional bracing.

Only 620 (67 %) of the 922 patients were able available for follow-up. Seventy-five percent were closed fractures. The remaining were open. Six percent of the open fractures and less than 2 % of the closed fractures had a non-union after bracing.

Only 565 patients had anteroposterior radiographs which were available and in 87 % of the these the fracture healed in less than 16° of varus angulation. Of the 546 who had a lateral X-ray 81 % healed in less than 16° of anterior angulation. At the time of brace removal, 98 % of the patients had limitation of shoulder motion of 25° or less. Most patients were unable to be followed up long term as they did not return to clinic after brace removal.

It was concluded that functional bracing for these fractures treatment results in high rate of union, particularly when used for closed fractures, and low rates of malunion.

Operative vs Non-operative Treatment

Denard A Jr, Richards JE, Obremskey WT, Tucker MC, Floyd M, Herzog GA. Outcome of non-operative vs operative treatment of humeral shaft fractures: a retrospective study of 213 patients. Orthopedics. 2010;33(8).

Two hundred and thirteen adult patients with a humeral shaft fracture who satisfied inclusion criteria were treated at 2 level 1 trauma centers with either a functional brace or compression plating. A retrospective analysis of times to union, non-union, malunion, infection, incidence of radial nerve palsy, and elbow range of motion (ROM) was performed.

Non-union (20.6 % vs 8.7 %) and malunion (12.7 % vs 1.3 %) was significantly more common in the non-operative group. There was no significant difference in infection rate. No difference in time to union or ultimate range of motion was found between the two groups.

It was concluded that closed treatment of humerus fractures had a significantly higher rate of non-union and malunion while operative intervention demonstrated no significant differences in time to union, infection, or iatrogenic radial nerve palsy.

Gosler MW, Testroote M, Morrenhof JW, Janzing HM. Surgical versus non-surgical interventions for treating humeral shaft fractures in adults. Cochrane Database Syst Rev. 2012;1:CD008832.

The purpose of this paper was to compare the effects of surgical versus non-surgical intervention for non-pathological fractures of the humeral shaft in adults. The intention was to include all randomised and quasi-randomised controlled trials that compared surgical with non-surgical intervention for humeral shaft fractures in adults. Based on their exclusion criteria the authors were not able to find any studies to include! They identified two potentially eligible ongoing studies. As a result they concluded that currently there is no evidence available from randomised controlled trials to ascertain whether surgical intervention of humeral shaft fractures gives a better or worse outcome than no surgery.

Bhandari M, Devereaux PJ, McKee MD, Schemitsch EH. Compression plating versus intramedullary nailing of humeral shaft fractures—a meta-analysis. Acta Orthop. 2006;77(2):279–84.

Review of the literature from 1969 to 2000 revealed 215 citations, however only 3 were included (involving 155 patients). Analysis suggested that plate fixation gave a lower relative risk of reoperation than intramedullary nailing. Plate fixation may reduce the risk of shoulder problems such as pain and impingement in comparison to intramedullary nails although the cumulative evidence remained weak. This article was updated in the following meta-analysis below.

Heineman DJ, Bhandari M, Nork SE, Ponsen KJ, Poolman RW. Treatment of humeral shaft fractures—meta-analysis reupdated. Acta Orthop. 2010;81(4):517.

Just after this original meta-analysis was accepted for publication a new randomized controlled trial was published comparing nails to plates. The authors conducted a cumulative meta-analysis to include these 34 patients. The primary outcome of the analysis changed a little and favoured plates over nails. The risk of a complication is lower when plating a fracture of the humeral shaft than when using an intramedullary nail.

Kurup H, Hossain M, Andrew JG. Dynamic compression plating versus locked intramedullary nailing for humeral shaft fractures in adults. Cochrane Database Syst Rev. 2011;(6):CD005959.

The objective of this paper was to compare compression plating and locked intramedullary nailing for primary surgical fixation in adults. Randomised and quasi-randomised controlled trials comparing compression plates and locked intramedullary nail fixation for humeral shaft fractures were reviewed. This included five trials with 260 fractures. There was no significant difference in fracture union between plating and nailing. There was a statistically significant increase in shoulder impingement following nailing when compared with plating. Intramedullary nails were removed significantly more frequently than plates. There was no difference in operating time, blood loss during surgery, iatrogenic radial nerve injury, return to occupation by 6 months or American Shoulder and Elbow Surgeons (ASES) scores.

Intramedullary nailing seems to be associated with an increased risk of shoulder impingement, decreased shoulder movement and the need for secondary surgery. There was insufficient evidence to determine any differences in functional outcome.

Radial Nerve Palsy

Shao YC, Harwood P, Grotz MR, Limb D, Giannoudis PV. Radial nerve palsy associated with fractures of the shaft of the humerus: a systematic review. J Bone Joint Surg Br. 2005;87(12):1647–52.

This study systematically reviewed the published evidence from the last 40 years and developed an algorithm to guide management of humeral shaft fractures with radial nerve injury. Of 391 papers identified initially, 35 papers met all the criteria for eligibility. They found a prevalence of radial nerve palsy after fracture of 11.8 %. Fractures of the middle and middle-distal parts of the shaft had a significantly higher association with radial nerve palsy than those in other parts. Transverse and spiral fractures were significantly more likely to be associated with radial nerve palsy than oblique and comminuted patterns of fracture. Overall rates of recovery were 88.1 %, with spontaneous recovery reaching 70.7 % (411 of 581) in patients treated conservatively.

The main conclusion is that there was no significant difference in the final results when comparing groups that were initially managed expectantly with those explored early, suggesting that the initial expectant treatment did not affect the extent of nerve recovery adversely and would avoid many unnecessary operations.

Wang JP, Shen WJ, Chen WM, Huang CK, Shen YS, Chen TH. Iatrogenic radial nerve palsy after operative management of humeral shaft fractures. J Trauma. 2009; 66(3):800–3.

There is no consensus with regard to the management of secondary radial nerve palsy, particularly when it is iatrogenic.

Seven hundred and seven humerus shaft fracture treated operatively over a 10-year period were identified. Of these, 30 patients sustained iatrogenic radial nerve palsy. Another 16 cases were referred from other institutions giving a total of 46 injuries. No recognized intraoperative injuries to the radial nerve were recorded in any case.

Of the 46 patients the median age was 40 years (range, 19–75 years). A total of 39 patients had been treated with dynamic compression plates and the rest with a variety of nails. Five cases were surgically explored and in all cases the nerve was in continuity with no macroscopic lesions. All cases eventually recovered grade 4 of five muscle strength or better. The median time to the beginning of clinical recovery was 16 weeks (range, 5–30 weeks).

The authors concluded that the timing and pattern of radial nerve recovery in this situation was similar to that seen in primary radial nerve palsy. There appears to be no advantage to early exploration of the radial nerve. In the absence of obviously 'misplaced instrumentation' or fracture displacement, the injury can be treated like a primary palsy and observed for a minimum of 4 months before exploration.

Reviews

Walker M, Palumbo B, Badman B, Brooks J, Van Gelderen J, Mighell M. Humeral shaft fractures: a review. J Shoulder Elbow Surg. 2011;20(5):833–44.

A good review of the current management of humeral shaft fractures including the results of non-operative and various modalities of operative management. They conclude that there are specific indications for operative intervention including polytrauma, open fractures and certain fracture patterns and failure to hold in an acceptable position. Plating has been the 'gold standard' of operative management but newer nail designs may prove effective. There is a paucity of RCT's comparing operative management. Radial nerve palsy remains a common comorbidity but most can be expected to recover.

Proximal Humeral Fractures

Handoll HH, Ollivere BJ, Rollins KE. Interventions for treating proximal humeral fractures in adults. Cochrane Database Syst Rev. 2012;12:CD000434.

The purpose of this study was to review the evidence supporting the various treatment and rehabilitation interventions for proximal humeral fractures. All randomised controlled trials pertinent to the management of proximal humeral fractures in adults up to January 2012 were selected. A limited meta-analysis was performed.

Twenty-three small randomised trials with a total of 1,238 participants were included. Eight trials evaluated conservative treatment. There was some evidence to support 'immediate' physiotherapy in people with undisplaced or stable fractures with better pain relief and no compromise in long term function. There remains insufficient evidence to inform the management of complex and unstable proximal humeral fractures. It remains unclear whether surgery, even for specific fracture types, is beneficial but it is likely to be associated with a higher risk of surgery-related complications and the need for further surgery. The authors also concluded that currently there is insufficient evidence to establish what is the best method of surgical treatment.

Fjalestad T, Hole MØ, Hovden IA, Blücher J, Strømsøe K. Surgical treatment with an angular stable plate for complex displaced proximal humeral fractures in elderly patients: a randomized controlled trial. J Orthop Trauma. 2012;26(2):98–106.

The objective of the study was to evaluate functional outcome, patient self-assessment, and radiographic outcome at 1 year in displaced three- and four-part proximal humeral fractures. Fifty patients aged 60 years or older with displaced three- or four-part proximal humeral fractures were randomized either to surgical treatment (angular stable plate) or to conservative treatment (manipulation was performed if the shaft was 50 % displaced on the shaft). Twenty-five patients were included in each group. Forty-eight patients completed 12-month follow-up. Two surgical patients died within 3 months. At 12 months, mean Constant scores favoured conservative treatment by but this was not significant. There was no difference in mean patient self-assessment.

This small study failed to provide evidence of a difference in functional outcome at 1-year follow-up between surgical treatment and conservative treatment of displaced proximal humeral fractures in elderly patients.

Thanasas C, Kontakis G, Angoules A, Limb D, Giannoudis P. Treatment of proximal humerus fractures with locking plates: a systematic review. J Shoulder Elbow Surg. 2009;18(6):837–44.

This was a systematic review of the literature to determine the efficacy and early to medium term functional results of locking plates for proximal humeral fractures. Criteria for eligibility were clinical studies with more than ten cases followed-up, and adequate data provided terms of implant related complications. Twelve studies including 791 patients met the inclusion criteria. The incidence of the reported complications was: avascular necrosis 7.9 % overall (14.5 % in 4 part fractures). Loss of reduction is relatively common at just over 12 % and is usually due to lack of medial support. Screw complications are common and screw cut-out occurred in 11.6 %, errors with plate position in just over 2 % and a re-operation rate 13.7 %. Some recommendations were made to help minimize these complications.

Olerud P, Ahrengart L, Ponzer S, Saving J, Tidermark J. Hemiarthroplasty versus non-operative treatment of displaced 4-part proximal humeral fractures in elderly patients: a randomized controlled trial. J Shoulder Elbow Surg. 2011;20(7):1025–33.

This study reported the 2-year outcome after a displaced 4-part fracture of the proximal humerus in elderly patients randomized to treatment with a hemiarthroplasty (HA) or non-operative treatment. A relatively small study of 55 patients with a mean age of 77 were assessed at regular periods postoperatively. The main outcome measures were the EQ-5D, Disabilities of Arm, Shoulder, and Hand (DASH) and Constant scores. At the final 2-year follow-up the measures of quality of life were significantly better in the HA group compared to the non-operative group. The results for DASH and pain assessment were both in favour (not significantly) of the HA group.

There were no significant differences regarding the Constant score or range of motion (ROM). Both groups achieved a mean flexion of approximately 90–95° and a mean abduction of 85–90°. The main advantage of HA appeared to be less pain while there were no differences in ROM.

Kontakis G, Koutras C, Tosounidis T, Giannoudis P. Early management of proximal humeral fractures with hemiarthroplasty: a systematic review. J Bone Joint Surg Br. 2008;90(11): 1407–13.

The outcome of humeral hemiarthroplasty depends on a number of factors including tuberosity healing, version and correct prosthetic height. This systematic review of the literature examines the role of hemiarthroplasty treatment of proximal humeral fractures. Sixteen studies were identified with 810 hemiarthroplasties in 808 patients with a mean age of 67.7 years and a mean follow-up of 3.7 years. The mean active anterior elevation was to 105.7° (10–180°) and the mean abduction to 92.4° (15–170°). The incidence of superficial and deep infection was 1.55 % and 0.64 %, respectively. Healing of the tuberosities is an important factor in determining outcome and complications related to tuberosity healing were seen in 11.15 %. The estimated incidence of heterotopic ossification was 8.8 % and that of proximal migration of the humeral head 6.8 %. The mean Constant score was only 56. No or only mild pain was experienced by most patients. The limitations to function persisted.

Boileau P, Krishnan SG, Tinsi L, Walch G, Coste JS, Molé D. Tuberosity malposition and migration: reasons for poor outcomes after hemiarthroplasty for displaced fractures of the proximal humerus. J Shoulder Elbow Surg. 2002;11(5): 401–12.

This was the first study to determine that tuberosity fixation and position was a major determinant of outcome in shoulder hemiarthroplasty for fractures of the proximal humerus. In a clinical and radiological study of 66 patients, they found that final tuberosity malposition occurred in 50 % and correlated with an unsatisfactory result, superior migration of the prosthesis, stiffness or weakness, and persistent pain. Factors associated with failure of tuberosity osteosynthesis were poor initial position of the prosthesis (specifically, excessive height and/or retroversion), poor position of the greater tuberosity, and women over age 75 years.

Taylor C, Cosker T, Smith C. Reverse the trend for proximal humeral fractures: a review of the evidence for the use of reverse shoulder replacement in acute trauma. Shoulder & Elbow. 2012;4(4):237–43.

This is a review of the use of the reverse shoulder replacements for acute proximal humeral fractures. The authors performed a systematic review of the literature and included studies with ten patients or more. The results were also compared to the most up to date literature for hemiarthroplasty. Eight papers of 178 patients met the full criteria.

The mean constant score for reverse shoulder replacement (RSR) was 54 % compared with an average of 57 % for hemiarthroplasty. There was an infection rate of 3 %, dislocation rate of 4 % and a reoperation rate of 5.6 %. In four of the studies the tuberosities are reattached, however this is technically difficult. There is a tendency to slightly greater forward flexion at 115° compared with 106° for HA. Mean abduction is similar for both groups however there is a tendency towards less external rotation with the RSR. Overall the literature is limited with only short term follow-up. There is also a tendency towards decreasing constant score and notching with time. At present clinical data on clinical effectiveness and cost effectiveness is not present.

Scapular and Glenoid Fractures

Anavian J, Gauger EM, Schroder LK, Wijdicks CA, Cole PA. Surgical and functional outcomes after operative management of complex and displaced intra-articular glenoid fractures. J Bone Joint Surg Am. 2012;94(7):645–53.

Although operative management is indicated for some fractures of the glenoid, little is known regarding functional outcomes. The aim of this study was to evaluate the functional results after fixation of displaced, high-energy, complex, intra-articular glenoid fractures. Thirty-three patients were treated surgically over a 7 year period up to 2009. The authors' indications for operative treatment included articular fracture gap or step-off of ≥4 mm. A posterior approach was utilized in 21 patients, an anterior approach in seven, and a combined approach in five. Functional outcomes, including Disabilities of the Arm, Shoulder and Hand (DASH) and Short Form-36 (SF-36) scores, shoulder motion and strength, and return to work and/or activities and were obtained for 31 patients (91 %).

At final follow-up all patients had radiographic union of the fracture. The mean DASH score was 10.8 (range, 0–42). All mean SF-36 subscores were comparable with those of the normal population. Eighty-seven percent were pain-free at the time of follow-up, and four had mild pain with prolonged activity. Ninety-percent returned to their preinjury level of work and/or activities. The authors suggest that surgical treatment for complex, displaced intra-articular glenoid fractures with or without involvement of the scapular neck and body can be associated with good functional outcomes and a low complication rate.

Cole PA, Gauger EM, Herrera DA, Anavian J, Tarkin IS. Radiographic follow-up of 84 operatively treated scapula neck and body fractures. Injury. 2012;43(3):327–33.

The purpose of this study was to determine the early radiographic follow-up of open reduction internal fixation (ORIF) for displaced, scapular fractures involving the glenoid neck and body. Eighty-four patients operated on over an 8 year period (up to 2010) with scapular body or neck fractures were retrospectively reviewed from a dedicated scapular database. The operated patients had fractures that met at least one of the author's criteria for operating. ($\geq$20 mm medial/lateral (M/L) displacement (lateral border offset), $\geq$45° of angular deformity on a scapular-Y X-ray, the combination of angulation $\geq$30° plus M/L displacement $\geq$15 mm, double disruptions of the superior shoulder suspensory complex both displaced $\geq$10 mm, glenopolar angle (GPA) $\leq$22° and open fractures). This is a single surgeon series and all fractures were stabilised with a posterior approach with five patients requiring a combined deltopectoral approach. Fixation consisted of lateral and vertebral border stabilisation with dynamic compression and reconstruction plates, respectively.

Union was achieved in all cases. There were three cases of malunion based on a GPA difference >10° from the uninjured shoulder. Re-operations included removal of the plates (seven patients) and manipulation under anaesthesia (three patients). There were no infections or wound dehiscence. The authors concluded that ORIF for displaced scapula fractures is a relatively safe and effective procedure for restoration of anatomy and promotion of union.

Jones CB, Sietsema DL. Analysis of operative versus non-operative treatment of displaced scapular fractures. Clin Orthop Relat Res. 2011;469(12):3379–89.

Operative indications for displaced scapular fractures have been controversial and decision making inconsistent. The purpose of this study was to evaluate the return to work, pain, and complications in patients with scapular fractures treated either non-operatively or operatively. This was a retrospective analysis of 182 scapular fractures treated between 2002 and 2005. Thirty-one patients were treated with open reduction internal fixation and matched by age, occupation, and gender to 31 patients treated non-operatively. The fracture types (AO/OTA) were similar in the two groups although the mean displacement, shortening, and angulation were greater in the operative group. Average follow-up was 1.5 years (14–32 months). All fractures healed and no differences were found in the return to work, pain or complications. The authors concluded that operative treatment results in similar results. They do not recommend operative intervention in any scapular neck or body fracture displaced less than 20 mm.

Elbow Trauma

David Hargreaves

Abstract This section deals with the common trauma challenges around the adult elbow. The bony injuries to the olecranon and the distal humerus are covered, with references addressing the treatment options and consideration of the mechanics and effects of fixation. The important topic of complex dislocation, leading to the concept of the terrible triad injury and instability is dealt with in detail, as is the difficult issue of biceps tendon rupture and its treatment.

Keywords Distal biceps rupture • Distal humeral fractures • Olecranon fractures • Complex elbow dislocation

D. Hargreaves, MBBS, FRCS (Orth)
Department of Orthopaedics,
University Hospital Southampton Trust,
Tremona Road, Southampton SO51 6YD, UK
e-mail: david.hargreaves@uhs.nhs.uk

G. Bowyer, A. Cole (eds.), *Selected References in Trauma and Orthopaedics*, DOI 10.1007/978-1-4471-4676-6_8,
© Springer-Verlag London 2014

Distal Biceps Rupture

Freeman CR, McCormick KR, Mahoney D, Baratz M, Lubahn JD. Non-operative treatment of distal biceps tendon ruptures compared with a historical control group. J Bone Joint Surg Am. 2009;91(10):2329–34.

Non-operative treatment has often been quoted as giving poor results, with significant weakness and arm cramps. The evidence for this has been lacking. This paper with large enough numbers (18 cases) and an average follow-up of 59 months has shown only a small difference. The average flexion strength measured 88 % and supination strength measured 74 % of the contralateral arm. Eight patients reported weakness on heavy lifting and six patients described weakness on activities that required supination. There were no cases of continued arm cramps. All patients had returned to work at an average of 12 weeks.

El-Hawary R, Macdermid JC, Faber KJ, Patterson SD, King GJ. Distal biceps tendon repair: comparison of surgical techniques. J Hand Surg Am. 2003;28(3):496–502.

A prospective study comparing the outcomes of nine surgical cases performed with a single incision technique using bone anchors to reattach the tendon to the bicipital tuberosity, against ten cases using the Morrey modified 2-incision technique (splitting extensor carpi ulnaris [ECU] and avoiding the ulna periosteum). The difference in outcomes between the two groups was relatively minor. The 2-incision group had a faster return to flexion strength and a significantly lower complication rate. This shows that either technique gives acceptable results with a slight preference towards the 2-incision technique.

Kelly EW, Morrey BF, O'Driscoll SW. Complications of repair of the distal biceps tendon with the modified two-incision technique. J Bone Joint Surg Am. 2000;82-A(11):1575–81.

This is a retrospective review of the modified 2-incision (Boyd-Anderson) technique. The paper gives particular reference to the complications. Seventy-eight cases were reviewed, of which 74 were primary repairs and 4 required an intercalary tendon graft. There was a 31 % complication rate (mostly transient neural deficits). This was more common if a large anterior exposure was required. There were no cases of radioulnar synostosis (but 4 cases of heterotopic ossification) using this muscle splitting approach which was specifically designed to reduce the risk of synostosis. The complication rate was much higher if the operation occurred more than 10 days post injury.

Distal Humeral Fractures

Ljungquist KL, Beran MC, Awan H. Effects of surgical approach on functional outcomes of open reduction and internal fixation of intra-articular distal humeral fractures: a systematic review. J Shoulder Elbow Surg. 2012;21(1): 126–35.

A systematic review of the literature comparing different surgical approaches. Paratricipital, Triceps split, Bryan-Morrey and Olecranon Osteotomy approaches were reviewed. All approaches required the elevation of triceps from the olecranon or the ulna. There was no significant difference in range of motion between any of the approaches but the least good arc of motion was in the olecranon osteotomy group. Patients with an olecranon osteotomy had a higher complication rate (36 %) and reoperation rate (14 %) than patients with any of the other soft tissue approaches.

Zalavras CG, Vercillo MT, Jun BJ, Otarodifard K, Itamura JM, Lee TQ. Biomechanical evaluation of parallel versus orthogonal plate fixation of intra-articular distal humerus fractures. J Shoulder Elbow Surg. 2011;20(1):12–20.

This human cadaver study assessed the biomechanics of the different plate configurations commonly used for fixation of distal humeral fractures (orthogonal and parallel). An unstable fracture model with a metaphyseal defect was created and fixed with two plates using unlocked screws. Cyclical loading and subsequent loading to failure was performed. Parallel plate configuration was found to have significantly higher stiffness. Screw loosening occurred in all posterior plates of orthogonal construct but in none of the parallel plates. This paper suggests that parallel plating is preferential to orthogonal plating for distal humeral fractures.

Kamineni S, Morrey BF. Distal humeral fractures treated with noncustom total elbow replacement. J Bone Joint Surg Am. 2004;86-A(5):940–7.

A large retrospective study of TER inserted primarily for distal humeral fracture. The indication was for acute complex fractures that were unable to be reconstructed either because of fracture comminution or because of poor quality bone in the older patient. Forty-three elbow replacements were followed up for an average of 7 years (minimum of 2 years). The average range of motion was from 24 to 131 degrees of flexion. Ten additional procedures, including five revision arthroplasties, were required in nine elbows. Sixty-five percent of cases had an uncomplicated recovery with no complication and no further surgery. This paper shows good long term outcome when TER is used for acute fracture treatment. This is now a standard treatment for the low demand, elderly patient.

Olecranon Fractures

van derLinden SC, van Kampen A, Jaarsma RL. K-wire position in tension-band wiring technique affects stability of wires and long-term outcome in surgical treatment of olecranon fractures. J Shoulder Elbow Surg. 2012;21(3):405–11.

This paper from Holland has shown that the back-out rate and fracture gap formation is higher if the K wires are positioned in the intramedullary canal rather than in a transcortical position. The consequence of the wires becoming loose is that this group had a higher incidence of radiological evidence of osteoarthritis. They also found that once metalwork was removed, a functional improvement was noted and thus they recommend a low threshold for advising removal of the wires and the tension band wire.

Gordon MJ, Budoff JE, Yeh ML, Luo ZP, Noble PC. Comminuted olecranon fractures: a comparison of plating methods. J Shoulder Elbow Surg. 2006;15(1):94–9.

This is a biomechanical study looking at different positions and plate configurations for a comminuted olecranon model. The study was performed on cadaver bone. The strength of dual medial-lateral plates and a single posterior plate with and without an intramedullary screw was evaluated. The strongest configuration was a posterior plate with a large intra-medullary screw passing through the plate and across the fracture. The authors concluded that this was their preferred technique.

Doornberg J, Ring D, Jupiter JB. Effective treatment of fracture-dislocations of the olecranon requires a stable trochlear notch. Clin Orthop Relat Res. 2004;(429):292–300.

Monteggia type fracture dislocations are often difficult to fix and sometimes are associated with a poor result. This paper showed that the stability of the coronoid was crucial to the outcome. Of 26 patients followed up for more than 3 years (average 6 years), 21 had a good or excellent result. The 5 poor results were as a consequence of inadequate fixation of the coronoid. These cases progressed on to arthrosis (3 cases) and proximal radio-ulna synostosis (3 cases).

Complex Elbow Dislocation

O'Driscoll SW, Morrey BF, Korinek S, An KN. Elbow subluxation and dislocation. A spectrum of instability. Clin Orthop Relat Res. 1992;(280):186–97.

This is a biomechanical cadaver study analyzing the mechanism of elbow dislocation. Thirteen cadaver elbows underwent sequential ligament release. Posterior dislocation of the elbow was shown to occur after three sequential stages of instability, starting with the lateral ligament complex and extending medially. In 12 of the 13 elbows, dislocation was achieved with the medial collateral ligament (MCL) still intact. It was postulated from this work that a posterior elbow dislocation following a fall on the outstretched hand occurs because of an external rotation/valgus force on a flexed elbow. This paper laid the foundation for the understanding of postero-lateral instability, and the mechanics of complex elbow dislocation (Terrible Triad).

Pugh DM, Wild LM, Schemitsch EH, King GJ, McKee MD. Standard surgical protocol to treat elbow dislocations with radial head and coronoid fractures. J Bone Joint Surg Am. 2004;86-A(6):1122–30.

This paper describes the current standard treatment protocol for terrible triad injuries and its results. Radial head fractures were either fixed or replaced. The coronoid fracture was reattached most commonly with a lasso type suture. The Lateral ulnar collateral ligament was always reattached. If further instability was noted then reattachment of the MCL was performed or a hinged external fixator was applied. Thirty-six elbows were followed up retrospectively with a mean of 34 months. They achieved an average arc of movement of 112°. There were only two cases of continuing instability. Seventy-eight percent of cases had a good or excellent result as measured by the Mayo Elbow Performance score. This paper has shown that the terrible triad is a treatable condition using the standard protocol described.

Doornberg JN, Ring D. Coronoid fracture patterns. J Hand Surg Am. 2006;31(1):45–52.

This paper correlated the type of coronoid fracture with the type of elbow instability. Coronoid fracture pattern was investigated in the four most common types of elbow fracture dislocation operated on by a single surgeon. They found that large coronoid fragments (>50 %) were usually associated with both anterior and posterior olecranon fracture dislocations (Monteggia Variant type injury), Small coronoid fragments (<50 %) were identified in all cases of Terrible triad injury. Anteromedial coronoid facet fractures were always present in Posteromedial rotatory instability.

This paper shows high statistical correlation between the type of instability and the type of coronoid fracture. It highlights that the type of coronoid fragment correlates with the type of elbow dislocation. The type of coronoid fracture will help the treating surgeon to identify the associated ligamentous injuries associated with each of the specific types of instability.

Doornberg JN, Linzel DS, Zurakowski D, Ring D. Reference points for radial head prosthesis size. J Hand Surg Am. 2006;31(1):53–7.

If the radial head is fractured and unreconstructable, the radial head will need to be replaced. The main complication from radial head replacement is inserting an implant too long ("overstuffing"). This paper assessed the normal position of the radial head in relation to the lateral edge and central ridge of the coronoid process. Using 3-dimensional computed tomography (CT), they showed that despite significant variability, the radial head articular surface lies approximately 1 mm proximal to the lateral edge of the coronoid articular surface. This defines the reference point for correct positioning of the radial head implant, in order to avoid overstuffing.

Sorensen AK, Søjberg JO. Treatment of persistent instability after posterior fracture-dislocation of the elbow: restoring stability and mobility by internal fixation and hinged external fixation. J Shoulder Elbow Surg. 2011;20(8):1300–9.

The main risk following an elbow dislocation is continuing instability with a further subluxation or dislocation. Such a situation has an increased risk of further re-dislocation and instability. The addition of a hinged external fixator to protect the repaired ligaments has been shown by this paper to prevent further instability but was associated with a 41 % complication rate. The end results were better in patients who underwent treatment within 6 weeks of injury compared to those having treatment later than 6 weeks post injury.

Pelvic and Lower Limb Trauma

Gavin Bowyer and Andrew Cole

Abstract This chapter deals with regional injuries from the pelvis and acetabulum down to the tibial shaft. Current thinking on the management and outcomes from these injuries is set out. Particular attention is paid to the management of life-threatening injuries, from polytrauma and pelvic haemorrhage. The very common, but still problematic and life-threatening, issue of proximal femoral fracture in the elderly is also examined with references setting out evidence for the treatment options and outcomes. Consideration is also given to the severe limb threatening injuries, the mangled limb, open fractures and compartment syndrome. The important work of the past two decades setting out the pathology, assessment, treatment and outcomes of these injuries is set out in detail. The assessment of periprosthetic fractures at the hip and knee, an increasing problem, is dealt with here, as is the management of fractures around the hip, knee and tibial shaft where there have been recent important reviews of treatment options and outcomes.

G. Bowyer, MA, MChir, FRCS (Orth) (✉)
A. Cole, BSc (Hons), MBBS, FRCS (Tr and Orth)
Department of Trauma and Orthopaedics,
University Hospital Southampton, NHS Trust,
Tremona Road, Southampton, Hampshire SO16 6YD, UK
e-mail: gwbowyer@aol.com

G. Bowyer, A. Cole (eds.), *Selected References in Trauma and Orthopaedics*, DOI 10.1007/978-1-4471-4676-6_9,
© Springer-Verlag London 2014

Keywords Pelvic fractures • Acetabular fractures • Proximal femoral fractures • Periprosthetic fractures • Distal femoral fractures • Tibial plateau fractures • Tibial shaft fractures • Open fractures • Limb salvage versus amputation • Compartment syndrome

Pelvic Fractures

Guthrie HC, Owens RW, Bircher MD. Fractures of the pelvis. J Bone Joint Surg Br. 2010;92(11):1481–8.

This excellent instructional article sets out the challenges associated with pelvic fractures. The treatment modalities of binders, angiographic embolization, packing and early internal fixation are all considered in the treatment of haemorrhage. Later definitive treatment seeks to reduce complications and prevent deformity. The most common modes of internal fixation are presented and the complications of delayed mortality, adverse functional outcome, sexual dysfunction and thromboembolism are all considered.

Moran CG, Forward DP. The early management of patients with multiple injuries: an evidence-based, practical guide for the orthopaedic surgeon. J Bone Joint Surg Br. 2012;94(4): 446–53.

This well written and well referenced review article shows how multi-trauma can now be managed, drawing on lessons from the organization of trauma systems in other countries and military experience.

Vallier HA, Cureton BA, Ekstein C, Oldenburg FP, Wilber JH. Early definitive stabilization of unstable pelvis and acetabulum fractures reduces morbidity. J Trauma. 2010;69(3): 677–84.

This study looks at 645 patients who were treated surgically for unstable fractures of the pelvic ring (251), acetabulum (359), or both (40). Definitive fixation was within 24 h of injury (early) in 233 patients and >24 h in 412 (late, mean

99.2 h). 12.4 % had complications after early fixation versus 19.7 % after late (statistically significant). In those with an injury severity score (ISS) > 18 (n = 165 early, 253 late), early fixation resulted in fewer pulmonary complications, less adult respiratory distress syndrome (ARDS) and less multi-organ failure (MOF) (1.8 % versus 4.3 %, p = 0.40). Rates of complications, pulmonary complications, deep vein thrombosis, and MOF were no different for patients with pelvis versus acetabulum fractures.

Shlamovitz GZ, Mower WR, Bergman J, Chuang KR, Crisp J, Hardy D, et al. How (un)useful is the pelvic ring stability examination in diagnosing mechanically unstable pelvic fractures in blunt trauma patients? J Trauma. 2009;66(3):815–20.

This retrospective review looked at the usefulness of clinical pelvic stability test in 1,502 consecutive blunt trauma patients, including 115 patients with pelvic fractures, 34 of whom had unstable pelvic fractures. Unstable pelvic ring on physical examination had a sensitivity and specificity of 8 % and 99 % respectively, for detection of any pelvic fracture and 26 % and 99.9 %, respectively, for detection of mechanically unstable pelvic fractures.

Comment: Another useful example of sensitivity and specificity for a test in widespread clinical usage.

Prasarn ML, Horodyski M, Conrad B, Rubery PT, Dubose D, Small J, et al. Comparison of external fixation versus the trauma pelvic orthotic device on unstable pelvic injuries: a cadaveric study of stability. J Trauma Acute Care Surg. 2012;72(6):1671–5.

This cadaveric study compared stability achieved with an external fixator (two pins in each crest) and the commercially available pelvic binder (trauma pelvic orthotic device [T-POD]).

There were no significant differences in stability conferred by an external fixator or a T-POD for unstable pelvic injuries.

Bonner TJ, Eardley WG, Newell N, Masouros S, Matthews JJ, Gibb I, et al. Accurate placement of a pelvic binder improves reduction of unstable fractures of the pelvic ring. J Bone Joint Surg Br. 2011;93(11):1524–8.

This paper reviewed X-rays of 167 patients with pelvic binders in situ. The binder positioning, optimally at the level of the greater trochanters or sub-optimally high or low was assessed, as was the state of pubic diastasis in those with this injury pattern (17 patients). Only 50 % were optimally placed, with 39 % being too high. The mean diastasis gap was 2.8 times greater (mean difference 22 mm) in the high group compared with the trochanteric group (p < 0.01).

Leslie MP, Baumgaertner MR. Osteoporotic pelvic ring injuries. Orthop Clin North Am. 2013;44(2):217–24.

This review article looks at osteoporotic pelvic ring injuries, which are rising in incidence. These injuries differ in their etiology, natural history, and treatment from the more recognizable patterns in young patients with high-energy pelvic ring injuries. Recognition of a potentially unstable fracture pattern, careful evaluation of the ambulatory and functional status of each patient before injury, and the potential pitfalls and benefits of operative versus non-operative care are critical to the effective treatment.

Shen C, Peng JP, Chen XD. Efficacy of treatment in peri-pelvic Morel-Lavallee lesion: a systematic review of the literature. Arch Orthop Trauma Surg. 2013;133(5):635–40.

Morel-Lavallee lesion (MLL) involves incomplete de-gloving with shearing of the skin and subcutaneous tissue from the underlying fascia of the peri-pelvic region. This literature review found that surgical intervention was better than conservative therapy. Sclerodesis method worked well in symptomatic MLL patients without fractures. Patients with peri-pelvic fractures could be managed with local suction drainage or open debridement with dead space closure technique during fracture fixation.

Comment: This is controversial; the flank de-gloving is associated with significant complications in pelvic and acetabular fixation.

Stover MD, Sims S, Matta J. What is the infection rate of the posterior approach to type C pelvic injuries? Clin Orthop Relat Res. 2012;470(8):2142–7.

This paper looked at the infective complications following posterior approach to the pelvis for unstable pelvic fracture patterns. Two hundred and thirty-six patients across several institutions were studied. Surgical site infection occurred in 3.4 %; none of these needed soft tissue reconstruction as a result of the infection. Treatment consisted of surgical débridement, wound closure, and antibiotics.

Manson TT, Perdue PW, Pollak AN, O'Toole RV. Embolization of pelvic arterial injury is a risk factor for deep infection after acetabular fracture surgery. J Orthop Trauma. 2013;27(1):11–5.

The combination of an acetabular fracture that requires open reduction and internal fixation (ORIF) and a pelvic arterial injury that requires angiographic embolization is rare. However, in this series there was a 58 % infection rate of the patients who underwent embolization before ORIF; this is an order of magnitude higher than typical historical controls (2–5 %) and significantly higher than that of the control group of patients who underwent angiography without embolization (14 %). In addition, a disproportionate number of the patients who developed infection had their entire internal iliac artery embolized.

Odutola AA, Sabri O, Halliday R, Chesser TJ, Ward AJ. High rates of sexual and urinary dysfunction after surgically treated displaced pelvic ring injuries. Clin Orthop Relat Res. 2012;470(8):2173–84.

Pelvic ring injuries may be associated with genitourinary injury (GUI) and result in urinary or sexual dysfunction. This paper presents a retrospective postal review of 151 patients who had surgically treated pelvic fractures, with or without GUI. New sexual dysfunction occurred in 43 % and urinary dysfunction in 41 % of responding patients. Neither new sexual nor urinary dysfunction was associated with gender or GUI. Lateral compression injury was less likely to result in new sexual or urinary dysfunction compared with anterior posterior (AP) type and vertical shear type injuries.

Vallier HA, Cureton BA, Schubeck D. Pregnancy outcomes after pelvic ring injury. J Orthop Trauma. 2012;26(5): 302–7.

This study looked retrospectively at the obstetric histories of 31 women who had pregnancies after healed pelvic fractures. Thirty-one women had 54 pregnancies after a mean 72 months follow-up. Sixteen women had 25 vaginal deliveries; 28 % after surgical treatment for their pelvic fracture with retained anterior (16 %) and/or posterior (16 %) hardware, including trans-symphyseal plating in three patients (12 %). Thirteen women had 26 Cesarean deliveries, 46 % after surgical treatment for their pelvis. Cesarean delivery was not related to age, fracture pattern, treatment type, or residual pelvic displacement. A trend for Cesarean delivery related to retained hardware was observed.

Laflamme GY, Delisle J, Rouleau D, Uzel AP, Leduc S. Lateral compression fractures of the superior pubic ramus with intra-articular extension. J Bone Joint Surg Br. 2009;91(9):1208–12.

This study of 30 patients with lateral compression fractures of the pelvis with intra-articular extension into the anterior column were followed for a mean of 4.2 years. Functional deficits were noted for the mental component summary score and in the social function domain of the Short Form-36 (SF-36), but there was no evidence of degenerative arthritis in the lateral-compression group.

Kanakaris NK, Angoules AG, Nikolaou VS, Kontakis G, Giannoudis PV. Treatment and outcomes of pelvic malunions and non-unions: a systematic review. Clin Orthop Relat Res. 2009;467(8):2112–24.

This systematic review found 437 malunions/non-unions reported in 25 studies. Treatment of these demanding complications appeared effective in the majority of the cases: overall union rates averaged 86.1 %, pain relief as much as 93 %, patient satisfaction 79 %, and return to a preinjury level of activities 50 %. Nevertheless, the patient should be informed about the incidence of perioperative complications, including neurologic injury (5.3 %), symptomatic vein thrombosis (5.0 %), pulmonary embolism (1.9 %), and deep wound infection(1.6 %).

Acetabular Fractures

Briffa N, Pearce R, Hill AM, Bircher M. Outcomes of acetabular fracture fixation with ten years' follow-up. J Bone Joint Surg Br. 2011;93(2):229–36.

This paper reports the outcome of 161 surgically fixed acetabular fractures from a single unit. The fracture pattern was simple in 42 % and associated fractures in 58 %. The result was excellent in 47 %, good in 25 %, fair in 7 % and poor in 20 %. Poor prognostic factors included increasing age, delay to surgery, quality of reduction and some fracture patterns. Complications were common in the medium- to long-term and functional outcome was variable.

Ohashi K, El-Khoury GY, Abu-Zahra KW, Berbaum KS. Interobserver agreement for Letournel acetabular fracture classification with multidetector CT: are standard Judet radiographs necessary? Radiology. 2006;241(2):386–91.

This analysis of 101 imaging studies of acetabular fractures looked at the interobserver agreement for Letournel acetabular fracture classification with radiography alone and multidetector computed tomography (CT) alone. There was substantial interobserver agreement for Letournel acetabular fracture classification with multiplanar reformatted and 3D multidetector CT images. Standard Judet pelvic radiographs add little information for changing the multidetector CT classification.

Burd TA, Hughes MS, Anglen JO. The floating hip: complications and outcomes. J Trauma. 2008;64(2):442–8.

This descriptive study deals with the problems associated with ipsilateral injuries to the femur and the pelvis or acetabulum ("floating hip"). These severe injuries are usually caused by high-energy trauma. The femur fracture will most commonly be addressed first. Delays of surgery were common because of severity of systemic trauma. There is a high incidence of sciatic nerve palsy (33 %) in this devastating combination of injuries. Other complications included deep vein thrombosis (DVT) (12 %), heterotopic ossification (34 %), femoral head avascular necrosis (AVN) (2 %), osteoarthritis (16 %).

Henry PD, Kreder HJ, Jenkinson RJ. The osteoporotic acetabular fracture. Orthop Clin North Am. 2013;44(2):201–15.

In elderly patients, these challenges of acetabular fractures are compounded by the complexity of fracture patterns, the poor biomechanics of osteoporotic bone, and comorbidities. Nonsurgical management is preferable when the fracture is stable enough to allow mobilization, and healing in a functional position can be expected. When significant displacement and/or hip instability are present, operative management is preferred in most patients, which may include open reduction and internal fixation with or without total hip arthroplasty.

Tannast M, Najibi S, Matta JM. Two to twenty-year survivorship of the hip in 810 patients with operatively treated acetabular fractures. J Bone Joint Surg Am. 2012; 94(17):1559–67.

This single surgeon study looked at 816 acetabular fractures treated with open reduction and internal fixation. The cumulative 20-year survivorship was 79 % at 20 years. Significant independent negative predictors were non-anatomical fracture reduction, an age of more than 40-years, anterior hip dislocation, postoperative incongruence of the acetabular roof, involvement of the posterior acetabular wall, acetabular impaction, a femoral head cartilage lesion, initial displacement of the articular surface of $\geq$20 mm, and utilization of the extended iliofemoral approach.

Moed BR, McMichael JC. Outcomes of posterior wall fractures of the acetabulum. J Bone Joint Surg Am. 2007;89(6): 1170–6.

This paper presents the outcomes for 46 patients with elementary posterior wall fractures of the acetabulum, managed operatively. At follow-up of 2-years or more there were significant functional restrictions and problems shown on the Musculoskeletal Function Assessment (MFA), with many limitations not directly related to hip function. The authors conclude that complete recovery after a posterior wall fracture of the acetabulum is uncommon.

Grimshaw CS, Moed BR. Outcomes of posterior wall fractures of the acetabulum treated non-operatively after diagnostic screening with dynamic stress examination under anesthesia. J Bone Joint Surg Am. 2010;92(17):2792–800.

In this study 21 patients with an acute posterior wall fracture of the acetabulum who were shown to have a stable hip joint by dynamic stress fluoroscopy while they were under general anesthesia were treated non-operatively. Fifteen patients had radiographic evaluation at a minimum of 2 years, and all were found to have a congruent joint with a normal joint space and no evidence of post-traumatic arthritis.

Gänsslen A, Hildebrand F, Krettek C. Conservative treatment of acetabular both column fractures: does the concept of secondary congruence work? Acta Chir Orthop Traumatol Cech. 2012;79(5):411–5.

Complete separation of all bony fragments around the acetabulum in both column fractures can lead to extra-anatomical orientation of these fragments around the femoral head with the potential of a "secondary congruence". This paper reviewed 35 patients in whom a both column fracture was treated non-operatively due to different reasons. Most patients had a multifragmentary anterior column but simple posterior column and 88 % healed with secondary congruence. Eighty percent of the patients had none or only slight pain and 77 % had an excellent or good functional result. The rate of joint failure due to non-union, femoral head necrosis, post-traumatic degenerative changes or pain was relatively low with 17 % after a mean of 5 years following trauma.

Giannoudis PV, Nikolaou VS, Kheir E, Mehta S, Stengel D, Roberts CS. Factors determining quality of life and level of sporting activity after internal fixation of an isolated acetabular fracture. J Bone Joint Surg Br. 2009;91(10):1354–9.

This study of 52 patients with an isolated acetabular fracture, operatively treated, looked at outcomes in terms of function and return to sporting activity. There was a significant reduction in level of activity, frequency of participation in sport and general quality of life scores in patients of all age groups compared to a normal English population. Forty-two percent were able to return to their previous level of activities: 67 % were able to take part in sport at some level.

Blokhuis TJ, Frölke JP. Is radiation superior to indomethacin to prevent heterotopic ossification in acetabular fractures?: a systematic review. Clin Orthop Relat Res. 2009;467(2):526–30.

Heterotopic ossification is a well-known complication after fixation of an acetabular fracture. Indomethacin and radiation therapy are used as prophylaxis to prevent heterotopic ossification. This systematic review found only five appropriate prospective studies and the quality of these made proper meta-analysis inappropriate. The findings suggested, however, that the incidence of heterotopic ossification was significantly lower in patients treated with radiation than in patients receiving indomethacin.

Proximal Femoral Fractures

Parker MJ, Pryor GA. The timing of surgery for proximal femoral fractures. J Bone Joint Surg Br. 1992;74(2):203–5.

This was a study of 765 patients with proximal femoral fractures to determine if the time interval between injury and surgery influenced the outcome. The analysis was between those stabilized with a dynamic hip screw (DHS) or had received a hemiarthroplasty. It excluded those with displaced fractures treated with internal fixation as this group were younger, fitter and more likely to be operated on earlier. Patients with a delay for medical reasons were also excluded leaving 468 in the study group. Four groups were compared. Those with surgery within 24 h, 24–47 h, 48–72 h and more than 72 h. Initial analysis failed to show any significant differences between the groups, but analysis of those that had surgery within 47 h and those that had surgery later showed a higher complication rate with pressure sores in those operated on early. There was a trend to longer hospital stay, pneumonia and pulmonary embolism (PE) in those treated after 48 h.

Orosz GM, Magaziner J, Hannan EL, Morrison RS, Koval K, Gilbert M, et al. Association of timing of surgery for hip fracture and patient outcomes. JAMA. 2004;291(14): 1738–43.

This was a study from four large centers and involving 1,206 patients. It was the first prospective trial associating timing of femoral neck and intertrochanteric hip fractures with outcomes. Fixation was performed either within 24 h of admission or after more than 24 h following admission. One-third had early surgery, with no improvement in mortality rates, no improvement in ambulation potential, and no difference in postoperative pain or length of stay after surgery. However, due to performing the procedure early, a decrease in duration of severe pain and overall length of stay was observed. The investigators concluded that early surgery is warranted in medically stable patients to reduce costs and control pain, although no functional improvement was seen at 6 months.

Moran CG, Wenn RT, Sikand M, Taylor AM. Early mortality after hip fracture: is delay before surgery important? J Bone Joint Surg Am. 2005;87(3):483–9.

This was a prospective, observational study of 2,660 patients who underwent surgical treatment of a hip fracture in one institution. Mortality rates were compared following the surgery in relation to the delay in the surgery and the acute medical comorbidities on admission. The overall mortality following the hip fracture surgery was 9 % (246 of 2,660) at 30 days, 19 % at 90 days, and 30 % at 12 months. Of the patients who had been declared fit for surgery, those operated on without delay had a 30-day mortality of 8.7 % and those for whom the surgery had been delayed between 1 and 4 days had a 30-day mortality of 7.3 % (p=0.51). The 30-day mortality for patients for whom the surgery had been delayed for more than 4 days was 10.7 %, and this small group had significantly increased mortality at 90 days and 1 year.

Patients who had been admitted with an acute medical comorbidity that required treatment prior to the surgery had a 30-day mortality of 17 %, which was nearly 2.5 times greater than that for patients who had been initially considered fit for surgery. Patients with medical comorbidities that delayed surgery had 2.5 times the risk of death within 30 days after the surgery compared with patients without comorbidities that delayed surgery.

Mortality was not increased when the surgery was delayed up to 4 days for patients who were otherwise fit for hip fracture surgery. However, a delay of more than 4 days significantly increased mortality.

Bottle A, Aylin P. Mortality associated with delay in operation after hip fracture: observational study. BMJ. 2006;332(7547): 947–51.

The purpose of this study was to estimate the number of deaths and readmissions associated with delay in operation after femoral fracture. There was an analysis of the inpatient hospital statistics within trusts in England with at least 100 admissions for fractured neck of femur (fnof) of people over the age of 65 during the study period of 3 years. There were 129,522 admissions within 28 days for fractured neck of femur in 151 trusts with 18,508 deaths in hospital (14.3 %). Delay in the operation was associated with an increased risk of death in hospital, which was reduced but persisted after adjustment for comorbidity. For all deaths in hospital, the odds ratio for more than 1 day's delay relative to 1 day or less was 1.27 (95 % confidence interval 1.23–1.32) after adjustment for comorbidity. The proportion with more than 2 days' delay ranged from 1.1 to 62.4 % between trusts. The authors concluded that if death rates in patients with at most 1 day's delay had been repeated throughout all 151 trusts in this study, there would have been an average of 581 (478–683) fewer total deaths per year (9.4 % of the total). There was little evidence of an association between delay and emergency readmission. Their conclusion was that a delay in operating is associated with an increased risk of death but not readmission after a fractured neck of femur, even with adjustment for comorbidity.

Jain R, Koo M, Kreder HJ, Schemitsch EH, Davey JR, Mahomed NN. Comparison of early and delayed fixation of subcapital hip fractures in patients sixty years of age or less. J Bone Joint Surg Am. 2002;84-A(9):1605–12.

The risk of avascular necrosis (AVN) in young patients sustaining femoral neck fractures is 30–35 %. It was thought that early anatomic reduction and decompression of the intracapsular hematoma were essential in reducing this risk. The timing of surgery remains unknown.

This study was a retrospective cohort of 38 patients and examined the effect of early versus delayed fixation of femoral neck fractures in patients 60 years of age or younger. Patients were followed for at least 2 years and consisted of an early and late cohort. Functional outcomes and AVN rates were compared. There was no difference in functional outcome score. There was a statistically significant increase in AVN in the late fixation group. However there were limitations in the size of the cohort and length of follow-up in the late cohort. It is also possible that the end results of increased AVN rates may not manifest for many years, warranting further study. Of the 29 femoral neck fractures in this study, decompression was performed in only one case, and no increase in AVN was observed. At present, the best conclusion that can be drawn is that early fixation for patients under 60 when feasible may reduce the rate of AVN, although this may not have any effect on outcome.

Ly TV, Swiontkowski MF. Treatment of femoral neck fractures in young adults. J Bone Joint Surg Am.2008; 90(10):2254–66.

This is an excellent review of the treatment of the femoral neck fractures in patients under the age of 65. The article deals with the surgical approach, timing and methods of fixation of these difficult fractures. The role of capsulotomy remains controversial. There are too few femoral neck fractures in young patients to allow the performance of randomized controlled trials of a sufficient sample size to evaluate the role of capsulotomy. The timing of surgery for femoral neck fractures also remains controversial, and the available data remain inconclusive. Osteonecrosis of the femoral head and non-union are the two most common and challenging complications associated with femoral neck fractures. Initial fracture displacement and disruption of the femoral head blood flow are the main contributing factors. It is suggested that the key factors in the treatment of femoral neck fractures include early diagnosis, early surgery, anatomic reduction, capsular decompression, and stable internal fixation.

Hopley C, Stengel D, Ekkernkamp A, Wich M. Primary total hip arthroplasty versus hemiarthroplasty for displaced intracapsular hip fractures in older patients: systematic review. BMJ. 2010;340:c2332.

This was a systematic review and meta-analysis to try to compile all available investigations of total hip arthroplasty compared with hemiarthroplasty for femoral neck fractures to determine whether total hip arthroplasty is associated with lower reoperation rates, mortality, and complications, and better function and quality of life than hemiarthroplasty for displaced fractures of the femoral neck in older patients. The review included randomized trials, quasi randomised trials and cohort studies.

Three thousand eight hundred and twenty-one references were identified. Of the 202 full papers inspected, 15 were included (four randomised controlled trials, three quasi randomised trials, and eight retrospective cohort studies, totalling 1,890 patients).

Meta-analysis of 14 studies showed a lower risk of reoperation after total hip arthroplasty compared with hemiarthroplasty (relative risk 0.57, 95 % confidence interval 0.34–0.96, risk difference 4.4 %, 95 % confidence interval 0.2–8.5 %). Total hip arthroplasty consistently showed better ratings in the Harris hip score after follow-up periods of 12–48 months, indicating a medium functional advantage of total hip arthroplasty over hemiarthroplasty. Total hip arthroplasty was associated with a slightly higher risk of dislocation and general complications. The authors concluded that total hip arthroplasty may lead to lower reoperation rates and better functional outcomes compared with hemiarthroplasty in older patients with displaced femoral neck fractures.

This paper has the usual disadvantages of a meta-analysis and the number of available studies was small, and with an overall sample size of fewer than 2,000 patients. These results do not allow for conclusive statements on the effectiveness of total hip arthroplasty and hemiarthroplasty for treating femoral neck fractures.

Burgers PT, Van Geene AR, Van den Bekerom MP, Van Lieshout EM, Blom B, Aleem IS, et al. Total hip arthroplasty versus hemiarthroplasty for displaced femoral neck fractures in the healthy elderly: a meta-analysis and systematic review of randomized trials. Int Orthop. 2012;36(8): 1549–60.

A further systematic review of the English literature was performed for this meta-analysis. Randomized controlled trials comparing all forms of total hip arthroplasty (THA) with hemiarthroplasty (HA) were included. Eight trials were identified with a total of 986 patients. Revision rates after THA were 4 % compared with 7 % for hemiarthroplasty. The 1 year mortality was equal in both groups at between 13 and 15 %. Dislocation rates were 9 % after THA versus 3 %

after HA. Equal rates were found for major and minor complications. Harris hip scores, pain scores and the Western Ontario and McMasters Universities Arthritis Index (WOMAC) score all favoured THA as did the EQ-5D. The authors concluded that Total hip arthroplasty for displaced femoral neck fractures in the fit elderly may lead to higher patient-based outcomes but has higher dislocation rates compared with hemiarthroplasty.

Further high-quality randomized clinical trials are needed to provide robust evidence and to definitively answer this clinical question.

Parker MJ, Handoll HH. Gamma and other cephalocondylic intramedullary nails versus extramedullary implants for extracapsular hip fractures in adults. Cochrane Database Syst Rev. 2008;(3):CD000093.

The purpose of this Cochrane review was to compare cephalocondylic intramedullary nails such as the Gamma nail with extramedullary implants (the sliding hip screw) for extracapsular hip fractures in adults. All randomised and quasi-randomised controlled trials comparing these implants for extracapsular hip fractures were included in the analysis.

There were 22 trials (3,871 participants) that compared the Gamma nail with the sliding hip screw (SHS). Overall the Gamma nail was associated with an increased risk of operative and later fracture of the femur and an increased reoperation rate. There were no major differences between implants in the wound infection, mortality or medical complications. Five trials (623 participants) compared the intramedullary hip screw (IMHS) with the SHS. Fracture fixation complications were more common in the IMHS group; all cases of operative and later fracture of the femur occurred in this group. Results for post-operative complications, mortality and functional outcomes were similar in the two groups. Three trials (394 participants) showed no difference in fracture fixation complications, reoperation, wound infection and length of hospital stay for proximal femoral nail (PFN) compared with the SHS. Single trials compared other types of plates and nail designs, however, these trials provided insufficient evidence to establish differences between these implants.

Two trials (65 participants with reverse and transverse fractures at the level of the lesser trochanter) found intramedullary nails (Gamma nail or PFN) were associated with better intra-operative results and fewer fracture fixation complications than extramedullary implants (a 90° blade plate or dynamic condylar screw) for these fractures.

The conclusion of the review is that given the lower complication rate of the SHS in comparison with intramedullary nails, SHS appears superior for trochanteric fractures. Further studies are required to determine if different types of intramedullary nail produce similar results, or if intramedullary nails have advantages for selected fracture types.

Frihagen F, Nordsletten L, Madsen JE. Hemiarthroplasty or internal fixation for intracapsular displaced femoral neck fractures: randomised controlled trial. BMJ 2007;335(7632): 1251–4.

A randomized prospective trial (RPT) of 222 patients; 165 (74 %) women, mean age 83 years. Inclusion criteria were age above 60, ability to walk before the fracture, and no major hip pathology, regardless of cognitive function. The aim was to compare the functional results after displaced fractures of the femoral neck treated with internal fixation or hemiarthroplasty. The intervention was either closed reduction and two parallel screws or bipolar cemented hemiarthroplasty. The main outcome measures were hip function (Harris hip score), health related quality of life (Eq-5d), activities of daily living (Barthel index). Complications occurred in 56 (50 %) patients in the internal fixation group and 16 (15 %) in the hemiarthroplasty group, $(P < 0.001)$. In each group 39 patients (35 %) died within 24 months. The authors concluded that hemiarthroplasty is associated with better functional outcome than internal fixation in treatment of displaced fractures of the femoral neck in elderly patients.

Bhandari M, Devereaux PJ, Swiontkowski MF, Tornetta P 3rd, Obremskey W, Koval KJ, et al. Internal fixation compared with arthroplasty for displaced fractures of the femoral neck. A meta-analysis. J Bone Joint Surg Am. 2003;85-A(9): 1673–81.

The objective of this study was to determine the effect of arthroplasty (hemiarthroplasty, bipolar arthroplasty, and total hip arthroplasty), compared with that of internal fixation, on rates of mortality, revision, pain, function, operating time, and wound infection in patients with a displaced femoral neck fracture.

Fourteen studies met all eligibility criteria. Nine trials, which included a total of 1,162 patients, provided detailed information on mortality rates over the first four postoperative months, which ranged from 0 to 20 %. There was a trend toward an increase in the relative risk of death in the first 4 months after arthroplasty compared with internal fixation. The risk of death after arthroplasty appeared to be higher than that after fixation with a compression screw and sideplate but not higher than that after internal fixation with use of screws only (rp < 0.05).

Fourteen trials that included a total of 1,901 patients provided data on revision surgery. The relative risk of revision surgery after arthroplasty compared with the risk after internal fixation was 0.23 (p = 0.0003) however, pain relief and the attainment of function were similar in patients treated with arthroplasty and those treated with internal fixation. Arthroplasty significantly increased the risk of infection (p = 0.009) with a range from 0 to 18 %. Patients who underwent arthroplasty had greater blood loss and longer operative times than those who were treated with internal fixation.

Their conclusions were that in comparison with internal fixation, arthroplasty for the treatment of a displaced femoral neck fracture significantly reduces the risk of revision surgery, at the cost of greater infection rates, blood loss, and operative time and possibly an increase in early mortality rates. Only larger trials will resolve the critical question of the impact on early mortality.

Periprosthetic Fractures

Zustin J, Krause M, Breer S, Hahn M, von Damarus C, Rüther W, et al. Morphologic analysis of periprosthetic fractures after hip resurfacing arthroplasty. J Bone Joint Surg Am. 2010;92(2):404–10.

This international multi-centre retrieval study analysed 107 femoral remnants and femoral components from five different manufacturers. Following analysis they noted three fracture modes: acute biomechanical – in the femoral neck (8 %), acute postnecrotic (51 %), chronic biomechanical (40 %); the latter two groups were predominantly in the bone inside the femoral component.

Erhardt JB, Grob K, Roderer G, Hoffmann A, Forster TN, Kuster MS. Treatment of periprosthetic femur fractures with the non-contact bridging plate: a new angular stable implant. Arch Orthop Trauma Surg 2008;128(4):409–16.

A series of 24 patients with peri-prosthetic femoral fractures treated with a plate combining both standard, locked and variable angle fixation achieving a 90 % union rate. The re-operation rate was 15 %.

Comment: Although a small study with short term follow-up this article illustrates the versatility of poly-axial screw fixation. This is particularly helpful gaining fixation around well fixed implants.

Ricci WM, Borrelli J Jr. Operative management of periprosthetic femur fractures in the elderly using biological fracture reduction and fixation techniques. Injury. 2007;38 Suppl 3:S53–8.

Retrospective review of 59 patients with acute fractures around well fixed hip or knee replacements. The study is carried out over a 5 year period and all fractures were treated with locked and non-locking plates, without bone graft or bone graft substitutes. All but 1 healed and 49 out of 59 returned to baseline function.

Masri BA, Meek RM, Duncan CP. Periprosthetic fractures evaluation and treatment. Clin Orthop Relat Res. 2004;(420): 80–95.

Excellent review article expanding on the original Vancouver classification and including intra-operative classifications, based on site of fracture, implant stability and bone stock. The treatment algorithm provides a logical approach to management, and shows that the surgeon needs access to various fixation and prosthetic devices plus allograft bone in some cases.

Franklin J, Malchau H. Risk factors for periprosthetic femoral fracture. Injury. 2007;38(6):655–60.

Review article drawing on outcomes from National Arthroplasty Databases and other studies demonstrating the factors associated with an increased risk of periprosthetic fracture. The authors conclude that the key to prevention of these periprosthetic femoral fractures is routine follow-up with radiographs.

Bhattacharyya T, Chang D, Meigs JB, Estok DM 2nd, Malchau H. Mortality after periprosthetic fracture of the femur. J Bone Joint Surg Am. 2007;89(12):2658–62.

This paper compares outcomes of periprosthetic fractures with matched groups of hip fractures and primary joint replacement. The mortality rates are similar between the periprosthetic and hip fracture groups at 1 year, 11 and 16.5 % respectively. The mortality for periprosthetic fractures increased with a delay of more than 2-days from admission to surgery. For Vancouver B fractures the mortality was much less in the group undergoing revision arthroplasty compared to fixation; mortality rates of 12 % versus 33 %.

Comment: This illustrates the frailty of this group of patients and suggests that their management should be on an equivalent to hip fracture patients, i.e. an emphasis on prompt surgery within a multi-disciplinary team setting, with revision arthroplasty preferred over ORIF for Vancouver B fractures.

Lindahl H, Malchau H, Odén A, Garellick G. Risk factors for failure after treatment of a periprosthetic fracture of the femur. J Bone Joint Surg Br. 2006;88(1):26–30.

A nationwide observation of a study using the Swedish national hip arthroplasty register reports of over 1,000 periprosthetic fractures of the femur a quarter of which required further surgery due to failure of initial treatment. Using the Vancouver classification B2 injuries treated by revision of the implant with or without open reduction and internal fixation reduced the failure rate.

The study highlighted the high risk of failure in B1 fractures with the use of only a single plate for fixation, a crucial point is made that it is likely many fractures initially classified as B1 are in reality B2 and loosening of the stem was not recognised at the initial assessment and planning: consider the prosthesis loose until proven otherwise.

Corten K, Vanrykel F, Bellemans J, Frederix PR, Simon JP, Broos PL. An algorithm for the surgical treatment of periprosthetic fractures of the femur around a well-fixed femoral component. J Bone Joint Surg Br. 2009;91(11): 1424–30.

Case series of 45 B1 periprosthetic fractures. Using this algorithm 97 % union rate was achieved at a mean of 6.4-months. Only one construct failed. The joint was dislocated at surgery and stability of the component "meticulously assessed". The fracture was suitable for single plate and cable graft fixation if the medial cortex could be restored.

Comment: This reiterates the importance of a systematic approach to the management of these fractures, in particular with a high index of suspicion to assess implant stability.

Egol KA, Kubiak EN, Fulkerson E, Kummer FJ, Koval KJ. Biomechanics of locked plates and screws. J Orthop Trauma. 2004;18(8):488–93.

Excellent review article examining the biomechanical principles comparing conventional and locked plates.

Comment: Although principally a trauma article, this is very relevant to understanding the use of locked plates in the management of periprosthetic fracture.

Distal Femoral Fractures

Papadokostakis G, Papakostidis C, Dimitriou R, Giannoudis PV. The role and efficacy of retrograding nailing for the treatment of diaphyseal and distal femoral fractures: a systematic review of the literature. Injury. 2005;36(7): 813–22.

The aim of this analysis has been to evaluate the efficacy of retrograde nailing in the treatment of distal femur and femoral shaft fractures. A systematic review was performed. Twenty-four articles were eligible for the final analysis, reviewing a total of 914 patients (mean age of 48.8 years) who sustained 963 distal and diaphyseal femoral fractures. The overall mortality rate was 5.3 %. The incidence of infection was 1.1 % and for septic arthritis of the knee was 0.18 %.

The analysis led the authors to conclude that that retrograde intramedullary nailing appears to be a reliable treatment option, mainly for distal femoral fractures. However, in the management of diaphyseal fractures, retrograde intramedullary nailing is associated with high rates of knee pain and lower rates of fracture union.

Wähnert D, Hoffmeier KL, von Oldenburg G, Fröber R, Hofmann GO, Mückley T. Internal fixation of type-C distal femoral fractures in osteoporotic bone. J Bone Joint Surg Am. 2010;92(6):1442–52.

The purpose of this study was to investigate the biomechanical stability of four different fixation devices for the treatment of comminuted distal femoral fractures in osteoporotic bone. They were tested in axial and torsional loading in an osteoporotic synthetic bone model. There were three intramedullary nails, differing in the mechanism of distal locking (with two lateral-to-medial screws in one construct, one screw and one spiral blade in another construct, and four screws and one angular stable plate). The angular stable plate constructs had significantly higher torsional stiffness than the other constructs; the intramedullary nail with four-screw distal locking achieved nearly comparable results. The four-screw distal locking construct had the greatest torsional strength and axial stiffness. For intramedullary nails the kind of distal locking affects the stabilization of distal femoral fractures. Four-screw distal locking provides the highest axial stability and nearly comparable torsional stability to that of the angular stable plate.

Henderson CE, Kuhl LL, Fitzpatrick DC, Marsh JL. Locking plates for distal femur fractures: is there a problem with fracture healing? J Orthop Trauma. 2011;25 Suppl 1: S8–14.

This article reviews the literature on distal femur fractures treated with locking plates to determine the reported rate of healing difficulties. Fifteen full-length publications and three abstracts were included. The rate of complications related to healing ranged from 0 to 32 % in these studies. Implant failures occurred late with 75 % of the failures occurring after 3 months and 50 % occurring after 6 months.

Thomson AB, Driver R, Kregor PJ, Obremskey WT. Long-term functional outcomes after intra-articular distal femur fractures: ORIF versus retrograde intramedullary nailing. Orthopedics. 2008;31(8):748–50.

This retrospective study evaluated the long-term clinical, functional, and radiographic outcomes of open reduction internal fixation (ORIF) versus limited open reduction with retrograde intramedullary nailing for supracondylar-intercondylar distal femur fractures (33-C type (AO)). Twenty-three fractures were followed in 22 patients for a mean follow-up of 80 months. Bone grafting and malunion were significantly higher in the ORIF group compared with the intramedullary nailing (IMN). A nonsignificant trend was noted for increased infection and non-union in the ORIF group.

Distal Femoral Fractures Around a Knee Replacement

Horneff JG 3rd, Scolaro JA, Jafari SM, Mirza A, Parvizi J, Mehta S. Intramedullary nailing versus locked plate for treating supracondylar periprosthetic femur fractures. Orthopedics. 2013;36(5):561–6.

This study compared locked supracondylar plating with retrograde intramedullary nailing for periprosthetic femur fractures around a total knee replacement. This was a retrospective review of 63 patients who sustained Rorabeck Type II periprosthetic femoral fractures. Patients were pooled from three academic institutions. Thirty-five patients were treated with intramedullary femoral nailing and 28 with a locking plate. The two groups were compared for radiographic union at 6, 12, 24, and 36 weeks. At 36 weeks, radiographic union was significantly greater in the locked screw-plate group. Time to full weight bearing was not significantly different. Perioperative blood transfusion was higher in the locked plating group but the overall reoperation rate was lower. The authors concluded that the results support the use of a laterally based locked plate in the treatment of Rorabeck type II distal femur periprosthetic fractures.

Ricci W. Classification and treatment of periprosthetic supracondylar femur fractures. J Knee Surg. 2013;26(1): 9–14.

This is a review and classification of periprosthetic supracondylar femur fractures. Periprosthetic distal femur fractures can be treated with locked plating and retrograde intramedullary devices. Each has relative benefits and potential pitfalls. This paper goes on to describe that appropriate patient selection is important and specific femoral component geometry are required to optimally choose between these two methods. Locked plating can be applied to most fracture types, however the specific pattern will dictate whether the technique will involve compression or bridging. Nailing obviously requires an open intercondylar box and a distal fragment of enough size to allow interlocking. With proper patient selection and proper techniques, good results can be obtained with either method.

Large TM, Kellam JF, Bosse MJ, Sims SH, Althausen P, Masonis JL. Locked plating of supracondylar periprosthetic femur fractures. J Arthroplasty. 2008;23(6 Suppl 1):115–20.

This was a review of 50 periprothetic fractures above a total knee replacement (TKR). Fractures were closed Lewis and Rorabeck type II with a stable prosthesis. Twenty-nine patients (group I), were treated with locked condylar plating and 21 (group II) were treated with non-locked plating systems or intramedullary fixation. The patients were followed up for a minimum of 1.7 years. In the plating group there was a 20 % malunion rate and no non-unions. In group II there was a 47 % malunion rate (p<0.5) and 16 % non-union rate. Complication rates were 12 % in group I, compared to 42 % in group II. Group I patients had less operative blood loss, healed in better alignment, and had greater knee motion. All seven patients treated with a retrograde intramedullary nail developed a malunion or non-union. The authors concluded that locked plating was reliable with a lower complication rate than other conventional treatments.

Herrera DA, Kregor PJ, Cole PA, Levy BA, Jönsson A, Zlowodzki M. Treatment of acute distal femur fractures above a total knee arthroplasty: systematic review of 415 cases (1981-2006). Acta Orthop. 2008;79(1):22–7.

A systematic review of the different fixation techniques in the management of distal femur fractures above a total knee arthroplasty (TKA). Twenty-nine case series with a total of 415 fractures were identified. Overall there was a 9 % non-union rate, a fixation failure rate of 4 %. Infection occurred in 3 % and the surgery was revised in 13 % Retrograde nailing was associated with relative risk reduction (RRR) of 87 % (p=0.01) for developing a non-union and 70 % (p=0.03) for requiring revision surgery compared to traditional (non-locking) plating methods. Risk reductions for locking plates compared to traditional plating were identified, although these were not statistically significant The results should be interpreted with caution, due to the lack of randomized controlled trials and the possible selection bias in case series.

Tibial Plateau Fractures

Canadian Orthopaedic Trauma Society. Open reduction and internal fixation compared with circular fixator application for bicondylar tibial plateau fractures. Results of a multicenter, prospective, randomized clinical trial. J Bone Joint Surg Am. 2006;88(12):2613–23.

This was one of the first studies comparing the two operative approaches of ORIF and minimally invasive techniques with circular frames in the treatment of bicondylartibial plateau fractures. This was a multicenter, prospective, randomized clinical trial in which standard open reduction and internal fixation with medial and lateral plates was compared with percutaneous and/or limited open fixation and application of a circular fixator for displaced bicondylartibial plateau fractures. Eighty-three fractures were randomized to ORIF and 43 to a circular frame. The patient demographics, mechanism of injury and fracture severity were the same in each group. Those treated with a circular frame had significantly less blood loss and spent less time in hospital. There was a trend for patients in the circular fixator group to have superior early outcome in terms of functional scores and return to pre injury activities. These outcomes were not significantly different at 2 years. At 2 years pain, stiffness and the functional scores were no different. Seven (18 %) of the 40 patients in the open reduction and internal fixation group had a deep infection. The number of unplanned repeat surgical interventions, and their severity, was significantly greater in the open reduction and internal fixation group. Both techniques provide a satisfactory quality of fracture reduction. Regardless of treatment method, patients with this injury have substantial residual limb-specific and general health deficits at 2 years of follow-up.

Colman M, Wright A, Gruen G, Siska P, Pape HC, Tarkin I. Prolonged operative time increases infection rate in tibial plateau fractures. Injury. 2013;44(2):249–52.

This was a retrospective controlled analysis of 309 consecutive unicondylar and bicondylar tibial plateau fractures treated with open plate osteosynthesis at a level I trauma centre over 5 years period. The operative times were recorded, as were the injury characteristics, surgical treatment, and need for operative debridement due to infection. Multivariable logistic regression analysis was performed to identify independent risk factors for postoperative infection. The authors found that operative times approaching 3 h and open fractures are related to an increased overall risk for surgical site infection after open plating of the tibial plateau. Dual incision approaches with bicolumnar plating do not appear to expose the patient to increased risk compared to single incision approaches.

Musahl V, Tarkin I, Kobbe P, Tzioupis C, Siska PA, Pape HC. New trends and techniques in open reduction and internal fixation of fractures of the tibial plateau. J Bone Joint Surg Br. 2009;91(4):426–33.

This is a review of the operative treatment of complex proximal tibial fractures and the different surgical techniques available. It reviews current surgical approaches and techniques, improved devices for internal fixation and the clinical outcome after utilisation of new methods for locked plating.

Egol KA, Tejwani NC, Capla EL, Wolinsky PL, Koval KJ. Staged management of high-energy proximal tibia fractures (OTA types 41): the results of a prospective, standardized protocol. J Orthop Trauma. 2005;19(7):448–55.

This study evaluated the use of a staged protocol involving temporary spanning external fixation and delayed formal definitive fixation in the management of high-energy proximal tibia fractures (OTA types 41). The study involved 57 high-energy tibial plateau fractures in 53 patients. After spanning external fixation the fractures underwent ORIF with a plate and screw construct or conversion to a ring fixator.

There were 42 Schatzker VI (74 %), 12 Schatzker V (21 %), 2 Schatzker IV (4 %), and 1 Schatzker II (2 %). Sixteen were open fractures. There was a 5 % deep wound infection rate, 4 % resulted in a non-union, 4 % had significant knee stiffness (<90°). Nine patients (16 %) underwent additional surgery after definitive skeletal stabilization related to their injury. The authors concluded that the benefits of temporizing spanning external fixation include osseous stabilization, access to soft tissues, and prevention of further articular damage. They recommended this technique on the basis of their low complication rate.

Stevens DG, Beharry R, McKee MD, Waddell JP, Schemitsch EH. The long-term functional outcome of operatively treated tibial plateau fractures. J Orthop Trauma. 2001;15(5):312–20.

This was a retrospective study of 47 displaced fractures of the tibial plateau in 46 patients were treated with open reduction, interfragmental screw fixation of the articular fragments, and buttress plate fixation and had a minimum of 5 years of follow-up. All aspects of their care, including tibial plateau fracture type, operative management and associated injuries, were documented. Preoperative and postoperative follow-up radiographs were analyzed for fracture classification and adequacy of reduction. All patients were contacted and given functional outcome questionnaires using both a generic health status scale (Short Form 36 [SF-36]) (18) and a disability scale relating to knee osteoarthritis (Western Ontario and McMaster Universities Osteoarthritis index [WOMAC]). Assessment scores were analyzed with respect to age, fracture type and severity, and were compared to standardized age and sex-matched scores for the healthy population. The average follow-up period was 8.3 years. Of the 47 fractures studied, 25 were classified as Schatzker types I, II, or III, and the remaining 22 were types IV, V, or VI.

Compared to the standardized SF-36 scores, there was no statistically significant difference between the healthy age-matched population and 24 of 26 of the under-age-40 group regardless of fracture type. With regard to the over-age-40 group, scores statistically similar to the control population were found in only 12 of 21 patients. The data revealed that presentation age was the most significant source of variation with respect to functional outcome.

Weigel DP, Marsh JL. High-energy fractures of the tibial plateau. Knee function after longer follow-up. J Bone Joint Surg Am. 2002;84-A(9):1541–51.

The purpose of this study was to assess the function of the knee and the development of arthrosis at a minimum of 5 years after injury in a consecutive series of patients in whom a high-energy fracture of the tibial plateau had been treated with a uniform technique of external fixation. Thirty patients with a total of 31 fractures of the tibial plateau were treated with a monolateral external fixator and limited internal fixation of the articular surface. Follow-up data was obtained at an average of 98 months and included the SF-36 and the Iowa knee score, general health survey and clinical examination. Weight bearing X-rays were performed. The range of motion was an average of 87 % of the total arc of the contralateral knee. The average Iowa Knee Score was 90 points (range, 72–100 points). Radiographs showed no evidence of arthrosis in 14 knees, grade-1 arthrosis in three, grade-2 in three, and grade-3 in two. Compared with the radiographic appearance 2–4 years after injury, there was no evidence of progression of arthrosis in 18 knees and one grade of progression in four. There was no deterioration in SF-36 scores. The authors concluded that patients with a high-energy fracture of the tibial plateau treated with external fixation have a good prognosis for satisfactory knee function in the second 5 years after injury. The rates of arthritic change are low.

Mahadeva D, Costa ML, Gaffey A. Open reduction and internal fixation versus hybrid fixation for bicondylar/severe tibial plateau fractures: a systematic review of the literature. Arch Orthop Trauma Surg. 2008;128(10):1169–75.

This study was a systematic analysis of the literature comparing two techniques of hybrid external fixation and internal fixation. Five studies contained data to directly compare the two techniques. Study designs and outcome measures were not consistent in all studies. The mechanical studies suggest that hybrid external fixation may have a benefit over internal fixation with respect to failure load. Two further papers presented only level 4 evidence. The final study was a multicentre randomized controlled trial (RCT) and it demonstrated a marginal non-significant benefit of hybrid external fixation over internal fixation. There is little evidence that hybrid external fixation is better and must be evaluated in the presence of newer locking plates.

Jiang R, Luo CF, Wang MC, Yang TY, Zeng BF. A comparative study of Less Invasive Stabilization System (LISS) fixation and two-incision double plating for the treatment of bicondylartibial plateau fractures. Knee. 2008;15(2):139–43.

The authors present a prospective study comparing the use of locked plates (LISS) and classic double plates in the treatment of 84 bicondylartibial plateau fractures. All patients were followed for a minimum of 24 months. Patient demographics were the same for both groups as was the mechanism of injury and fracture type. No differences in the surgical time, bony union rate or radiographic healing times were observed between the two groups. Also the functional scores and incidences of complications were all similar in both groups. The size of the incision was significantly less in the LISS group as was the blood loss however in this group there was a significantly higher incidence of post-operative malalignment of the proximal tibia (P = 0.041).

Higgins TF, Klatt J, Bachus KN. Biomechanical analysis of bicondylartibial plateau fixation: how does lateral locking plate fixation compare to dual plate fixation? J Orthop Trauma. 2007;21(5):301–6.

A lateral-only locked plate was compared to medial and lateral non-locked plating in a cadaveric model of a bicondylar proximal tibial plateau fracture in ten matched pairs of human cadaveric proximal tibia. Cyclic loading and the maximum load to failure on the medial condyle for both plate constructs was measured. The results of this study demonstrated that dual-plate fixation allows less subsidence in this bicondylar tibial plateau cadaveric model when compared to isolated locked lateral plates raising concern about the widespread use of isolated lateral locked plate constructs in bicondylar tibial plateau fractures.

Catagni MA, Ottaviani G, Maggioni M. Treatment strategies for complex fractures of the tibial plateau with external circular fixation and limited internal fixation. J Trauma. 2007;63(5):1043–53.

This was a retrospective review of treatment over a 10 years period. The authors treated 59 patients with proximal tibial fractures Schatzker types V and VI, (age from 23 to 63 years). All patients were treated with external circular fixation. Five of these fractures were open. Three different strategies were used, ring fixator confined to the tibia when soft tissues and stability allowed or the fixator was extended onto the femur with the proximal tibial ring at joint level or when soft tissue was compromised the tibial ring was lower down the tibia bypassing the fracture. Their results were evaluated as excellent in 30 patients (50.85 %), good in 27 patients (45.76 %), fair in 1 patient (1.695 %), and poor in another 1 (1.695 %). The patients' satisfaction was significantly correlated with the functional results.

Haidukewych G, Sems SA, Huebner D, Horwitz D, Levy B. Results of polyaxial locked-plate fixation of periarticular fractures of the knee. J Bone Joint Surg Am. 2007;89(3): 614–20.

The purpose of this study was to evaluate the clinical performance of a variable-axis locking plate in a multicenter series of periarticular fractures about the knee. Fifty-four patients with a total of 56 fractures were treated with a poly-axial locked-plate fixation system. There were 20 male patients and 34 female patients with a mean age of 57 years. There were 25 distal femoral fractures and 31 proximal tibial fractures. Twelve of the fractures were open. Ninety-four percent of the 52 fractures united. There were no mechanical complications. Most importantly, there was no evidence of varus collapse as a result of polyaxial screw failure. There were three deep infections and one aseptic non-union. No plate fractured, and no screw cut out. The authors concluded that variable axis plates had similar complications to other plates but offered more versatility.

Zura RD, Adams SB Jr, Jeray KJ, Obremskey WT, Stinnett SS, Olson SA, et al. Timing of definitive fixation of severe tibial plateau fractures with compartment syndrome does not have an effect on the rate of infection. J Trauma. 2010;69(6):1523–6.

The objective of this study was to analyze whether there is an association between infection and the timing of definitive fracture fixation in relation to fasciotomy closure or coverage. Eighty-one tibial plateau fractures, complicated by compartment syndrome, were treated with four-compartment fasciotomies and definitive fracture fixation before, at, or after fasciotomy closure. Thirty were treated with fixation before the fasciotomy and 23 % developed infection. Thirty-two percent (26 fractures) were treated with definitive fixation at the time of fasciotomy closure and 12 % developed an infection. The remainder (25 fractures), were treated after the fasciotomy closure and 16 % developed an infection. There was no significant difference between the groups and it would seem that the timing of definitive fixation can be determined by the preference of the surgeon.

Hak DJ, Lee M, Gotham DR. Influence of prior fasciotomy on infection after open reduction and internal fixation of tibial plateau fractures. J Trauma. 2010;69(4):886–8.

The purpose of this study was to compare the rate of infection after internal fixation of tibial plateau fractures in patients requiring fasciotomy for compartment syndrome with patients in whom a fasciotomy was not required. It was a retrospective review of 142 tibial plateau fractures. Fourteen required a fasciotomy. Operative treatment of their plateau fracture, follow-up surgical procedures, follow-up complications, and length of follow-up were reviewed. In the fasciotomy group, two patients developed cellulitis that was treated with a short course on oral antibiotics. There were no documented deep infections. In the no fasciotomy group, eight patients (6.25 %) had a documented culture-positive deep infection. Additionally, six patients had documented occurrences of cellulitis. The conclusion reached was that definitive internal fixation of tibial plateau fractures in the presence of open fasciotomy wounds does not seem to be associated with an increased infection risk.

Tibial Shaft Fractures

Reamed and Unreamed Intramedullary Nailing

Study to Prospectively Evaluate Reamed Intramedullary Nails in Patients with Tibial Fractures Investigators, Bhandari M, Guyatt G, Tornetta P 3rd, Schemitsch EH, Swiontkowski M, Sanders D, et al. Randomized trial of reamed and unreamed intramedullary nailing of tibial shaft fractures. J Bone Joint Surg Am. 2008;90(12):2567–78.

This was a very large multicentre, blinded and randomized trial of 1,319 adults with a tibial shaft fracture. The fracture was treated with either a reamed or an un-reamed nail. All perioperative care was standardized. The outcomes measured at 12 months were exchange of the nail, bone grafting and dynamization with a fracture gap of <1 cm (primary outcome). Infection and fasciotomy were considered as part of the composite outcome, irrespective of the postoperative gap.

Ninety-three percent completed 1 year of follow-up. Of these, 622 patients were randomized to reamed nailing and 604 patients were randomized to unreamed nailing. Among all patients 4.6 % had exchange of the nail or bone grafting because of non-union. Among all patients, almost 17 % of the reamed nailing group and 19 % of the unreamed nailing group experienced a primary outcome event (relative risk, 0.90; 95 % confidence interval, 0.71–1.15). In patients with closed fractures, 45 (11 %) of 416 in the reamed nailing group and 68 (17 %) of 410 in the unreamed nailing group experienced a primary event (relative risk, 0.67; 95 % confidence interval, 0.47–0.96; p = 0.03). This difference was largely due to differences in dynamization. In patients with open fractures, 29 % of 206 in the reamed nailing group and 24 % of 194 in the unreamed nailing group experienced a primary event (relative risk, 1.27; 95 % confidence interval, 0.91–1.78; p=0.16). The authors concluded that there is a possible benefit for reamed nailing in closed tibial shaft fractures. There appears to be no difference with open fractures. Delaying reoperation for at least 6 months may decrease the need for reoperation.

Schemitsch EH, Bhandari M, Guyatt G, Sanders DW, Swiontkowski M, Tornetta P, et al. Prognostic factors for predicting outcomes after intramedullary nailing of the tibia. J Bone Joint Surg Am. 2012;94(19):1786–93.

Using the same data from the trial above the authors attempted to look at baseline and surgical factor to determine if they could make associations with adverse events within a year of intramedullary nailing. Fifteen different factors were investigated.

The investigators found that there was a increased risk of negative events in high energy fracture, a stainless steel compared with a titanium nail, the presence of a fracture gap and full weight-bearing status after surgery. The use of nonsteroidal anti-inflammatory agents, late or early time to surgery, or smoking status did not appear to be associated with negative events.

Open fractures had a higher risk of events among patients treated with reamed nailing but not in patients treated with unreamed nailing. Patients with open fractures who had wound debridement either without any additional procedures or with delayed primary closure had a decreased risk of events compared with patients who required subsequent, more complex reconstruction.

Duan X, Al-Qwbani M, Zeng Y, Zhang W, Xiang Z. Intramedullary nailing for tibial shaft fractures in adults. Cochrane Database Syst Rev. 2012;1:CD008241.

This was a Cochrane review and a systematic analysis of the literature (up to September 2011) to assess the effects of different methods and types of intramedullary nailing for treating tibial shaft fractures in adults. Randomised and quasi-randomised controlled clinical studies evaluating different methods and types of intramedullary nailing for treating tibial shaft fractures in adults were included. Primary outcomes were health-related quality of life, patient-reported function and re-operation for treatment failure or complications. Eleven studies (9 randomised and 2 quasi-randomised clinical trials), involving a total of 2,093 participants with 2,123 fractures, were included.

The trials evaluated five different comparisons of interventions: reamed versus unreamed intramedullary nailing (six trials); Ender nail versus interlocking nail (two trials); expandable nail versus interlocking nail (one trial); interlocking nail with one distal screw versus with two distal screws (one trial); and closed nailing via the transtendinous approach versus the paratendinous approach (one trial).

There is moderate level evidence to suggest that there is no difference between the reamed and unreamed nailing groups in 'major' re-operations or in the secondary outcomes of non-union, pain, deep infection, malunion and compartment syndrome. Subgroup analysis provides 'low' level evidence that reamed nailing is more likely to reduce the incidence of major re-operations related to non-union in closed fractures than in open fractures. Implant failure, such as broken screws, occurred less often in the reamed nailing group.

There was insufficient evidence established to determine the effects of interlocking nail with one distal screw versus with two distal screws, interlocking nail versus expandable nail and paratendinous approach versus transtendinous approach for treating tibial shaft fractures in adults. The Ender nail has poorer results in terms of re-operation and malunion than an interlocking nail. In the one trial evaluated there is no difference in the non-union rate between using one distal or two distal screws. There were however significantly more implant failures in the single screw group. One trial found no statistically significant differences in functional outcomes or anterior knee pain at 3 year follow-up between the transtendinous approach and the paratendinous approach for nail insertion.

Comment: The evidence was dominated by one large multicentre trial of 1,319 participants. Both quasi-randomised trials were at high risk of selection bias. There were very few data on functional outcomes and often incomplete data on re-operations.

Lam SW, Teraa M, Leenen LP, van der Heijden GJ. Systematic review shows lowered risk of non-union after reamed nailing in patients with closed tibial shaft fractures. Injury. 2010;41(7):671–5.

Non-union after intramedullary nailing (IMN) in patients with tibial shaft fractures occurs in up to 16 %. This systematic review of the literature aimed to compare the non-union rate in patients with a tibial shaft fracture treated by either a reamed or an unreamed intramedullary device. The publications selected were RCT's and seven studies were identified. The insertion of a reamed IMN resulted in a reduced non-union rate (compared to reamed) in closed fractures. The difference between the two treatments for open tibial shaft fractures was not clinically relevant. The evidence showed a consistent trend of reduced non-union rate in closed tibial shaft fracture treated with reamed compared to unreamed IMN.

Finkemeier CG, Schmidt AH, Kyle RF, Templeman DC, Varecka TF. A prospective, randomized study of intramedullary nails inserted with and without reaming for the treatment of open and closed fractures of the tibial shaft. J Orthop Trauma. 2000;14(3):187–93.

A prospective surgeon randomized comparative study in 94 patients with closed and open tibial fractures. Patients were randomized to a reamed or unreamed IMN. The study was to determine differences in healing, complications and secondary procedures required to obtain healing. (Anderson and Gustillo IIIb and IIIC were excluded). For open fractures, there were no significant differences in the time to union or number of additional procedures performed to obtain union in patients with reamed nail insertion compared with those without reamed insertion. In the closed fracture group a higher percentage of fractures had healed at 4 months compared to the unreamed group. There was no difference at 6 and 12 months. More secondary procedures were needed to obtain union after unreamed nail insertion for the treatment of closed tibia fractures, but the difference was not statistically significant given the limited power of the study. There were no differences in rates of infection or compartment syndrome.

Foster PA, Barton SB, Jones SC, Morrison RJ, Britten S. The treatment of complex tibial shaft fractures by the Ilizarov method. J Bone Joint Surg Br. 2012;94(12):1678–83.

This study reports on the use of the Ilizarov method to treat 40 consecutive fractures of the tibial shaft (35 AO 42C fractures and five AO 42B3 fractures) in adults. The series included 19 open fractures (six Gustilo grade 3A and 13 grade 3B) and 21 closed injuries. The mean time from injury to application of definitive Ilizarov frame was 8 days (0–35) with 36 fractures successfully uniting without the need for any bone-stimulating procedure. Four patients required a second frame to stimulate union. There were no deep infections, amputations or significant malunions, requiring further intervention. Time to healing was from injury to the date of frame removal, with a median of 166 days (mean 187, (87–370)). Twenty-three percent had minor complications. Functional scores were available in 32/40 patients (Olerud and Molander ankle, Lysholm knee, Tegner activity, and SF36). The authors concluded that the Ilizarov method is a safe and reliable way of treating complex tibial shaft fractures with a high rate of primary union.

Open Fractures

British Association of Plastic, Reconstructive and Aesthetic Surgeons (BAPRAS) and British Orthopaedic Association (BOA). Standards for the management of open fractures of the lower limb. London: BAPRAS and BOA; 2009 [cited 28 2013 May 28]. Available from: http://www.boa.ac.uk/ Publications/Documents/Lower%20Limb%20Guide.pdf

This clear, concise and evidence-based publication sets out standards for the management of open lower limb fractures, advocating co-operation between orthopaedic and plastic surgeons. It deals with care of these injuries from the Emergency Department onwards, and offers advice on what to do with the complications that may arise.

The publications are available from the British Orthopaedic Association (BOA) and British Association of Plastic, Reconstructive and Aesthetic Surgeons (BAPRAS) – the short guide is available to download, the full guide offers details of the supporting evidence behind the standards.

Keating JF, Blachut PA, O'Brien PJ, Court-Brown CM. Reamed nailing of Gustilo grade-IIIB tibial fractures. J Bone Joint Surg Br. 2000;82(8):1113–6.

This paper analysed the effectiveness of reamed intramedullary nailing on 57 (55 patients) Gustillo and Anderson grade III-B open tibial fractures. After debridement, there was substantial bone loss in 49 % of the fractures. The mean time to union was 43 weeks (14–94). When there was no bone loss, the mean time to union was 32 weeks; it was 45 weeks if there was bone loss. The presence of infection which occurred in 17.5 % delayed union to a mean of 53 weeks. Twenty-three percent required exchange nailing and 26 % were bone grafted. In the group that got infected 9/10 were successfully treated, one ended up with an amputation. The authors concluded that these results indicate that reamed intramedullary nailing is a satisfactory treatment for Gustilo grade-III tibial fractures.

Keating JF, O'Brien PJ, Blachut PA, Meek RN, Broekhuyse HM. Locking intramedullary nailing with and without reaming for open fractures of the tibial shaft. A prospective, randomized study. J Bone Joint Surg Am. 1997;79(3): 334–41.

Ninety-four open fractures (in 91 patients) were randomized to receive either a reamed intramedullary nail or an IMN without reaming. There were no differences in the patient demographics or fracture types. Average nail diameter was 11.5 mm in the reamed group and 9.2 in the group without reaming. No differences were identified in the rate of early postoperative complications. The average time to union was 30 weeks (13–72) in the group treated with reaming and 29 weeks

(13–50) in the group treated without reaming. Nine percent of the fractures treated with reaming and 12 % of the fractures treated without reaming did not unite, this was not a significant difference. The rate of infection was the same. Significantly more screws broke in the group treated without reaming (29 %) than in the group treated with reaming (9 %). Functional difference was similar in the two groups as measured by knee pain, range of motion, return to work and recreational activity. In conclusion the results are similar but the rate of screw failure in the unreamed group is significantly higher.

Larsen LB, Madsen JE, Høiness PR, Øvre S. Should insertion of intramedullary nails for tibial fractures be with or without reaming? A prospective, randomized study with 3.8 years' follow-up. J Orthop Trauma. 2004;18(3):144–9.

In this study 45 patients with open fractures grade I-IIIA were randomized into the two treatment groups. Two different nails were used, either a slotted stainless steel reamed nail or a titanium unreamed nail. The average time to fracture healing was 16.7 weeks in the reamed group and 25.7 weeks in the unreamed group. The difference was statistically significant (P=0.004). All the non-unions occurred in the unreamed group. There were two malunions in the reamed group and four malunions in the unreamed group. There were no differences for all other outcome measurements. It was concluded that unreamed nails may be associated with higher rates on non-union and the need for secondary intervention with longer times to healing.

Limb Salvage Versus Amputation

Probe RA. Orthopaedic trauma myth busters: is limb salvage the preferred method of treatment for the mangled lower extremity? Instr Course Lect. 2013;62:35–40.

Comment: This thoughtful and well-referenced review sets out the understanding of limb salvage versus amputation based on up to date evidence. It makes the point that functional outcomes for amputation and salvage are similar in the severely injured lower limb. Whilst technical and biological advances might mean that salvage is possible, this is not necessarily the optimum pathway as those undergoing limb salvage have more hospital episodes and prolonged treatment times.

MacKenzie EJ, Bosse MJ, Kellam JF, Burgess AR, Webb LX, Swiontkowski MF, et al. Factors influencing the decision to amputate or reconstruct after high-energy lower extremity trauma. J Trauma. 2002;52(4):641–9.

This North American multi-centre prospective study of severe lower limb injury recruited 527 patients. Eligible patients were between the ages of 16 and 69 with Gustilo type IIIB and IIIC tibial fractures, dysvascular limbs resulting from trauma, type IIIB ankle fractures, or severe open mid-foot or hindfoot injuries. Four hundred and eight left the hospital with a salvaged limb. Of the 119 amputations performed, 55 were immediate and 64 were delayed. Soft tissue injury severity had the greatest impact on decision making regarding limb salvage versus amputation.

Comment: This publication from The Lower Extremity Assessment Project (LEAP) looked at the indications for amputation and the reconstructive efforts made in the 1990s. This paper, and those that followed, offer useful insights in to the assessment of lower limb trauma and the outcomes following either amputation or salvage.

Busse JW, Jacobs CL, Swiontkowski MF, Bosse MJ, Bhandari M; Evidence-Based Orthopaedic Trauma Working Group. Complex limb salvage or early amputation for severe lower-limb injury: a meta-analysis of observational studies. J Orthop Trauma. 2007;21(1):70–6.

This meta-analysis found 9 observational studies comparing the outcomes of amputation and limb salvage in severe lower limb injury. The evidence suggested that length of hospital stay is similar for limb salvage and primary amputation, but length of rehabilitation and total costs are higher for limb salvage patients. Long-term functional outcomes (up to 7 years post injury) are equivalent between limb salvage and primary amputation; both are associated with high rates of self-reported disability (40 %; to 50 %;), and functional status worsens over time. Report of pain following limb salvage or primary amputation is similar. Return to work is essentially the same between limb salvage and primary amputation groups, with approximately half returning to competitive employment at 2 years post injury.

Bosse MJ, MacKenzie EJ, Kellam JF, Burgess AR, Webb LX, Swiontkowski MF, et al. A prospective evaluation of the clinical utility of the lower-extremity injury-severity scores. J Bone Joint Surg Am. 2001;83-A(1):3–14.

This paper from the LEAP study looked at 556 high energy lower limb injuries, assessed with the established scoring systems: Mangled Extremity Severity Score (MESS); the Limb Salvage Index (LSI); the Predictive Salvage Index (PSI); the Nerve Injury, Ischemia, Soft-Tissue Injury, Skeletal Injury, Shock, and Age of Patient Score (NISSSA); and the Hannover Fracture Scale-97 (HFS-97). Four hundred and seven limbs were still on the salvage/reconstruction pathway 6-months after injury. Analysis of the 5 scoring systems showed high specificity of the scores: low scores could be used to predict limb-salvage potential. The converse, however, was not true. There was low sensitivity of the scores, which could not be used as predictors of amputation.

Comment: Scoring systems might be used to guide our assessment of the severity of injury, but cannot be used to predict the non-salvagable limb.

Ly TV, Travison TG, Castillo RC, Bosse MJ, MacKenzie EJ; LEAP Study Group. Ability of lower-extremity injury severity scores to predict functional outcome after limb salvage. J Bone Joint Surg Am. 2008;90(8):1738–43.

This paper from the LEAP (Lower Extremity Assessment Project) study group looked at the subset of 407 patients who had undergone successful lower limb salvage and reconstruction. Their limb injury severity was assessed with common scoring systems: Mangled Extremity Severity Score (MESS); the Limb Salvage Index (LSI); the Predictive Salvage Index (PSI); the Nerve Injury, Ischemia, Soft-Tissue

Injury, Skeletal Injury, Shock, and Age of Patient Score (NISSSA); and the Hannover Fracture Scale-98 (HFS-98). Functional outcomes were measured using Sickness Impact Profile (SIP). None of the scoring systems was usefully predictive of the SIP at 6 or 24 months.

Bosse MJ, McCarthy ML, Jones AL, Webb LX, Sims SH, Sanders RW, et al. The insensate foot following severe lower extremity trauma: an indication for amputation? J Bone Joint Surg Am. 2005;87(12):2601–8.

This LEAP paper looked at the subset of 55 patients who had an insensate foot at presentation. Twenty-six had amputation and 29 had limb salvage – of this latter group 55 % had normal plantar sensation at 2 years after injury, and only one had a total loss of plantar sensation at this point. Outcome was not adversely affected by limb salvage, despite the presence of an insensate foot at the time of presentation. Initial plantar sensation is not prognostic of long-term plantar sensory status or functional outcomes and should not be a component of a limb-salvage decision algorithm.

MacKenzie EJ, Bosse MJ. Factors influencing outcome following limb-threatening lower limb trauma: lessons learned from the Lower Extremity Assessment Project (LEAP). J Am Acad Orthop Surg. 2006;14(10 Spec No.):S205–10.

This analysis based on the LEAP study showed no difference in functional outcome between those undergoing limb salvage or amputation at 2 and 7 year follow-up after severe lower limb trauma. It also showed wide-ranging variations in outcome in these patients with many having significant disability. The importance of the patient's socio-economic and personal resources are often more important than initial treatment of the injury.

Ellington JK, Bosse MJ, Castillo RC, MacKenzie EJ; LEAP Study Group. The mangled foot and ankle: results from a 2-year prospective study. J Orthop Trauma. 2013;27(1):43–8.

This analysis of the LEAP study looked at the 174 severe open hindfoot or ankle injuries, of which 116 had salvage and

58 had a below knee amputation (BKA). When compared to patients treated with standard BKA, salvage patients who required free flaps and/or ankle arthrodesis had significantly worse 2-year outcomes.

Akula M, Gella S, Shaw CJ, McShane P, Mohsen AM. A meta-analysis of amputation versus limb salvage in mangled lower limb injuries—the patient perspective. Injury. 2011; 42(11):1194–7.

This is a meta-analysis of studies evaluating quality of life for patients having limb salvage or amputation after lower limb injuries. There were 11 suitable studies. The pooled data showed that lower limb salvage was psychologically more acceptable to the patient compared with amputation despite similar physical outcomes for both treatments.

O'Toole RV, Castillo RC, Pollak AN, MacKenzie EJ, Bosse MJ; LEAP Study Group. Determinants of patient satisfaction after severe lower-extremity injuries. J Bone Joint Surg Am. 2008;90(6):1206–11.

The LEAP data analysed here show that patient satisfaction after surgical treatment of lower-extremity injury is predicted more by function, pain, and the presence of depression at 2-years than by any underlying characteristic of the patient, injury, or treatment.

MacKenzie EJ, Bosse MJ, Castillo RC, Smith DG, Webb LX, Kellam JF, et al. Functional outcomes following trauma-related lower-extremity amputation. J Bone Joint Surg Am. 2004;86-A(8):1636–45.

This analysis of 161 lower limb amputees in the LEAP study found no significant differences between Sickness Impact Profiles of those with above knee amputations (AKA) versus below knee amputations (BKA). The BKA group had faster walking speed than those with an AKA Those who had a through knee amputation fared worse than either the AKA or BKA groups and often had problems with coverage of the end of the stump. In general, the state of soft tissue coverage and sophistication of the prosthesis did not correlate with outcome; amputees, in general, had severe disabilities.

Compartment Syndrome

Pearse MF, Harry L, Nanchahal J. Acute compartment syndrome of the leg. BMJ. 2002;325(7364):557–8.

Comment: Well written and available free online from PubMed. A review article setting out the understanding of acute compartment syndrome and its management a decade ago - but not much has changed and the recommendations in this paper were incorporated in the later "Standards for the Management of Open Lower Limb Fractures" by British Orthopaedic Association and British Association of Plastic, Reconstructive and Aesthetic Surgeons.

McQueen MM, Court-Brown CM. Compartment monitoring in tibial fractures. The pressure threshold for decompression. J Bone Joint Surg Br. 1996;78(1):99–104.

A prospective study of 116 patients with tibial diaphyseal fractures who had continuous monitoring of anterior compartment pressure for 24 h. A differential pressure (diastolic minus compartment pressure) of less than 30 mmHg as a threshold for fasciotomy led to no missed cases of acute compartment syndrome.

Al-Dadah OQ, Darrah C, Cooper A, Donell ST, Patel AD. Continuous compartment pressure monitoring vs. clinical monitoring in tibial diaphyseal fractures. Injury. 2008;39(10): 1204–9.

A cohort of 109 consecutive patients with a tibial fracture who underwent continuous compartment pressure monitoring of the anterior compartment of the leg were reviewed and compared to a historical control group of the immediate previous 109 patients who were clinically monitored. The fasciotomy rate of patients who underwent continuous compartment pressure monitoring was 15.6 %. Patients who were not monitored had a fasciotomy rate of 14.7 %. The mean time delay from injury to fasciotomy was 22 h in the monitored group and 23 h in the non-monitored group. Continuous compartment pressure monitoring did not increase the rate of unnecessary fasciotomies. We could not demonstrate a significant difference in terms of clinical outcome and time delay from injury to fasciotomy.

McQueen MM, Duckworth AD, Aitken SA, Court-Brown CM. The estimated sensitivity and specificity of compartment pressure monitoring for acute compartment syndrome. J Bone Joint Surg Am. 2013;95(8):673–7.

This retrospective review of a prospective trauma database identified 1,184 patients who had sustained a tibial diaphyseal fracture. A diagnosis of acute compartment syndrome was made if there was escape of muscles at fasciotomy and/or color change in the muscles or muscle necrosis intraoperatively. A diagnosis of acute compartment syndrome was considered incorrect if it was possible to close the fasciotomy wounds primarily at 48-h. The absence of acute compartment syndrome was confirmed by the absence of neurological abnormality or contracture at the time of the latest follow-up.

There were 850 patients satisfying the inclusion criteria; 17.9 % underwent fasciotomy for the treatment of acute compartment syndrome: 141 had acute compartment syndrome (true positives), six did not have it (false positives), and five underwent fasciotomy despite having a normal differential pressure reading, with subsequent operative findings consistent with acute compartment syndrome (false negatives). Of the 698 patients (82.1 %) who did not undergo fasciotomy, 689 had no evidence of any late sequelae of acute compartment syndrome (true negatives) at a mean follow-up time of 59 weeks. The estimated sensitivity of intracompartmental pressure monitoring for suspected acute compartment syndrome was 94 %, with an estimated specificity of 98 %, an estimated positive predictive value of 93 %, and an estimated negative predictive value of 99 %.

Comment: This is an important paper regarding compartment syndrome and tibial fractures, but also serves as a very clear example of sensitivity, specificity, positive and negative predictive values (rather than talking about fire alarms!)

Ferlic PW, Singer G, Kraus T, Eberl R. The acute compartment syndrome following fractures of the lower leg in children. Injury. 2012;43(10):1743–6.

This paper looks at 1,028 fractures of the lower leg in children. Thirty-one patients(3 %) with a median age of 14.6 years (range 7.3–17.1 years) developed an acute compartment syndrome (ACS). In the group of patients younger than 12 years the incidence was even lower (1.3 %). Eighty-one percent of injuries leading to ACS were caused by high-energy trauma, with motorcycle accidents being the most common (45 %). The diagnosis of an ACS was primarily based on clinical symptoms. In 23 cases an intracompartmental pressure of median 55 mmHg were measured. ACS was diagnosed after 19 h mean. There was a tendency that the ACS occurred earlier after high-energy trauma than after low energy trauma (mean 16.9 vs. mean 28 h). No complications linked to the compartment syndrome were observed.

McQueen MM, Gaston P, Court-Brown CM. Acute compartment syndrome. Who is at risk? J Bone Joint Surg Br. 2000;82(2):200–3.

This paper analysed associated factors in 164 patients with acute compartment syndrome. In 69 % there was an associated fracture, about half of which were of the tibial shaft. Most patients were men, usually under 35 years of age. Acute compartment syndrome of the forearm, with associated fracture of the distal end of the radius, was again seen most commonly in young men. Injury to soft tissues, without fracture, was the second most common cause of the syndrome and one-tenth of the patients had a bleeding disorder or were taking anticoagulant drugs.

Hope MJ, McQueen MM. Acute compartment syndrome in the absence of fracture. J Orthop Trauma. 2004;18(4):220–4.

This study examines 38 cases of acute compartment syndrome with no fracture and excluding those with a crush syndrome. These patients were older and with more co-morbidities than those who had a compartment syndrome associated with a fracture. There was also a longer delay to fasciotomy and a greater incidence of muscle necrosis in this group compared to those with acute compartment syndrome associated with a fracture. The authors conclude that referral of swollen limbs without fracture for an orthopaedic opinion should not be delayed.

Court-Brown C, McQueen M. Compartment syndrome delays tibial union. Acta Orthop Scand. 1987;58(3):249–52.

This retrospective survey of the results of the treatment of closed and Grade I tibial fractures complicated by compartment syndrome was undertaken. There was a significant delay in fracture union in patients over 18 years of age, but not in younger patients.

White TO, Howell GE, Will EM, Court-Brown CM, McQueen MM. Elevated intramuscular compartment pressures do not influence outcome after tibial fracture. J Trauma. 2003;55(6):1133–8.

The differential compartment pressures (Delta P) after tibial fractures is generally accepted as the important variable in determining the need for fasciotomy. Some, however, are concerned about the absolute compartment pressures. In this study 41 patients had elevated intramuscular pressures of over 30 mmHg for more than 6 h continuously, despite an acceptable delta P. These patients were compared with a control group of 60 patients who had pressures of less than 30 mmHg throughout. No significant differences were found in muscular power or return to function between the two groups at 1 year.

Fitzgerald AM, Gaston P, Wilson Y, Quaba A, McQueen MM. Long-term sequelae of fasciotomy wounds. Br J Plast Surg. 2000;53(8):690–3.

A retrospective study of patients requiring fasciotomies, of either upper or lower limb. Sixty patients were studied, of which 49 had an underlying fracture. Ongoing symptoms such as pain related to the wound occurred in 10 % and altered sensation within the margins of the wound occurred in 77 %. Problems with the wounds were common: 40 % with dry scaly skin, 33 % with pruritus, 30 % with discoloured wounds, 25 % with swollen limbs, 26 % with tethered scars, 13 % with recurrent ulceration, 13 % with muscle herniation and 7 % with tethered tendons. The appearance of the scars affected patients such that 23 % kept the wound covered, 28 % changed hobbies and 12 % changed occupation. This study reveals a significant morbidity associated with fasciotomy wounds.

Foot and Ankle Trauma

Gavin Bowyer

Abstract This section covers fractures and associated ligamentous injuries to the ankle, hindfoot and mid-foot/forefoot junction (the Lisfranc injuries). Particular consideration is given to the current understanding of ankle instability and the treatment options. The up-to-date understanding of the talar blood supply helps to make sense of the management and outcome of talar fractures. The controversy over the value of operative fixation of calcaneal fractures continues, but some recent studies shed light on this.

Keywords Achilles tendon rupture • Ankle instability • Ankle fractures • Talar fractures • Talar blood supply • Calcaneal fractures • Lisfranc injury

G. Bowyer, MA, MChir, FRCS (Orth)
Department of Trauma and Orthopaedics,
University Hospital Southampton, NHS Trust, Tremona Road,
Southampton, Hampshire SO16 6YD, UK
e-mail: gwbowyer@aol.com

G. Bowyer, A. Cole (eds.), *Selected References in Trauma and Orthopaedics*, DOI 10.1007/978-1-4471-4676-6_10,

221

Achilles Tendon Rupture

Jiang N, Wang B, Chen A, Dong F, Yu B. Operative versus non-operative treatment for acute Achilles tendon rupture: a meta-analysis based on current evidence. Int Orthop. 2012; 36(4):765–73.

This meta-analysis looks at the clinical effectiveness of operative treatment vs non-operative treatment for acute Achilles tendon rupture. Ten randomized controlled trials (RCTs) with a total of 894 patients were screened. These showed that operative treatment was superior to non-operative treatment regarding lower risk of re-rupture and shorter time for sick leave but inferior to non-operative treatment regarding complication risks. No significant difference was identified between the two methods regarding the return to pre-injury sports, deep infection or deep vein thrombosis.

Khan RJ, Carey Smith RL. Surgical interventions for treating acute Achilles tendon ruptures. Cochrane Database Syst Rev. 2010;(9):CD003674.

This Cochrane Review included 12 trials involving 844 participants, although the methodology of the included trials was often poor. Open surgical treatment had a lower re-rupture risk compared to non-operative intervention, but had an increased risk of infection and numbness. Open repair was not conclusively different from percutaneous or minimally invasive repair, other than carrying a higher risk of infection; numbers involved were small and conclusions were guarded.

Kearney RS, McGuinness KR, Achten J, Costa ML. A systematic review of early rehabilitation methods following a rupture of the Achilles tendon. Physiotherapy. 2012;98(1):24–32.

Advances have led to the development of immediate weight bearing rehabilitation. This meta-analysis identifies nine relevant papers with a range of rehabilitation protocols.

It concludes that the efficacy of different immediate weight bearing rehabilitation remains unclear.

Park YS, Sung KS. Surgical reconstruction of chronic Achilles tendon ruptures using various methods. Orthopedics. 2012;35(2): 273–5.

Chronic Achilles tendon ruptures can be reconstructed using a variety of local tissues, depending on the extent of the gap at presentation; Achilles allograft might be considered with large gaps. The outcome is favourable (improved post-operative American Orthopedic Foot & Ankle Society [AOFAS] scores).

Comment: Flexor hallucislongus (FHL) transfer/reconstruction is currently popular, when the gap is more than 2.5 cm, precluding direct repair.

Ankle Instability

Kerkhoffs GM, Handoll HH, de Bie R, Rowe BH, Struijs PA. Surgical versus conservative treatment for acute injuries of the lateral ligament complex of the ankle in adults. Cochrane Database Syst Rev. 2007;(2):CD000380.

This systematic review of the literature compared surgical versus conservative treatment for acute injuries of the lateral ligament complex of the ankle in adults. Twenty trials, all with methodological weaknesses, were included. There is insufficient evidence available from RCTs to determine the relative effectiveness of surgical and conservative treatment for acute injuries of the lateral ligament complex of the ankle.

Loudon JK, Santos MJ, Franks L, Liu W. The effectiveness of active exercise as an intervention for functional ankle instability: a systematic review. Sports Med. 2008;38(7):553–63.

This is a systematic review of the literature on exercise interventions in functional ankle instability (FAI) – the ankle that easily 'gives way' with activity. Sixteen papers were analysed, covering conservative treatment interventions including balance, proprioceptive and muscle strengthening exercises. It concludes that these are effective for patients with FAI in decreasing the incidence of giving-way episodes, improving balance stability, and improving function.

Urgüden M, Söyüncü Y, Ozdemir H, Sekban H, Akyildiz FF, Aydin AT. Arthroscopic treatment of anterolateral soft tissue impingement of the ankle: evaluation of factors affecting outcome. Arthroscopy. 2005;21(3):317–22.

Forty-one patients underwent operative arthroscopy for anterolateral impingement of the ankle following inversion injury to the ankle. The most frequent preoperative complaints were tenderness localized to the anterolateral aspect of the ankle, swelling, crepitation, and pain at weight-bearing. All patients had failed to respond to at least 3 months of conservative treatment. There were excellent results in 21 patients, good in 16, fair in 2, and poor in 2. The mean AOFAS score was 89.6 points (range, 60–100) at follow-up. Four different soft tissue pathologies causing impingement were described.

deVries JS, Krips R, Sierevelt IN, Blankevoort L, van Dijk CN. Interventions for treating chronic ankle instability. Cochrane Database Syst Rev. 2011;(8):CD004124.

This systematic review compared conservative or surgical treatment for chronic lateral ankle instability. Ten randomised controlled trials were included. There were limitations of trial design, and only limited pooling of data was possible. Neuromuscular training alone appears effective in the short term. There is insufficient evidence to support any one surgical intervention over another but it is likely that there are limitations to the use of dynamic tenodesis. After surgical reconstruction, early functional rehabilitation appears to be superior to 6 weeks immobilisation in restoring early function.

Hua Y, Chen S, Li Y, Chen J, Li H. Combination of modified Broström procedure with ankle arthroscopy for chronic ankle instability accompanied by intra-articular symptoms. Arthroscopy. 2010;26(4):524–8.

This trial evaluated the effectiveness of the modified Broström procedure combined with ankle arthroscopy for chronic ankle instability (CAI) accompanied by intra-articular symptoms, in 85 patients. Ankle arthroscopy dealt with any intra-articular lesions. This was followed by the modified Broström procedure shortening of the anterior talofibular ligament and/or calcaneofibular ligament, as well as extensor retinaculum augmentation. The mean AOFAS score improved from 46.6 ± 8.1 preoperatively to 86.5 ± 7.6 postoperatively (P < .05). Improvements in AOFAS scores after surgery were significantly greater in patients without chondral lesions than in those with chondral lesions.

Barg A, Tochigi Y, Amendola A, Phisitkul P, Hintermann B, Saltzman CL. Subtalar instability: diagnosis and treatment. Foot Ankle Int. 2012;33(2):151–60.

Subtalar instability is challenging to diagnose. It can be suggested by the patient's feeling of ankle instability, easy "rolling over," and a need to look at the ground constantly when walking. Clinical measures for inversion and eversion do not accurately reflect isolated subtalar motion. Stress radiographs have high false positive rates. Magnetic resonance imaging can show injured or disorganized ligaments but are not dynamic and cannot alone diagnose instability. Operative treatment, when elected, should focus on determining the source of the problem. Generally direct repair of the lateral ligaments is sufficient.

Bare A, Ferkel RD. Peroneal tendon tears: associated arthroscopic findings and results after repair. Arthroscopy. 2009;25(11):1288–97.

This study sought to identify the intra-articular pathology associated with peroneal tendon tears and report the outcomes after tendon repair or tenodesis with arthroscopic treatment.

Thirty-two patients had a total of 60 intra-articular lesions, treated arthroscopically: 47 lesions (78 %) were discovered during arthroscopy rather than on pre-operative clinical assessment. All patients with peroneal tendon tears had associated intra-articular pathology, with the majority of patients having two or more intra-articular lesions. Correction of the tendon tears and arthroscopic treatment of the intra-articular lesions produced statistically significantly improved results and patient satisfaction.

Ankle Fractures

Sanders DW, Tieszer C, Corbett B; Canadian Orthopedic Trauma Society. Operative versus non-operative treatment of unstable lateral malleolar fractures: a randomized multicenter trial. J Orthop Trauma. 2012;26(3):129–34.

Six trauma centres contributed 81 patients with undisplaced, unstable, isolated fibula fractures (confirmed by an external rotation stress examination). Forty-one had open reduction and internal fixation (ORIF), 40 had short leg cast or brace and protected weight bearing for 6 weeks. There were no statistically significant differences in functional outcome scores or pace of recovery between the operative and non-operative groups. Complications in the non-operative group included eight patients with a medial clear space ≥5 mm and eight patients with delayed union or non-union. In the operative group, five patients had a surgical site infection and five patients required hardware removal.

Pakarinen H, Flinkkilä T, Ohtonen P, Hyvönen P, Lakovaara M, Leppilahti J, et al. Intraoperative assessment of the stability of the distal tibiofibular joint in supination-external rotation injuries of the ankle: sensitivity, specificity, and reliability of two clinical tests. J Bone Joint Surg Am. 2011;93(22):2057–61.

This is a prospective study of 140 patients with an unstable unilateral ankle fracture resulting from a supination-external rotation mechanism. After internal fixation of the malleolar fracture, a hook test and an external rotation stress test under fluoroscopy were performed; these were compared with a standardized 7.5-Nm external rotation stress test of each ankle under fluoroscopy (as the reference standard). Interobserver agreement for the hook test and the clinical stress test was excellent, and the specificity was high (0.98 and 0.96 respectively) but the sensitivity of these tests (0.25 and 0.58 respectively) was insufficient to adequately detect instability of the syndesmosis intraoperatively.

Shibuya N, Frost CH, Campbell JD, Davis ML, Jupiter DC. Incidence of acute deep vein thrombosis and pulmonary embolism in foot and ankle trauma: analysis of the National Trauma Data Bank. J Foot Ankle Surg. 2012;51(1):63–8.

The (US) National Trauma Data Bank data set (2007–2009) was used to evaluate the incidence of thromboembolism in foot and ankle trauma. The incidence of deep vein thrombosis (DVT) and pulmonary embolism (PE) was 0.28 and 0.21 %, respectively. The risk factors statistically significantly associated and clinically relevant for both DVT and PE in foot and ankle trauma were older age, obesity, and higher injury severity score. Owing to the low incidence, routine pharmacologic thromboprophylaxis might be contraindicated in foot and ankle trauma. Instead, careful, individualized assessment of the risk factors associated with DVT/PE is important.

Nåsell H, Ottosson C, Törnqvist H, Lindé J, Ponzer S. The impact of smoking on complications after operatively treated ankle fractures—a follow-up study of 906 patients. J Orthop Trauma. 2011;25(12):748–55.

This study of 906 operatively treated ankle fracture patients comprised 721 nonsmokers and 185 smokers. Follow-up data at 6 weeks were available for 98.2 % of the patients.

Postoperative complications of any kind (30.1 % versus 20.3 %, P=0.005) as well as deep wound infections (4.9 % versus 0.8 %, P<0.001) were more common among smokers than nonsmokers. Multivariable analyses showed that smokers had six times higher odds of developing a deep infection compared with nonsmokers. A more complicated fracture, associated diabetes mellitus, and unsatisfactory operative fracture reduction also enhanced the risk of postoperative complications.

Shivarathre DG, Chandran P, Platt SR. Operative fixation of unstable ankle fractures in patients aged over 80 years. Foot Ankle Int. 2011;32(6):599–602.

Ninety-two consecutive patients, 80 females and 12 males, above 80 years of age had open reduction and internal fixation for unstable ankle fractures. The superficial wound infection rate was 7 % (six cases) and the deep infection rate was 4.6 %. The 30 day postoperative mortality was 5.4 % (five cases). Eighty-six percent (75 out of 87 cases) were able to return back to their pre injury mobility at the last follow-up. Diabetes, dementia, peripheral vascular disease and smoking were found to be statistically significant risk factors associated with wound complications.

Schepers T. To retain or remove the syndesmotic screw: a review of literature. Arch Orthop Trauma Surg. 2011;131(7): 879–83.

In this study, the recent literature is reviewed concerning the need for removal of the syndesmotic screw placed to stabilize the syndesmosis in ankle fractures. A total of seven studies were identified. Most studies found no difference in outcome between retained or removed screws. Patients with screws that were broken, or showed loosening, had similar or improved outcome compared to patients with removed screws. Removal of the syndesmotic screws, when deemed necessary, is usually not performed before 8–12 weeks.

Stufkens SA, Knupp M, Horisberger M, Lampert C, Hintermann B. Cartilage lesions and the development of osteoarthritis after internal fixation of ankle fractures: a prospective study. J Bone Joint Surg Am. 2010;92(2):279–86.

A prospective study of 288 ankle fractures that were treated operatively. Arthroscopy had been performed in all cases to classify the extent and location of cartilage damage. Forty-seven percent were available for follow-up after a mean of 12.9 years.

Initial cartilage damage seen arthroscopically following an ankle fracture is an independent predictor of the development of post-traumatic osteoarthritis. Specifically, lesions on the anterior and lateral aspects of the talus and on the medial malleolus correlate with an unfavourable clinical outcome.

Wukich DK, Kline AJ. The management of ankle fractures in patients with diabetes. J Bone Joint Surg Am. 2008;90(7): 1570–8.

Patients with diabetes mellitus have higher complication rates following both open and closed management of ankle fractures. Unstable ankle fractures in diabetic patients without neuropathy or vasculopathy are best treated with open reduction and internal fixation with use of standard techniques. Patients with neuropathy or vasculopathy are at increased risk for both soft-tissue and osseous complications, including delayed union and non-union. Careful soft-tissue management as well as stable, rigid internal fixation are crucial to obtaining a good outcome. Prolonged non-weight-bearing and subsequently protected weight-bearing are recommended following both operative and non-operative management of ankle fractures in patients with diabetes.

Egol KA, Tejwani NC, Walsh MG, Capla EL, Koval KJ. Predictors of short-term functional outcome following ankle fracture surgery. J Bone Joint Surg Am. 2006;88(5):974–9.

Two hundred and thirty-two patients who sustained a fracture of the ankle and were treated surgically. Complete follow-up data were available for 198 patients (85 %). At 1 year, 174 (88 %) of the patients had either no or mild ankle pain and 178 (90 %) had either no limitations or limitations only in recreational activities. According to the AOFAS ankle-hindfoot score, 178 (90 %) of the patients had ≥90 % functional recovery. Patients at 1 year have a significant improvement in function compared with 6 months after the surgery. Younger age, male sex, absence of diabetes, and a lower American Society of Anesthesiologists (ASA) class are predictive of functional recovery at 1 year following ankle fracture surgery.

Talar Fractures

Babu N, Schuberth JM. Partial avascular necrosis after talar neck fracture. Foot Ankle Int. 2010;31(9):777–80.

Recently, it has been shown that avascular necrosis of the talus can occur in only a portion of the talar body. There is little information regarding the anatomic location of the avascular segment and the clinical significance of an incomplete avascular process. This paper looked at seven patients with partial avascular necrosis after Hawkins type II or III fracture dislocations, evaluated with magnetic resonance imaging (MRI). The avascular segment of the talar body was located predominantly in the anterior lateral and superior portion in six of the seven patients. Collapse occurred in three of the patients in the area of avascular process.

Vallier HA, Nork SE, Barei DP, Benirschke SK, Sangeorzan BJ. Talar neck fractures: results and outcomes. J Bone Joint Surg Am. 2004;86-A(8):1616–24.

This is a retrospective study of 102 fractures of the talar neck; all were treated with ORIF. Sixty fractures were evaluated at an average of 36 months after surgery, but only 39 had complete radiographic data. Osteonecrosis was seen in 49 % of those with radiographic follow-up, however, 37 % of these patients demonstrated revascularization of the talar dome without collapse. Osteonecrosis was seen in 39 % of Hawkins II fractures and 64 % of 14 Hawkins III fractures. The mean time to fixation was 3.4 days for patients who developed of osteonecrosis, compared with 5.0 days for patients who did not development of osteonecrosis.

Osteonecrosis and post-traumatic arthritis were each associated with higher energy injuries (comminution of the talar neck and/or open fracture). Those with comminuted fractures also had worse functional outcome scores.

The authors recommend urgent reduction of dislocations and treatment of open injuries, then proceeding with definitive rigid internal fixation of talar neck fractures after soft-tissue swelling has subsided.

Vallier HA, Nork SE, Benirschke SK, Sangeorzan BJ. Surgical treatment of talar body fractures. J Bone Joint Surg Am. 2003;85-A(9):1716–24.

This is a retrospective study of 57 talar body fractures; all were treated with ORIF. Twenty-three had a concomitant talar neck fracture. Thirty-eight patients were evaluated after an average of 33-months. Early complications occurred in eight patients and most patients developed radiographic evidence of osteonecrosis and/or post-traumatic arthritis. Associated talar neck fractures and open fractures more commonly resulted in osteonecrosis or advanced arthritis. Advanced post-traumatic arthritis and osteonecrosis that progresses to collapse were associated with poorer functional outcome.

Lindvall E, Haidukewych G, DiPasquale T, Herscovici D Jr, Sanders R. Open reduction and stable fixation of isolated, displaced talar neck and body fractures. J Bone Joint Surg Am. 2004;86-A(10):2229–34.

This is a retrospective review of 26 displaced fractures isolated to the talus, treated with ORIF and followed for a minimum of 48 months after the injury. The overall union rate was 88 %. All closed, displaced talar neck fractures healed, regardless of the time delay until surgical intervention. Post-traumatic arthritis of the subtalar joint occurred in all patients, 16 of whom had involvement of more than one joint. Osteonecrosis occurred in 50 % overall and after six of the seven open fractures.

The authors advise that patients with a displaced fracture of the talus should be counselled that post-traumatic arthritis and chronic pain are expected outcomes even after anatomic reduction and stable fixation.

Talar Blood Supply

This topic also often arises in Basic Sciences section of the FRCS (Tr & Orth) examination.

Miller AN, Prasarn ML, Dyke JP, Helfet DL, Lorich DG. Quantitative assessment of the vascularity of the talus with gadolinium-enhanced magnetic resonance imaging. J Bone Joint Surg Am. 2011;93(12):1116–21.

The arterial anatomy of the talus was studied in ten pairs of cadaver limbs with use of gadolinium-enhanced MRI in addition to gross dissection following latex injection. MRI proved useful to confirm the presence of specific arterial branches in situ as well as to demonstrate the rich anastomosis network in and around the talus. The peroneal artery contributed 16.9 % of the blood supply to the talus; the anterior tibial artery, 36.2 %; and the posterior tibial artery, 47.0 %. In contrast to the findings in previous studies, a substantial portion of the talar blood supply can enter posteriorly.

The paper goes on to assess the contribution of each artery to the vascularity of the four quadrants of the talus.

Comment: easy to remember approximately 1/6 from the peroneal artery, 2/6 from the anterior tibial artery and 3/6 from the posterior tibial artery.

Tezval M, Dumont C, Stürmer KM. Prognostic reliability of the Hawkins sign in fractures of the talus. J Orthop Trauma. 2007;21(8):538–43.

The Hawkins sign is a subchondral radiolucent band in the talar dome, seen on anterior posterior (AP) X-ray, that is indicative of viability at 6–8 weeks after a talus fracture. The prognostic reliability of the Hawkin sign was assessed in this study of 41 displaced talar fractures. The Hawkins sign (if present) appeared between the sixth and the ninth week after trauma. No Hawkins sign was found in the five patients who developed avascular necrosis (AVN) of the talus. In the

26 patients who did not develop AVN, a positive (full) Hawkins sign was observed 11 times, a partially positive Hawkins sign 4 times, and a negative Hawkins sign 11 times. The Hawkins sign thus showed a sensitivity of 100 % and a specificity of 57.7 %.

Comment: a useful example of sensitivity, specificity, positive predictive value etc.

Calcaneal Fractures

Buckley R, Tough S, McCormack R, Pate G, Leighton R, Petrie D, et al. Operative compared with non-operative treatment of displaced intra-articular calcaneal fractures: a prospective, randomized, controlled multicenter trial. J Bone Joint Surg Am. 2002;84-A(10):1733–44.

The purpose of this multicenter study was to determine whether open reduction and internal fixation of displaced intra-articular calcaneal fractures results in better general and disease-specific health outcomes at 2 years after the injury compared with those after non-operative management.

Without stratification of the groups, the functional results after non-operative care of displaced intra-articular calcaneal fractures were equivalent to those after operative care. However, after unmasking the data by removal of the patients who were receiving Workers' Compensation, the outcomes were significantly better in some groups of surgically treated patients.

Barla J, Buckley R, McCormack R, Pate G, Leighton R, Petrie D, et al. Displaced intraarticular calcaneal fractures: long-term outcome in women. Foot Ankle Int. 2004;25(12): 853–6.

Operative treatment of the fractures showed statistically significant better results when compared to non-operative treatment in women.

Csizy M, Buckley R, Tough S, Leighton R, Smith J, McCormack R, et al. Displaced intra-articular calcaneal fractures: variables predicting late subtalar fusion. J Orthop Trauma. 2003;17(2):106–12.

This study demonstrates that there is a distinct patient group with a displaced intra-articular calcaneal fracture who are at high risk of subtalar fusion. These include male Worker's Compensation Board patients who participate in heavy labor work with a fracture pattern with Böhler angle less than 0°. If their initial treatment was non-operative, the likelihood of requiring late subtalar fusion was significantly increased. Initial ORIF of patients with displaced intra-articular calcaneal fracture minimized the likelihood that subtalar fusion would be required.

Comment: The Canadian multi-centre trial came out in 2002, and cast doubt on the value of ORIF in displaced intra-articular calcaneal fractures. The subsequent stratification raised further controversy, but supports the principle of restoring calcaneal morphology and articular surfaces. The following papers bring results up to date.

Jiang N, Lin QR, Diao XC, Wu L, Yu B. Surgical versus non-surgical treatment of displaced intra-articular calcaneal fracture: a meta-analysis of current evidence base. Int Orthop. 2012;36(8):1615–22.

Controversy still surrounds the optimal treatment for patients with displaced intra-articular calcaneal fractures (DIACF). An up-to-date meta-analysis was performed to evaluate clinical effectiveness of surgical treatment versus nonsurgical treatment. Ten studies (six RCTs and four clinical controlled trials [CCTs]) with a total of 891 participants were screened. Results showed that surgical treatment was superior to nonsurgical treatment in better recovery of the Böhler angle, more stable calcaneal height and width. Moreover, fewer surgically treated patients needed increased shoe size and more were able to resume pre-injury work than the nonsurgical patients. No significant difference was identified between the two methods regarding the incidence of residual pain. However, operative management was associated with a higher risk of complications.

Schepers T. The primary arthrodesis for severely comminuted intra-articular fractures of the calcaneus: a systematic review. Foot Ankle Surg. 2012;18(2):84–8.

This systematic review assessed the functional outcome of primary arthrodesis in the management of comminuted displaced intra-articular calcaneal fractures. Seven case series and one abstract were identified, reporting on 120 patients with 128 severely comminuted calcaneal fractures. Average follow-up time was 28 months and union rate 97 %. Functional outcome was assessed using the modified AOFAS score in seven studies; with a weighted average of 77.4 (range 72.4–88). Three studies reported on return to work, ranging from 75 to 100 %. Overall reported wound complications occurred in 19.4 %.

Makki D, Alnajjar HM, Walkay S, Ramkumar U, Watson AJ, Allen PW. Osteosynthesis of displaced intra-articular fractures of the calcaneum: along-term review of 47 cases. J Bone Joint Surg Br. 2010;92(5):693–700.

A retrospective review of 47 intra-articular fractures of the calcaneum treated by open reduction and internal fixation in 45 patients. The mean follow-up was for 10 years (7–15). There were 18 excellent (38.3 %), 17 good (36.2 %), 3 fair (6.3 %) and 9 poor (19.2 %) results. Five patients had a superficial wound infection and five others eventually had a subtalar arthrodesis because of continuing pain. Restoration of Böhler's angle was associated with a better outcome. The degree of arthritic change in the subtalar joint did not correlate with the outcome scores or Sanders' classification.

Gurkan V, Dursun M, Orhun H, Sari F, Bulbul M, Aydogan M. Long-term results of conservative treatment of Sanders type 4 fractures of the calcaneum: a series of 64 cases. J Bone Joint Surg Br. 2011;93(7):975–9.

This study assessed the long-term outcome of 83 Sanders type 4 comminuted intra-articular fractures of the calcaneum in 64 patients who underwent non-operative treatment. Each fracture was treated by closed reduction and immobilisation in a long leg cast. At a mean follow-up of 51 months (24–70) the mean AOFAS score was 72 (52–92). Osteoarthritis was evident in the subtalar joints of 75 (90 %) on X-ray and in all ankles on computed tomography (CT) scans.

Bhattacharya R, Vassan UT, Finn P, Port A. Sanders classification of fractures of the oscalcis. An analysis of inter- and intra-observer variability. J Bone Joint Surg Br. 2005; 87(2):205–8.

This study examined the inter- and intra-observer variability of the classification system of Sanders for calcaneal fractures. Results show that, despite its popularity, the classification system of Sanders has only fair agreement among users.

Strauss EJ, Petrucelli G, Bong M, Koval KJ, Egol KA. Blisters associated with lower-extremity fracture: results of a prospective treatment protocol. J Orthop Trauma. 2006;20(9): 618–22.

Forty-seven patients who had sustained a closed lower-extremity fracture with early development of fracture blisters in the zone of injury were treated with a standardized regime: blisters were unroofed, and antibiotic cream (silver sulfadiazine) was applied twice daily until the blister bed had re-epithelialized. Mean delay in definitive surgical care was 7.7 days. Thirty-seven of the 45 patients (82.3 %) available for follow-up at a mean of 27 weeks had an uncomplicated post-operative course, and fracture union was achieved in 95.6 %. The soft-tissue complication rate was 13.3 %: three cases of minor soft-tissue breakdown, one superficial infection, and two major complications directly related to the presence of fracture blisters. Both major complications involved full-thickness skin breakdown at the base of fracture blisters in diabetics.

Comment: This paper sets out a protocol for fracture blister management which is applicable to this problem throughout the lower limb, particularly pilon and calcaneal fractures.

Lisfranc Injury

Watson TS, Shurnas PS, Denker J. Treatment of Lisfranc joint injury: current concepts. J Am Acad Orthop Surg. 2010;18(12):718–28.

This is a review and instructional paper. Injuries to the tarsometatarsal joint complex, also known as the Lisfranc joint, are relatively uncommon. However, the importance of an accurate diagnosis cannot be overstated. These injuries, especially when missed, may result in considerable long-term disability as the result of post-traumatic arthritis. A high level of suspicion, recognition of the clinical signs of injury, and appropriate radiographic studies are needed for correct diagnosis. When surgery is indicated, closed reduction with percutaneous screw fixation should be attempted. If reduction is questionable, open reduction should be performed. Screw fixation remains the traditional fixation technique.

Sheibani-Rad S, Coetzee JC, Giveans MR, DiGiovanni C. Arthrodesis versus ORIF for Lisfranc fractures. Orthopedics. 2012;35(6):e868–73.

This systematic review of the literature compared the two most common procedures for Lisfranc fractures: primary arthrodesis and open reduction and internal fixation (ORIF). Six articles with a total of 193 patients met the inclusion criteria. There was no significant effect of treatment group on the percentage on patients who had an anatomic reduction. Both procedures yield satisfactory and equivalent results. A slight advantage may exist in performing a primary arthrodesis for Lisfranc joint injuries in terms of clinical outcomes.

Pearse EO, Klass B, Bendall SP. The 'ABC' of examining foot radiographs. Ann R Coll Surg Engl. 2005;87(6):449–51.

Comment: This paper describes a systematic approach to examining foot X-rays, akin to the advanced trauma and life support (ATLS) method for the cervical spine. The authors show that the ability of junior doctors to spot abnormalities is significantly increased if this systematic approach, looking at alignment of features in three views, is used.

Mann RA, Prieskorn D, Sobel M. Mid-tarsal and tarsometatarsal arthrodesis for primary degenerative osteoarthrosis or osteoarthrosis after trauma. J Bone Joint Surg Am. 1996;78(9):1376–85.

Arthrodesis of the mid-tarsal and tarsometatarsal joints was performed for osteoarthrosis after dislocation with or without ± a fracture (17 patients), for primary degenerative osteoarthrosis (21 patients), or for inflammatory arthritis (2 patients). All 40 patients had a severe loss of function because of pain. Thirty-seven patients (38 ft; 93 %) were satisfied with the results of the procedure after an average duration of 6 years. Union was achieved after 176 (98 %) of the 179 attempted arthrodeses, and only one of the three nonunions necessitated an operative repair. A stress fracture of the second metatarsal developed in three patients, but all three fractures responded to immobilization of the foot.

Part III
Children's Orthopaedics

Children's Orthopaedics (Including Paediatric Orthopaedic Trauma)

Christopher J. Kershaw

Abstract The common and important topics in children's orthopaedics are covered in two sections in this chapter, elective or developmental, and traumatic. References are provided that give an understanding of the pathology, presentation and treatment options for the developing skeleton in the child with osteogenesis imperfect, cerebral palsy, scoliosis, muscular dystrophy and diaphyseal aclasis. The important hip conditions manifesting in childhood, developmental dysplasia, septic arthritis, Perthes disease and slipped upper femoral epiphysis are considered, with the patterns of presentation, current thoughts on management and evidence of outcome. Foot deformities are similarly addressed with key references taking account of the latest thinking on club foot non-operative management and its effectiveness, and diagnosis and treatment of tarsal coalition. An approach to gait analysis and the management of leg length discrepancy in the child is dealt with.

The trauma topics focus on the effects of trauma to the growth plate, and in particular the range of fractures around the elbow, the forearm and the femur. The treatment options

C.J. Kershaw, MBCHB, FRCS (Ed), FRCS
Department of Trauma and Orthopaedics,
Leicester Royal Infirmary, Infirmary Square,
Leicester LE1 5WW, UK
e-mail: christopher.j.kershaw@uhl-tr.hs.uk

G. Bowyer, A. Cole (eds.), *Selected References in Trauma and Orthopaedics*, DOI 10.1007/978-1-4471-4676-6_11,
© Springer-Verlag London 2014

are described, some of the orthodox thinking is challenged and outcomes are reported.

Keywords Children's orthopaedics • Gait analysis • Osteogenesis imperfecta • Cerebral palsy • Osteomyelitis • Septic arthritis • Physeal injury • Leg length discrepancy • Developmental dysplasia of the hip • Tarsal coalition • Talipes equinovarus • Legg-Calve-Perthes disease • Slipped upper femoral epiphysis • Scoliosis • Muscular dystrophy • Diaphyseal aclasis • Elbow fractures • Femoral fractures • Supracondylar humeral fractures • Radius and ulna fractures

Gait Analysis

Gage JR, Deluca PA, Renshaw TS. Gait analysis: principles and applications. Emphasis on its use in cerebral palsy. J Bone Joint Surg Am. 1995;77-A(10):1607–23.

A review of the role that gait analysis plays in preoperatively assessing specific pathologies and postoperatively, providing an accurate assessment of outcome. The importance of re-establishing normal gait pre-requisites, reducing energy expenditure, lever arm action, the role and importance of 2-joint muscles, and the need to separate primary abnormalities from coping mechanisms are all discussed.

DeLuca PA, Davis RB 3rd, Ounpuu S, Rose S, Sirkin R. Alterations in surgical decision making in patients with cerebral palsy based on three-dimensional gait analysis. J Pediatr Orthop. 1997;17(5):608–14.

A comparison of surgical recommendations based on clinical examination with videotape compared to those made when additional kinematic, kinetic and electromyographic data are provided. Ninety-one patients were assessed and changes to the initial plan were made in 52 % of patients after kinematics, kinetic and electromyography (EMG) data was reviewed. This extra information from gait analysis reduced the number of surgical procedures and reduced cost. Operations on gastrocnemius and rectus femoris were more often recommended but operations on the hamstrings, gastrocnemius, psoas, femur and tibia were reduced in frequency.

Narayanan UG. The role of gait analysis in the orthopaedic management of ambulatory cerebral palsy. Curr Opin Pediatr. 2007;19(1):38–43.

This review article examines the best evidence for the use of gait analysis in ambulatory cerebral palsy. Gait analysis provides a superior objective record of gait and can be used to describe pathological gait. There is however, little evidence that gait analysis leads to better patient outcomes.

Osteogenesis Imperfecta

Cole WG. Advances in osteogenesis imperfecta. Clin Orthop Relat Res. 2002;(401):6–16.

This review article covers in some detail, classification, aetiology, pathogenesis (including a thorough account of the genetics), natural history and treatments. In medium-term studies, bisphosphonate treatment has been shown to be the first method of treatment to improve the clinical course of the disease. Somatic cell therapy, using allogeneic bone marrow and mesenchymal stromal cell transplantation, are in the early phases of development. Somatic gene therapy, which aims to inactivate the mutation, is being evaluated in vitro.

Nicolaou N, Bowe JD, Wilkinson JM, Fernandes JA, Bell MJ. Use of the Sheffield telescopic intramedullary rod system for the management of osteogenesis imperfecta: clinical outcomes at an average follow-up of nineteen years. J Bone Joint Surg Am. 2011;93(21):1994–2000.

This is a long-term retrospective review (average 19 years follow-up) of 22 patients who had undergone 66 intramedullary rodding procedures for recurrent long bone fractures. Thirty-five percent of rods required exchange, 15 % because of disengagement or potential disengagement of the rods, 7 % because of rod bending after re-fracture and 15 % because of infection or rod migration. There were no cases of premature physeal arrest. All patients were wheelchair bound or required walking aids preoperatively and 15 were able to go on to independent walking, most maintaining this ability to the time of final review. Reoperation rates are high but are most commonly related to the patient outgrowing the rods. Proximal femoral fixation was the main problem with the implant.

Bajpai A, Kabra M, Gupta N, Sharda S, Ghosh M. Intravenous pamidronate therapy in osteogenesis imperfecta: response to treatment and factors influencing outcome. J Pediatr Orthop. 2007;27(2):225–7.

A prospective trial of 20 patients, showing significant improvements of bone density and reduction in fracture rate with bisphosphonate treatment. Treatment in infancy showed the greatest bone density improvement. Walking ability doubled (88 % after treatment vs 45 % before treatment). Almost half achieved bone densities within normal range. There was one case of hypocalcaemic seizures requiring calcium infusion and one developed temporary liver dysfunction.

Esposito P, Plotkin H. Surgical treatment of osteogenesis imperfecta: current concepts. Curr Opin Pediatr. 2008; 20(1): 52–7.

This paper describes the multidisciplinary team approach to the treatment of osteogenesis. Medical treatment with bisphosphonates has allowed for safer, more effective surgical management of these children. Intramedullary fixation rather than plating is preferred, allowing early protected weight bearing and rehabilitation of children with ambulatory potential. Several new intramedullary rodding surgical techniques and modifications of older techniques have been developed to correct deformities of the long bones whilst limiting postoperative immobilization, enabling earlier rehabilitation, and allowing for treatment of multiple bones simultaneously.

Castillo H, Samson-Fang L, American Academy for Cerebral Palsy and Developmental Medicine Treatment Outcomes Committee Review Panel. Effects of bisphosphonates in children with osteogenesis imperfecta: an AACPDM systematic review. Dev Med Child Neurol. 2008;51(1):17–29.

This is a systematic review of the effects of bisphoshonates on children with osteogenesis imperfecta conducted by the American Academy for Cerebral Palsy and Developmental Medicine. It reviews 85 studies but only 8 studies with sufficient internal validity were found. There was evidence for increases in bone density, enhanced growth and a reduced fracture rate with the use of bisphosphonates.

Cerebral Palsy

Kerr Graham H, Selber P. Musculoskeletal aspects of cerebral palsy. J Bone Joint Surg Br. 2003;85(2):157–66.

This is a review article describing the patho-physiology and management of children with cerebral palsy. The role of orthopaedic surgery in flexion contractures, spastic hemiplegia, spastic diplegia and spastic quadriplegia are all described. Orthopaedic surgery has much to offer in the management of cerebral palsy, however, evidence for the efficacy of most orthopaedic operations is lacking with focus on the measurement of deformity and disability and not enough on validated functional outcome measures. This review suggests that we must improve the evidence for the value of orthopaedic surgery for children with cerebral palsy by appropriate clinical trials and by applying comprehensive, balanced, validated outcome measures.

Sussman MD, Aiona MD. Treatment of spastic diplegia in patients with cerebral palsy: Part I. J Pediatr Orthop B. 2004; 13(2):S1–12.

Sussman MD, Aiona MD. Treatment of spastic diplegia in patients with cerebral palsy: Part II. J Pediatr Orthop B. 2004;13(2):S13–38.

The function of children with cerebral palsy can be improved by orthopaedic surgery, physical and occupational therapy, recreational therapy, orthotics, and assistive devices. Intramuscular injections of botulinum toxin, and constant intrathecal administration of Baclofen via an implanted pump may also be of benefit. Orthopaedic surgery can enhance function, and the challenge for the surgeon is to identify which combination of procedures is appropriate for each individual patient and at what point during development to implement them. Some surgeons prefer to wait until patients are older (8–10 years) and perform all of their surgical interventions in one sitting. The authors favour an approach they call 'Staged Multilevel Interventions in the Lower Extremity' or 'SMILE'. This paper presents the rationale for this approach.

Chin TYP, Duncan JA, Johnstone BR, Kerr Graham H. Management of the upper limb in cerebral palsy. J Pediatr Orthop B. 2005;14(6):389–404.

This review article considers the difficult problem of upper limb spasticity in cerebral palsy. It details the assessment, classification and management options. The use of physiotherapy, neuro-developmental therapy, and spasticity management with botulinum toxin treatment are discussed. Botulinum toxin A therapy has been shown to relieve spasticity and improve function in the short term. Surgery is also effective but requires careful patient selection. Occupational therapy and physiotherapy have small treatment effects alone but are essential adjuncts to medical and surgical management. Specific surgery for shoulder, elbow, wrist, fingers and thumb problems are examined in detail and treatments recommended.

Kerr Graham H, Boyd R, Carlin JB, Dobson F, Lowe K, Nattrass G, Thomason P, Wolfe R, Reddihough D. Does botulinum toxin A combined with bracing prevent hip displacement in children with cerebral palsy and "hips at risk"? A randomized, controlled trial. J Bone Joint Surg Am. 2008;90(1):23–33.

This article reports a randomized controlled trial of 90 patients with bilateral cerebral palsy and "hips at risk". Progressive hip displacement was assessed by radiographs measuring migration percentage. The rate of displacement was reduced in the treatment group by a mean of 1.4 % per year over a 3 year period. There is a small but significant benefit from combined botulinum toxin injections and abduction bracing, but displacement continued and this treatment method is not recommended.

Osteomyelitis

El-Shanti HI, Ferguson PJ. Chronic recurrent multifocal osteomyelitis: a concise review and genetic update. Clin Orthop Relat Res. 2007;462:11–19.

This review article discusses the possible aetiology, clinical features, diagnosis and treatment based on 100 articles. A further section reviews the possible genetic causes of this autoinflammatory disorder. With an obscure aetiology, the diagnosis is based on clinical criteria (bone pain and fever, a course of exacerbations and remissions, and a frequent association with other inflammatory conditions) and empirical treatment is often unsuccessful. Several observations suggest a contribution of genetic factors to the etiology of chronic recurrent multifocal osteomyelitis.

Jagodzinski NA, Kanwar R, Graham K, Bache CE. Prospective evaluation of a shortened regimen of treatment for acute osteomyelitis and septic arthritis in children. J Pediatr Orthop. 2009;29(5):518–25.

A prospective two-centre trial of 70 consecutive children to establish if a 3 day course of intravenous antibiotics and a

3 week course of oral therapy would safely treat acute bone and joint infections. Children with underlying disease were excluded. All 33 patients with septic arthritis underwent joint washout. Eighty percent of these involved the knee or hip. Fifty-nine percent could stop intravenous antibiotics by day 3 and 86 % by day 5. Oral treatment continued for 3 weeks. Three patients did not respond and required surgery. After 3 weeks oral treatment 83 % stopped antibiotics and 14 % continued for a further period until clinical and haematological parameters resolved. All patients were well with normal X-rays at 1 year.

Dartnell J, Ramachandran M, Katchburian M. Haematogenous acute and subacute paediatric osteomyelitis: a systematic review of the literature. J Bone Joint Surg Br. 2012; 94(5):584–95.

This review article sought papers dealing with paediatric osteomyelitis: 1,854 papers were identified, 132 of which were examined in detail. On admission 40 % of children are afebrile. The tibia and femur are the most commonly affected long bones. Clinical examination, blood and radiological tests are only reliable for diagnosis in combination. Staph aureus is the most common organism detected, but isolation of Kingella kingae is increasing. Antibiotic treatment is usually sufficient to eradicate the infection, with a short course intravenously and early conversion to oral treatment. Surgery is indicated only in specific situations. The article presents evidence-based algorithms for accurate and early diagnosis and effective treatment.

Septic Arthritis

Kocher MS, Zurakowski D, Kasser JR. Differentiating between septic arthritis and transient synovitis of the hip in children: an evidence-based clinical prediction algorithm. J Bone Joint Surg Am. 1999;81(12):1662–70.

This is a retrospective review of 282 admissions with a diagnosis of irritable hip to identify features that differentiate acute septic arthritis from transient synovitis. Four independent clinical predictors were identified to differentiate the possible diagnoses; history of fever, weight-bearing, erythrocyte sedimentation rate (ESR) over 40 mm/h and white blood cell count >12,000/cm³. Increasing number of predictors present increases probability of septic arthritis.

Kang S-N, Sanghera T, Mangwani J, Paterson JMH, Ramachandran M. The management of septic arthritis in children: systematic review of the English language literature. J Bone Joint Surg Br. 2009;91-B(9):1127–33.

This paper examined 2,236 citations and included 154 articles that met agreed criteria. Changing bacteriological profiles are emerging and positive identification of pathogens from blood and synovial cultures is often difficult. No single investigation, including joint aspiration, is sufficiently reliable to diagnose conclusively joint infection. There is no agreement on antibiotic choice, duration of course or the role of surgery. Poor prognosis was associated with young age, delay in treatment, staphylococcal infection and the hip as the site of infection. Further large-scale, multi-centre studies are needed to delineate the optimal management of paediatric septic arthritis.

Paakkonen M, Kallio MJT, Peltola H, Kallio PE. Paediatric septic hip with or without arthrotomy: retrospective analysis of 62 consecutive non-neonatal culture-positive cases. J Pediatr Orthop B. 2010;19(3):264–9.

A multicentre review of 62 cases of septic hip arthritis. Staphylococcus was isolated in 71 %. Arthrotomy was only undertaken if progress was delayed. Patients were reviewed a year after discharge from hospital and all had recovered fully. The authors suggest that arthrotomy is only required if the clinical progress, monitored by set criteria, is not satisfactory. They avoided arthrotomy in 81 % of cases.

Singhal R, Perry DC, Khan FN, Cohen D, Stevenson HL, James LA, et al. The use of CRP within a clinical prediction algorithm for the differentiation of septic arthritis and transient synovitis in children. J Bone Joint Surg Br. 2011; 93-B(11): 1556–61.

This large retrospective review of 311 children presenting with an acute, new-onset atraumatic limp and hip effusion confirmed on ultrasound. C-reactive protein (CRP) was used instead of ESR as an adaptation of the Kocher algorithm for differentiating acute septic arthritis from transient synovitis. A CRP>20 mm/h was the strongest independent predictor for septic arthritis. If CRP and weight-bearing were normal there was a <1 % chance of septic arthritis. If both were present, the probability of septic arthritis was 74 %. A two-variable algorithm is an excellent negative predictor.

Physeal Injury

Mizuta T, Benson WM, Foster BK, Paterson DC, Morris LL. Statistical analysis of the incidence of physeal injuries. J Pediatr Orthop. 1987;7(5):518–23.

One thousand nine hundred and seventy-four fractures were reviewed and physeal injuries were recorded in 18 %. The incidence of growth arrest was 1 %. Fracture frequency and Salter-Harris classification are recorded for the major epiphyses. The site of fracture was more predictive of growth arrest than Salter-Harris Classification. Physeal injuries were more common among adolescents and in the upper limb.

Ecklund K, Jaramillo D. Patterns of premature physeal arrest: MR imaging of 111 children. Am J Roentgenol. 2002;178(4):967–72.

One hundred and eleven physeal bone bridges were assessed by magnetic resonance imaging (MRI). Post-traumatic bone bridges were usually distal and those involving the distal tibia (43/111) were usually anteromedial. Distal femoral physeal bridges were usually central. Oblique recovery lines were only seen in peripheral injuries and in smaller, potentially resectable bridges.

Marsh JS, Polzhofer GK. Arthroscopically assisted central physeal bar resection. J Pediatr Orthop. 2006;26(2):255–9.

This article describes the technique used in the management of 37 cases of central physeal arrest. The outcomes of 32 cases at skeletal maturity or physeal closure showed 70 % regained adequate longitudinal growth. In 13 % bar resection failed. 17 % required osteotomy, lengthening or epiphyseodesis in addition to bar excision. The technique offers excellent visualisation of the bar with little morbidity.

Arkader A, Warner WC Jr, Horn D, Shaw RN, Wells L. Predicting the outcome of physeal fractures of the distal femur. J Pediatr Orthop. 2007;27(6):703–8.

This uncommon fracture has a high rate of complication, the commonest being growth arrest. Seventy-three fractures were reviewed. Fifty-nine percent were Salter Harris type II and 59 % were displaced. Complications occurred in 40 %. Displacement, degree of displacement and Salter-Harris classification correlated with complications.

Leary JT, Handling M, Talerico M, Yong L, Bowe JA. Physeal fractures of the distal tibia: predictive factors of premature physeal closure and growth arrest. J Pediatr Orthop. 2009;29(4):356–61.

This is a retrospective review of 124 patients with distal tibial fractures. Fifteen fractures developed partial physeal closure (PPC). There is an association between method of injury (higher in motor vehicle accidents) and partial physeal closure and between degree of initial fracture displacement and incidence of PPC.

Leg Length Discrepancy

Ilizarov GA. Clinical application of the tension-stress effect on limb lengthening. Clin Orthop Relat Res. 1990;(250): 8–26.

This article describes the experimental biology of limb lengthening and techniques using circular frame external fixation. Mechanisms to stimulate new osseous tissue formation are discussed. Important factors for neo-osteogenesis after osteotomy include preservation of extraosseous and medullary blood supply and stable external fixation. There should be a delay prior to distraction with a distraction rate of 1 mm/day in frequent small steps combined with a period of stable neutral fixation after lengthening.

Paley D. Problems, obstacles, and complications of limb lengthening by the Ilizarov technique. Clin Orthop Relat Res. 1990;(250):81–104.

This classic paper on the Ilizarov limb lengthening technique introduced the concept that difficulties during limb lengthening could be subclassified into problems, obstacles, and complications. Problems represented difficulties that required no operative intervention to resolve, while obstacles represented difficulties that required an operative intervention. All intraoperative injuries were considered true complications, and all problems during limb lengthening that were not resolved before the end of treatment were considered true complications. The difficulties that occurred during limb lengthening include muscle contractures, joint luxation, axial deviation, neurologic injury, vascular injury, premature consolidation, delayed consolidation, non-union, pin site problems, and hardware failure. Late complications are those of loss of length, late bowing, and refracture. Joint stiffness may also be a permanent residual complication. Pain and difficulty sleeping are other problems that arise during limb lengthening, especially in the more extensive cases.

The problems, obstacles and complications from 60 limb-lengthenings are detailed in this paper. The original goals of surgery were achieved in 57 of the 60 limb segments treated.

Vitale MA, Choe JC, Sesko AM, Hyman JE, Lee FY, Roye DP Jr, et al. The effect of limb length discrepancy on health-related quality of life: is the "2 cm rule" appropriate? J Pediatr Orthop B. 2006;15(1):1–5.

Using the Child Health Questionnaire the parents of 76 children with limb length discrepancies were asked about quality of life issues related to their limb difference. Differences in quality of life increased with limb length difference. Although a discrepancy of over 2 cm or more was associated with greater problems there was no discrete cut off.

Rozbruch SR, Kleinman D, Fragomen AT, Ilizarov S. Limb lengthening and then insertion of an intramedullary nail. A case-matched comparison. Clin Orthop Relat Res. 2008;466(12):2923–32.

Seventy-three segments were lengthened according to two protocols; one with classic use external fixator through distraction and consolidation and the second with external fixator for lengthening and then nailing (LATN) with an intramedullary nail. There were 34 and 39 segments respectively in the two groups and LATN conferred a lower external fixation time (12 v 29 weeks) and a lower bone healing index (0.8 v 1.9). LATN confers advantages over the classic method: shorter time in external fixation, quicker healing and a lower refracture rate.

Ilharreborde B, Gaumetou E, Souchet P, Fitoussi F, Presedo A, Penneçot GF, et al. Efficacy and late complications of percutaneous epiphysiodesis with transphyseal screws. J Bone Joint Surg Br. 2012;94-B(2):270–5.

This technique has been developed to eliminate the need for open epiphysiodesis. Forty-five patients were included in the study and followed to maturity. The technique is quick and reliable in the femur but revision in the tibia is high. The arrest of growth was delayed and the final loss of growth at maturity was only 66 % of that predicted preoperatively. The technique has a role but the pre-operative planning needs to consider possible delay in growth arrest. The complication rate in the tibia led the authors to abandon the technique in that bone.

Developmental Dysplasia of the Hip

Mankey MG, Arntz CT, Staheli LT. Open reduction through a medial approach for congenital dislocation of the hip: a critical review of the Ludloff approach in sixty-six hips. J Bone Joint Surg Am. 1993; 75-A(9):1334–45.

A retrospective review of 66 hip dislocations treated by medial open reduction and reviewed for a mean of 6 years. Avascular necrosis was recorded in 14 % (3 % pre-operatively) and redislocation and subluxation occurred in 4.5 %. One-third of patients required further surgery with pelvic osteotomy. The review suggested that the procedure is safe in children under 2 years of age and in whom a concentric closed reduction could not be achieved with less than 60° abduction. The paper discusses in detail reduction, acetabular development and avascular necrosis.

Segal LS, Boal DK, Borthwick L, Clark MW, Localio AR, Schwentker EP. Avascular necrosis after treatment of DDH: the protective influence of the ossific nucleus. J Pediatr Orthop. 1999;19(2):177–84.

This is a retrospective analysis of 57 hip dislocations to identify if timing of closed or open reduction influenced the development of avascular necrosis. No variable other than the presence of the ossific nucleus (on X-ray or on ultrasound) was significant in determining the development of avascular necrosis. The presence of the ossific nucleus was protective.

Bache CE, Clegg J, Herron M. Risk factors for developmental dysplasia of the hip: ultrasonographic findings in the neonatal period. J Pediatr Orthop B. 2002;11(3): 212–8.

A review of 29,323 babies screened neonatally by ultrasound for developmental dysplasia of the hip (DDH). 6.6 % were abnormal on ultrasound (3,866) but only 92 required Pavlik harness treatment. Sixty-three of these were bilateral giving 155 hips. Only one-third of these had risk factors. Clinical examination detected abnormalities in 39 hips and had a sensitivity of only 20 %. The overall rate of Pavlik harness treatment is 0.31 % and no case of late dislocation presented from the screened population.

Holman J, Carroll, KL, Murray KA, MacLeod LM, Roach JW. Long-term follow-up of open reduction surgery for developmental dislocation of the hip. J Pediatr Orthop. 2012;32(2):121–4.

This study aimed to find out the long-term results of open reduction surgery and to identify an age threshold over which surgery would not be recommended. One hundred and forty-eight patients, treated mainly by anterior open reduction had surgery prior to 1996 and 53 could be traced. One-third had Severin IV hips or worse and 7 had already undergone total hip replacement. Outcomes deteriorated over age 3 at time of index surgery. Half the hips had required surgery for residual dysplasia. Hips that were "normal" during childhood deteriorated and developed dysplasia as teenagers.

Tarsal Coalition

Gantsoudes GD, Roocraft JH, Mubarak SJ. Treatment of talocalcaneal coalitions. J Pediatr Orthop. 2012:32(3): 301–7.

This is a retrospective review of 49 feet treated by surgery for talo-calcaneal coalition and with a minimum 12 month follow-up. There is a description of the surgical techniques (excision of coalition and fat graft interposition) and a review of the literature on this subject. Assessment was by American Orthopedic Foot & Ankle Society (AOFAS) scores and the average was 90/100 (excellent) and computed tomography (CT) scans in 20 feet showed only one recurrence. Twenty-two percent of the feet required secondary procedures.

Mubarak SJ, Patel PN, Upasani VV, Moor MA, Wenger DR. Calcaneonavicular coalition: treatment by excision and fat graft. J Pediatr Orthop. 2009;29(5):418–26.

This is a retrospective review of 69 feet treated surgically for calcaneo-navicular coalition by excision of the bony bar. Seventy-five percent had an improved range of subtalar movement and pain scores improved from mean 6.7 to mean 0.3. Nine percent of patients complained of persistent pain at rest and three underwent revision surgery. Extensor digitorum interposition graft was shown to fill only 60 % of the defect in cadaveric studies leading to the use of fat as the interposition.

Nalaboff KM, Schweitzer ME. MRI of tarsal coalition: frequency, distribution, and innovative signs. Bull NYU Hosp Jt Dis. 2008;66(1):14–21.

This paper incorporates a retrospective review of 101 of 169 MRI scans reported as having tarsal coalition from over 27,000 ankle MRI scans. Seventy-five percent were calcaneonavicular coalitions and the most common feature was the "reverse anteater sign" in 24 %, talar "beaks" in 19 % and "anteater signs" in 10 %. The majority of the talocalcaneal coalitions showed the "drunken waiter" sign (a dysplastic sustentaculum). Prospectively 667 consecutive MRI scans were examined for evidence of coalitions. They were present as cartilaginous or fibrous bars in 11 %. Tarsal coalitions appear to be more common than previously thought, but almost always non-osseous.

Talipes Equinovarus

Ponseti IV, Zhivkov M, Davis N, Sinclair M, Dobbs MB, Morcuende JA. Treatment of the complex idiopathic clubfoot. Clin Orthop Relat Res. 2006;451:171–6.

Treatment with the Ponseti method corrects congenital idiopathic clubfeet in the majority of patients. However, some feet do not respond to the standard treatment protocol. This level IV paper documents retrospectively the treatment of 50 such patients with atypical clubfoot. The clinical features of atypical clubfoot are severe equinus and supination, shortness, and adducted and plantar flexed metatarsals. The difficulties in management and an adjusted Ponseti management regime are described. With this modified technique correction was achieved in all patients. However it required an average of five casts (range, 1–10 casts). Four percent had a posterior release with tendo Achilles lengthening. There were seven relapses that responded to casting. Three patients had a second tenotomy. Modifying the treatment protocol for complex clubfeet successfully corrected the deformity without the need for extensive corrective surgery.

Siapkara A, Duncan R. Congenital talipes equinovarus: a review of current management. J Bone Joint Surg Br. 2007; 89-B(8):995–1000.

Talipes equinovarus is one of the more common congenital abnormalities affecting the lower limb and can be challenging to manage. This review provides a comprehensive update on idiopathic congenital talipes equinovarus including aetiology, epidemiology, classification, imaging and treatment options, with emphasis on the initial treatment. The initial results of treatment with the Ponseti regimen are encouraging, but longer term studies are needed. In this paper the clinical results of 46 patients with clubfoot were assessed using both traditional radiological and patient generic and disease-specific measures 16 years after surgery. Radiographs are not good indicators of outcome.

Richards BS, Faulks S, Rathjen KE, Karol LA, Johnston CE, Jones SA. A comparison of two non-operative methods of idiopathic clubfoot correction: the Ponseti method and the French functional (physiotherapy) method. J Bone Joint Surg Am. 2008;90(11):2313–21.

This is a report of a large prospective non-randomised parent-selected study from the Texas Scottish Rite Hospital. Two hundred and sixty-seven patients were treated by Ponseti method and 80 patients were treated by French functional method. Relapses occurred in 37 % and 29 % respectively. Treatment outcomes were similar, but with a tendency for the 2 year outcomes to favour the Ponseti method.

Halanski MA, Davison JE, Huang J-C, Walker CG, Walsh SJ, Crawford HA. Ponseti method compared with surgical treatment of clubfoot: a prospective comparison. J Bone Joint Surg Am. 2010;92(2):270–8.

A prospective study of two treatment groups, 40 feet treated by Ponseti method and 46 by posteromedial release. Relapse occurred in about a third of patients in both groups, with high non-compliance rates in the Ponseti group. Only three patients in the Ponseti group required posteromedial release. Despite high non-compliance with abduction bracing, surgical intervention and number of cast changes was significantly less in the Ponseti group.

Jowett CR, Morcuende JA, Ramachandran M. Management of congenital talipes equinovarus using the Ponseti method: a systematic review. J Bone Joint Surg Br. 2011;93-B(9): 1160–4.

A review of 74 full-text papers, commenting on epidemiology, treatment and results. These papers showed an initial correction rate of 90 % in idiopathic talipes. Non-compliance varied from 0 to 51 % and relapse rates were related to compliance. Comparison with other techniques showed advantages in results and ease of performing the treatment in favour of the Ponseti method.

Ponseti IV, Campos J. The classic. Observations on pathogenesis and treatment of congenital clubfoot. Clin Orthop Relat Res. 2009;467(5):1124–32.

Ponseti IV, Smoley EN. The classic. Congenital club foot. The results of treatment. Clin Orthop Relat Res. 2009; 467(5):1133–45.

These two papers, reprints of the originals produced over 35 years previously, meticulously explain the rationale, treatment and results of Ponseti management of clubfoot.

Legg-Calve-Perthes Disease

Kim HKW. Legg-Calve-Perthes disease: etiology, pathogenesis, and biology. J Pediatr Orthop. 2011;31(2 Suppl):S141–6.

Legg-Calve-Perthes disease is a complex paediatric hip disorder which still lacks clarity in many aspects. Various theories on its etiology have been proposed but none have been validated conclusively. Experimental studies give some insight into the pathogenesis of the femoral head deformity in this condition following ischemic necrosis; mechanical and biological factors contribute to the deformity.

Herring JA. Legg-Calve-Perthes disease at 100: a review of evidence-based treatment. J Pediatr Orthop. 2011;31 (2 Suppl):S137–140.

This paper summarizes evidence previously published and discussed at several world conferences. Factors related to outcome in patients treated for Legg-Calve-Perthes disease (LCPD) are the age at onset, the classification of severity of femoral head involvement, and the type of treatment. In patients over the age of 8 at onset who had lateral pillar B or B/C border class involvement, surgical treatment with femoral varus osteotomy or Salter innominate osteotomy was associated with improved Stulberg outcomes compared with non-operative treatment. Outcomes of LCPD in lateral pillar A hips are between 70 and 100 % excellent with

Stulberg I and II hip morphology. Lateral pillar B hips will achieve 51–70 % Stulberg I and II. Lateral pillar C will achieve 13–30 % excellent Stulberg outcomes.

Little DG, Kim HKW. Potential for bisphosphonate treatment in Legg-Calve-Perthes Disease. J Pediatr Orthop. 2011:31(2 Suppl):S182–8.

This paper describes the latest research into bisphosphonates as treatment to prevent femoral head collapse in LCPD. Animal and clinical research is described. Bisphosphonates have been shown to decrease femoral head deformity in animal studies, delay resorption of necrotic bone potentially allowing more time for revascularization and maintain trabeculae. Clinical studies have shown benefit in adolescents treated with bisphosphonates when they had sustained hip fracture or slipped upper femoral epiphysis but no radiographic improvement in chemotherapy induced osteonecrosis. Potential hazards of bisphosphonate treatment are discussed.

Slipped Upper Femoral Epiphysis

Yildirim Y, Bautista S, Davidson RS. Chondrolysis, osteonecrosis, and slip severity in patients with subsequent contralateral slipped capital femoral epiphysis. J Bone Joint Surg Am. 2008;90(3):485–92.

A 10 year cohort of patients with a unilateral slipped upper femoral epiphysis at a single hospital was retrospectively reviewed. There was a strong possibility of a subsequent contralateral slip (36 % of a series of 227 patients). Over a fifth of this group developed a moderate to severe slip (8 % of 227 patients). Five patients with a contralateral slip developed avascular necrosis or osteolysis (2 % of 227 patients). Contralateral pinning was recommended.

Dewnany G, Radford P. Prophylactic contralateral fixation in slipped upper femoral epiphysis: is it safe? J Pediatr Orthop B. 2005;14(6):429–33.

A retrospective analysis of 65 patients that had contralateral hip pinning using a single cannulated cancellous screw. The only complication was a superficial wound infection. There were no cases of avascular necrosis or chondrolysis. Contralateral pinning was regarded as safe and desirable.

Kalogrianitis S, Khoon Tan C, Kemp GJ, Bass A, Bruce C. Does unstable slipped capital femoral epiphysis require urgent stabilization? J Pediatr Orthop B. 2007;16(1):6–9.

A retrospective study of 117 consecutive slips was undertaken and 16 of these were unstable. Of these eight developed avascular necrosis. An "unsafe window", when surgery seemed to be associated with an increased risk of avascular necrosis was identified between 24 h and 7 days, when seven of the eight avascular necrosis (AVN) cases occurred. Avoidance of this period for any surgical intervention was recommended.

Huber H, Dora C, Ramseier LE, Buck F, Dierauer S. Adolescent slipped capital femoral epiphysis treated by a modified Dunn osteotomy with surgical hip dislocation. J Bone Joint Surg Br. 2011;93-B(6):833–8.

Thirty cases of slipped capital femoral epiphysis were treated by surgical hip dislocation with an avascular necrosis rate of 3 % and a fixation complication rate of 13 %. Excellent results (according to Harris Hip Scores) were achieved in 28 of the 30 hips and mean slip angles were improved from 45° to 5°. The ability to determine the vascularity of the head per-operatively and the direct visualization of the prominent posterior bone buttress were thought particular benefits of this technique.

Larson AN, Sierra RJ, Yu EM, Trousdale RT, Stans AA. Outcomes of slipped capital femoral epiphysis treated with in situ pinning. J Pediatr Orthop. 2012;32(2):125–30.

A follow-up study of 146 patients (176 hips) from 2 to 43 years after in-situ pinning of a slipped upper femoral epiphysis. Ten percent of hips had undergone reconstructive surgery within 10 years and a further 17 % scored only poor or fair on Harris Hip scores. Less good patient reported outcomes were associated with slip instability. Reconstruction surgery was associated with more severe slips.

Scoliosis

Asher MA, Burton DC. Adolescent idiopathic scoliosis: natural history and long term treatment effects. Scoliosis. 2006;1(1):2.

This paper reviews 71 articles relating to the natural history of scoliosis, untreated and treated. Idiopathic scoliosis does not increase mortality rate, although thoracic curves >80° may be associated with respiratory symptoms. Bracing may reduce progression in about a third of patients. Surgery virtually eliminates large thoracic curves, but a significant number of surgically managed patients will develop decrease in function and increase in pain by 20 years post surgery.

Lenke LG, Dobbs MB. Management of juvenile idiopathic scoliosis. J Bone Joint Surg Am. 2007;89-A(Suppl 1):55–63.

An extensive review of the natural history, epidemiology and treatments available for children with scoliosis between 3 and 10 years of age.

Weiss H-R, Goodall D. Rate of complications in scoliosis surgery—a systematic review of the Pub Med literature. Scoliosis. 2008;3:9.

254 papers are reviewed to establish complications of scoliosis surgery, occurring in the different scoliosis aetiologies. Rates of mortality, pseudarthrosis, infection, neurological

complications, implant misplacement are detailed as well as post-operative pain, patient satisfaction and the need for revision surgery. Scoliosis surgery has a varying but high rate of complications and the rate of complications may even be higher than reported. A medical indication for this treatment cannot be established in view of the lack of evidence. Long-term risks of scoliosis surgery have not yet been reported.

Weinstein SL, Dolan LA, Cheng JCY, Danielsson A, Morcuende JA. Adolescent idiopathic scoliosis. Lancet. 2008;371(9623):1527–37.

This is a detailed review of the literature on adolescent idiopathic scoliosis (AIS). The disease affects 1–3 % of children aged 10–16 years. The aetiology and pathogenesis remain unclear. Non-surgical treatments try to reduce the number of operations by preventing curve progression. Although bracing and physiotherapy are common treatments in much of the world, their effectiveness has never been rigorously assessed. Technological advances have much improved the ability of surgeons to safely correct the deformity while maintaining sagittal and coronal balance. However, we do not have long-term results of these changing surgical treatments. Despite this review of 145 papers, much has yet to be learned about the general health, quality of life, and self-image of both treated and untreated patients with AIS.

Muscular Dystrophy

Bushby K, Bourke J, Bullock R, Eagle M, Gibson M, Quinby J. The multidisciplinary management of Duchenne muscular dystrophy. Curr Paediatr. 2005;15(4):292–300.

This review article describes the genetics, diagnosis and natural history of Duchenne muscular dystrophy and the way in which this determines a rational, multidisciplinary treatment plan. It discusses practical points of management across orthopaedics, respiratory medicine and other disciplines to maximize the quality and length of life.

Kinali M, Messina S, Mercuri E, Lehovsky J, Edge G, Manzur AY, et al. Management of scoliosis in Duchenne muscular dystrophy: a large 10-year retrospective study. Dev Med Child Neurol. 2006;48(6):513–8.

A 10 year retrospective study of 123 patients with Duchenne muscular dystrophy showed 90 % had a scoliosis, and in 77 % this was progressive. Thirteen percent were unfit for surgery and 7 % showed slowing of their scoliosis progression and surgery was avoided. At 17 years there was no difference in the survival, respiratory impairment or sitting comfort of those treated conservatively and those undergoing surgery. The article aids decision making by families considering surgery.

Karol LA. Scoliosis in patients with Duchenne muscular dystrophy. J Bone Joint Surg Am. 2007;89-A(Suppl 1):155–62.

This review article describes the natural history, treatment options and surgical considerations in the management of Duchenne muscular dystrophy (DMD) scoliosis. It reviews the controversies surrounding the selection of patients and the outcomes of scoliosis surgery. Ninety percent of boys with DMD will develop scoliosis. Once identified, full assessment and discussion of the options for surgery is indicated. Scoliosis surgery in DMD can be effective in correcting scoliosis, preventing further deformity and in promoting better seating posture. There is probably not a significant effect on respiratory function, which continues to decline because of the intrinsic weakness of the respiratory musculature. The role of physiotherapy and orthotics is discussed.

Diab M, Darras BT, Shapiro F. Scapulothoracic fusion for facioscapulohumeral muscular dystrophy. J Bone Joint Surg Am. 2005;87-A(10):2267–75.

A medium-term review of 11 patients following scapular stabilization. All patients showed an improvement in function, pain and movement initially and two-thirds maintained that improvement to a mean of 6 years post-operatively. The surgical technique is described in detail and the procedure was effective and safe. Early stabilization was recommended, before deltoid power reduced and functional gain diminished.

Diaphyseal Aclasis

Peterson HA. Deformities and problems of the forearm in children with multiple hereditary osteochondromata. J Pediatr Orthop. 1994;14(1):92–100.

This article discusses the possible treatments able to be employed to manage ulnar shortening, bowing, increased radial articular angle, radial head dislocation and carpal slip. Excision of osteochondromas is recommended as soon as they begin to cause growth problems, pain or restrictions of movement.

Wirganowicz PZ, Watts HG. Surgical risk for elective excision of benign exostoses. J Pediatr Orthop. 1997;17(4): 455–9.

This is a retrospective review of 285 osteochondroma excisions. Four percent of excisions resulted in complications, most commonly peroneal neurapraxia (2.5 %). One patient had an arterial laceration, one developed a compartment syndrome and one a fractured fibula. All complications took place in the lower limb osteochondroma excisions (which comprised three-quarters of the operations).

Porter DE, Lonie L, Fraser M, Dobson-Stone C, Porter JR, Monaco AP, et al. Severity of disease and risk of malignant change in hereditary multiple exostoses. A genotype-phenotype study. J Bone Joint Surg Br. 2004;86-B(7):1041–6.

This prospective study of genotype and phenotypes in 172 individuals used molecular screening to identify the genetic mutations and assessed severity of disease by stature, deformity and functional scores. EXT1 and EXT 2 genes were both present in about 40 % of the study group. EXT 1 gene mutations were associated with greater severity of disease and had seven times more risk of the development of chondrosarcoma than the EXT2 group.

Elbow Fractures

Medial

Farsetti P, Potenza V, Caterini R, Ippolito E. Long-term results of treatment of fractures of the medial humeral epicondyle in children. J Bone Joint Surg Am. 2001;83-A(9): 1299–305.

This paper reviewed the outcomes of treatment of 42 patients who had sustained displaced (>5 mm) medial epicondyle fractures as children, Review took place over 30 years after the injury. The results of patients treated by above elbow cast and those treated by open reduction and internal fixation were mostly good with normal or near normal movement, grip and stability. Patients who had excision of the medial epicondyle and reattachment of the soft tissues did not obtain good results.

Kamath AF, Baldwin K, Horneff J, Hosalkar HS. Operative versus non-operative management of paediatric medial epicondyle fractures: a systematic review. J Child Orthop. 2009;3(5):345–57.

Fourteen studies comprising 498 patients were evaluated. The average age was 11.93 years and follow-up ranged from 6 to 216 months. The operative group had a much higher chance of union (9.33 times) but there was no difference in pain at final follow-up or ulnar nerve symptoms between the groups.

Patel NM, Ganley TJ. Medial epicondyle fractures of the humerus: how to evaluate and when to operate. J Pediatr Orthop. 2012;32(Suppl 1):S10–13.

The problems of diagnosis because of poor reliability of X-rays compared to MRI are discussed. The assessment of radiographs in deciding borderline cases is problematic and the lack of any clear benefit from operative treatment is described. The clear indications for surgery are reported as open fractures, gross instability, incarceration of fracture fragments and ulnar nerve symptoms.

Lateral

Song KS, Kang CH, Min BW, Bae KC, Cho CH, Lee JH. Closed reduction and internal fixation of displaced unstable lateral condylar fractures of the humerus in children. J Bone Joint Surg Am. 2008;90(12):2673–81.

Sixty-three unstable fractures were treated prospectively and 73 % of displaced fractures were treated by closed reduction with residual displacement 2 mm or less. The remaining cases were treated by open reduction and fixation – the whole group had no major complications such as osteonecrosis, non-union or physeal arrest. The importance of the internal oblique X-ray is stressed and a classification based on this is proposed. High levels of interobserver reliability using this X-ray were reported.

Song KS, Waters PM. Lateral condylar humerus fractures: which ones should we fix? J Pediatr Orthop. 2012;32 (Suppl 1):S5–9.

This paper gives clear and succinct guidelines on the indications for non-operative and operative treatment and the techniques to be used. The roles of oblique X-rays for diagnosis, arthrograms to assess articular displacement, and closed reduction with percutaneous pinning in appropriate cases are advocated. Operative intervention with closed reduction and percutaneous pinning or open reduction internal fixation are indicated for a malaligned articular surface and/or an unstable fracture.

Femoral Fractures

Ligier JN, Metaizeau JP, Prévot J, Lascombes P. Elastic stable intramedullary nailing of femoral shaft fractures in children. J Bone Joint Surg Br. 1988;70(1):74–7.

This is a report of 123 femoral fractures that were stabilized with elastic nails. More than half of the fractures were unstable. All but one case united with the nails in situ and there were no refractures. Thirteen cases required adjustments to the nails (10 %) and one deep infection occurred in a case with paraplegia and required nail extraction and cast immobilization. Two cases later required epiphyseodesis because of leg length difference greater than 2 cm. Compared with conservative treatment, elastic nailing reduces the need for prolonged bed rest with an average stay of 4.5 days.

Moroz LA, Launay F, Kocher MS, Newton PO, Frick SL, Sponseller PD, et al. Titanium elastic nailing of fractures of the femur in children. Predictors of complications and poor outcome. J Bone Joint Surg Br. 2006;88-B(10):1361–6.

A multicentre retrospective review of 234 fractures treated by titanium elastic nails. Complications occurred in 33 % and outcomes were poor in 10 % and fair in 25 %. Poor outcomes were due to leg length discrepancy (2 %), unacceptable angulation (7 %) and failure of fixation (0.4 %). Complications were almost four times commoner in children 11 years and older compared to those 10 and younger. The heavier children had more complications; a poor outcome was five times more likely if the child weighed 50 kg or more.

Ferguson J, Nicol RO. Early spica treatment of paediatric femoral shaft fractures. J Pediatr Orthop. 2000;20(2): 189–92.

A prospective trial of early spica treatment in children under 11 years old. One hundred and two fractures were treated and spica treatment was abandoned or unsuitable in eight fractures. Plaster spicas were applied under general anaesthetic with the knee flexed 90°, 50 % within 24 h of admission. Twelve spicas required wedging to attain satisfactory alignment. Average bed stay was 7 days with readmission for mobilization in 26 % for a further 4 days. Angular alignment within 10° was achieved in 93 % and rotational alignment was abnormally external in 7 %.

Song K-S. Displaced fractures of the femoral neck in children: open versus closed reduction. J Bone Joint Surg Br. 2010;92-B(8):1148–51.

This is a retrospective review of 27 fractures. Fifteen were treated operatively. Anatomic reduction was achieved in 93 %. There was a good outcome in 93 % and fair in 7 %. In the group of 12 managed with closed reduction, an anatomical reduction was achieved in only 3. Outcomes were good in 7 (58 %) and poor in 3 (25 %). In addition 5 patients in this group had complications including non-union (2), avascular necrosis (2) and coxavara (2). There were no complications in the operative group. Open reduction through a Watson-Jones approach is recommended.

Supracondylar Humeral Fractures

Omid R, Choi PD, Skaggs DL. Supracondylar humeral fractures in children. J Bone Joint Surg Am. 2008;90-A(5): 1121–32.

A thorough review of pathoanatomy, classification, clinical and radiographic findings and treatment. Lateral pins are recommended to avoid ulnar nerve injury (which occurs in 5 % of medial pinned fractures). Medial comminution is a potential problem. Operative fixation is recommended for Gartland Type 2 and 3 fractures. Fracture reduction is advocated before angiography if the limb is pulseless, as realignment usually corrects the vascular problem.

Slongo T, Schmid T, Wilkins K, Joeris A. Lateral external fixation — a new surgical technique for displaced unreducible supracondylar humeral fractures in children. J Bone Joint Surg Am. 2008;90-A(8):1690–7.

A small external fixator is advocated for unstable fractures that are irreducible. This represented 18 % of a retrospective analysis of 170 displaced supracondylar humeral fractures. In this subgroup they achieved a success rate of 90 %, producing a satisfactory closed reduction with maintenance of position in 25 cases and only one with a mild varus deformity. Ninety-seven percent regained normal movement or less than 10° fixed flexion by 3 months after fixator removal.

Mangat KS, Martin AG, Bache CE. The 'pulseless pink' hand following supracondylar fracture of the humerus in children: the predictive value of nerve palsy. J Bone Joint Surg Br. 2009;91(11):1521–5.

This paper compared two management strategies for the perfused but pulseless hand after stabilisation of a Gartland type III supracondylar fracture (19 patients). Of those treated conservatively after closed reduction, 4 required secondary exploration, and were found to have tethering or entrapment of both nerve and vessel at the fracture site.

In six of the eight patients who were explored early the vessel was tethered at the fracture site. The authors recommend early exploration of a Gartland type III supracondylar fracture in patients who present with a coexisting anterior interosseous or median nerve palsy, as these appear to be strongly predictive of nerve and vessel entrapment.

Blakey CM, Biant LC, Birch R. Ischaemia and the pink, pulseless hand complicating supracondylar fractures of the humerus in childhood: long-term follow-up. J Bone Joint Surg Br. 2009;91(11):1487–92.

This paper documents a series of 26 children (mean age 8.6 years (2–12)) referred to a specialist unit with a 'pink pulseless hand' following a supracondylar fracture of the distal humerus after a mean period of 3 months (4 days to 12 months). They were followed up for a mean of 15.5 years (4–26). The neurovascular injuries and resulting impairment in function and salvage procedures were recorded. Only 4 of the 26 patients had undergone immediate surgical exploration before referral. Three of these had a satisfactory outcome. As a result 23 of the 26 children presented with established ischaemic contracture of the forearm and hand. Two responded to conservative stretching. In the remaining 21 the antecubital fossa was explored. Based on their results the authors recommend urgent exploration of the vessels and nerves in a child with a 'pink pulseless hand', not relieved by reduction of a supracondylar fracture of the distal humerus and presenting with persistent and increasing pain suggestive of a deepening nerve lesion and critical ischaemia.

Edmonds EW, Roocroft JH, Mubarak SJ. Treatment of displaced paediatric supracondylar humerus fracture patterns requiring medial fixation: a reliable and safer cross-pinning technique. J Pediatr Orthop. 2012;32(4):346–51.

A retrospective analysis of 381 displaced supracondylar fractures over a 7 year period. One hundred and eighty-seven underwent cross pinning and 194 lateral entry pinning. There was no significant difference in the incidence of ulnar nerve injury. The technique for reducing the risk of ulnar nerve injury in medial pinning is described. This technique is recommended (1) for high supracondylar fractures, (2) when there is medial comminution and (3) if here is initial cubitusvarus and medial instability.

Radius and Ulna Fractures

Jubel A, Andermahr J, Isenberg J, Issavand A, Prokop A, Rehm KE. Outcomes and complications of elastic stable intramedullary nailing for forearm fractures in children. J Pediatr Orthop B. 2005;14(5):375–80.

A prospective study of 51 children with displaced forearm shaft fractures treated by elastic stable intramedullary nailing. Forty-three were followed up for more than a year. 93 % were rated excellent and 7 % good results. There were eight cases of soft tissue irritation at nail site insertion and three cases required revision wire shortening. Two patients had transient radial nerve branch injuries and four had minimal rotation deficits. All returned to full activities.

Clement ND, Yousif F, Duckwoth AD, Teoh KH, Porter DE. Retention of forearm plates: risks and benefits in a paediatric population. J Bone Joint Surg Br. 2012; 94-B(1):134–7.

This prospective series of 82 patients with 116 plates were reviewed. Eighty-five percent of the plates were retained with 7.3 % needing removal because of pain or stiffness and 7.3 % sustained implant related fractures at a later stage. Compared to complications of implant removal (9 % and also a 7 % re-fracture rate reported by Kim et al.) the results are similar. Ulnar plates were most likely to cause pain-requiring removal. Although elastic nails are the preferred choice for forearm fractures, if plate fixation is required then routine removal is not necessary and should only be performed if indicated.

Weiss JM, Mencio GA. Forearm shaft fractures: does fixation improve outcome? J Pediatr Orthop. 2012;32(Suppl 1): S22–4.

A brief review of acceptable alignment and angulation guidelines, indications for surgery and operative options. Plating is associated with more severe complications than intramedullary (IM) fixation as well as increased operating times, duration of hospitalization and scarring. Compartment syndrome is more common in operated fractures, but injury severities for reported groups are probably not matched.

Part IV
Hand and Upper Limb

Elbow

David Hargreaves

Abstract The stiff and arthritic elbow is covered in this chapter, with references including the current thinking on total elbow replacement, its indications, outcomes and the consequences of failed arthroplasty. Nerve problems around the elbow, with compressive neuropathy, or the consequences of radial nerve injury on the forearm wrist and hand are dealt with in terms of diagnosis and treatment options.

Keywords Compressive neuropathies • Osteoarthritis • Radial nerve injury • Stiff elbow • Total elbow replacement

Compressive Neuropathies

Roles NC, Maudsley RH. Radial tunnel syndrome: resistant tennis elbow as a nerve entrapment. J Bone Joint Surg Br. 1972; 54(3):499–508.

This is the "classic" paper describing the pathology, clinical signs and the treatment of radial tunnel syndrome. The anatomy of the radial tunnel is described and the proximity

D. Hargreaves, MBBS, FRCS (Orth)
Department of Orthopaedics,
University Hospital Southampton Trust,
Tremona Road, Southampton SO51 6YD, UK
e-mail: david.hargreaves@uhs.nhs.uk

G. Bowyer, A. Cole (eds.), *Selected References in Trauma and Orthopaedics*, DOI 10.1007/978-1-4471-4676-6_12, © Springer-Verlag London 2014

of the free edge of extensor carpi radialis brevis (ECRB) to the posterior interosseous nerve (PIN) is documented. The clinical sign of pain on active resistance of middle finger extension was first described (Maudsley Sign). The operative technique, using an anterior muscle splitting approach, highlights the importance of releasing the free edge of ECRB as well as the arcade of Frohse (fibrous edge of supinator). Ninety-two percent of the 38 elbows reviewed had a good or excellent result. Little has changed since this paper.

Nabhan A, Ahlhelm F, Kelm J, Reith W, Schwerdtfeger K, Steudel W. Simple decompression or subcutaneous anterior transposition of the ulnar nerve for cubital tunnel syndrome. J Hand Surg Br. 2005;30(5):521–4.

This prospective randomised controlled study comparing the two most commonly performed operations for ulnar neuropathy at the elbow shows that both are effective. The outcomes of simple decompression and anterior subcutaneous transposition are equivalent. Because the intervention is simpler and associated with fewer complications, simple decompression is advised. The main indications for transposition are if there is a structural cause for the compression such as cubitus valgus or nerve subluxation.

Hartz CR, Linscheid RL, Gramse RR, Daube JR. The pronator teres syndrome: compressive neuropathy of the median nerve. J Bone Joint Surg Am. 1981;63(6):885–90.

Forearm compression of the median nerve is more common in clinical examinations than it is in clinical practice! Pronator Syndrome is a misnomer as there are many more different structures that can cause compression of the median nerve in the proximal forearm than just the two heads of pronator teres. This paper, which included 36 operative releases, highlights this as well as the often, vague symptoms of forearm pain, the lack of forearm motor weakness (differentiating it from Anterior Interosseous syndrome), and the similar sensory alteration to carpal tunnel syndrome.

Osteoarthritis

Stanley D. Prevalence and etiology of symptomatic elbow osteoarthritis. J Shoulder Elbow Surg. 1994;3(6):386–9.

One thousand patients were reviewed from a fracture clinic setting. The prevalence of symptomatic degeneration of the elbow was 2 %. They found an association between heavy manual workers and the development of elbow osteoarthritis. This corresponded with previous papers, which have found a statistical association between steel foundry workers and elbow osteoarthritis. The mechanism by which the degeneration occurred was not discussed, but this is an important association.

Cohen AP, Redden JF, Stanley D. Treatment of osteoarthritis of the elbow: a comparison of open and arthroscopic debridement. Arthroscopy. 2000;16(7):701–6.

Cohen et al. compared outcomes after open debridement of the elbow for osteoarthritis (using the Outerbridge-Kashiwagi procedure) and arthroscopic debridement. Both patient groups demonstrated improved range of elbow flexion, decrease in pain, and a high level of satisfaction. Increases in elbow extension, although improved in both groups, were more modest; however, neither procedure included capsular release. Comparison between the open and arthroscopic procedures demonstrated that the open procedure might be more effective in improving flexion, whereas the arthroscopic procedure seemed to provide more pain relief. No significant differences between overall effectiveness of the two procedures were noted.

Giannicola G, Angeloni R, Mantovani A, Rebuzzi E, Merolla G, Greco A, et al. Open debridement and radiocapitellar replacement in primary and post-traumatic arthritis of the elbow: a multicenter study. J Shoulder Elbow Surg. 2012;21(4):456–63.

Early osteoarthritis of the elbow often starts with degeneration and symptoms from the radio-capitellar articulation. Resurfacing replacements for the lateral column have recently been developed. This is a multi-centre prospective study showing the early results (mean follow-up of 22 months) in 20 cases. Most patients had a painfree functional range of motion. The main complication was of malpositioning of the implants and especially mild overstuffing. Radio-capitellar replacement is a procedure that is still in its infancy, but may become increasingly common over the next decade.

Radial Nerve Injury

Shao YC, Harwood P, Grotz MR, Limb D, Giannoudis PV. Radial nerve palsy associated with fractures of the shaft of humerus: a systematic review. J Bone Joint Surg Br. 2005;87(12): 1647–52.

Twenty-one papers were reviewed showing a prevalence of radial nerve palsy after humeral shaft fractures to be 11.8 %. Transverse and spiral fractures were confirmed to be the most likely type of fracture to cause a radial nerve palsy. The final outcomes of nerve function were the same whether the patient was treated with early surgical exploration or with a limited period of conservative treatment initially. The issue of the length of period to wait prior to exploring a non-recovering nerve was unanswered, but as the mean time to recovery was 7.3 weeks it is reasonable to wait between 7 weeks and 6 months to see if the nerve starts to have spontaneous recovery. If there are no signs of recovery at this stage then surgical exploration of the nerve should be performed. Continuing deterioration of nerve function warrants immediate surgical exploration.

Shergill G, Bonney G, Munshi P, Birch R. The radial and posterior interosseous nerves. Results of 260 repairs. J Bone Joint Surg Br. 2001;83(5):646–9.

Of all injury types, 42 % of repairs failed to give recovery of nerve function. In the group of open tidy injuries that underwent repair, 79 % achieved a good or fair result. Other types of injury faired less well. Poor prognostic features for outcome were length of defect that required grafting and delay in surgical repair. All defects more than 10 cm failed to recover. Repairs performed within 14 days of injury did better than delayed ones. All repairs performed after 12 months failed. Repairs of the posterior interosseous nerve were more successful, probably because of its proximity to the end target organ.

Ropars M, Dréano T, Siret P, Belot N, Langlais F. Long-term results of tendon transfers in radial and posterior interosseous nerve paralysis. J Hand Surg Br. 2006;31(5):502–6.

Over 50 modifications of tendon transfers for radialnerve palsy have been described. In many situations, the outcomes of tendon transfer are better than for primary nerve repair. The lengths of rehabilitation following tendon transfers are much shorter than for nerve repair. This paper shows good results with long term follow-up. It advocates the use of Pronator Teres being transferred to ECRB to give wrist extension. Finger extension being restored with flexor carpi radialis (FCR) rather than flexor carpi ulnaris (FCU) as the loss of FCU allows the wrist to deviate radially. Palmaris Longus was used to reconstruct extensor pollicic longus (EPL) function when available. An alternative, in the absence of the palmaris tendon, is flexor digitorum superficialis to the ring finger. Simply reconstructing EPL is not enough for the thumb function, a tenodesis of abductor pollicis longus (APL) to Brachioradialis is also needed to regain thumb abduction.

Stiff Elbow

Myden C, Hildebrand K. Elbow joint contracture after traumatic injury. J Shoulder Elbow Joint 2011;20:39–44.

Twenty-five cases with significant elbow pathology were prospectively reviewed for 1 year following their injuries. Injuries included fractures, fracture-dislocation, dislocation and biceps tendon ruptures. The range of motion was assessed and 12 % were found to have an arc of movement less than the functional range (100° arc). The deficit of movement was enough to warrant surgical release. Range of motion continued to improve up to 1 year following the index injury. They found that failure to improve 3 months after injury was a poor prognostic sign and was a sign of impending joint contracture.

Nguyen D, Proper SI, MacDermid JC, King GJ, Faber KJ. Functional outcomes of arthroscopic capsular release of the elbow. Arthroscopy. 2006;22(8):842–9.

Arthroscopic contracture release has recently become more common but is not always appropriate in all cases of stiffness. This paper reviews the results of a series of 22 patients with a follow-up of more than 1 year. Twenty patients had a capsulectomy and two patients had a capsulotomy. The improvement in arc of motion was 38° (±23°). There were no significant complications. This paper confirms a role for arthroscopic release. It should be appreciated, though, that arthroscopic release of the elbow is technically very challenging and carries a significant risk of nerve injury.

Ring D, Hotchkiss RN, Guss D, Jupiter JB. Hinged elbow external fixation for severe elbow contracture. J Bone Joint Surg Am. 2005;87(6):1293–6.

When initially introduced it was hoped that the use of the hinged external fixation with a built-in gear mechanism for applying passive motion and static progressive stretch by turning a dial would improve the arc of movement following open surgical arthrolysis. Nineteen patients underwent arthrolysis without the use of a hinged fixator. Twenty-three patients had arthrolysis and static progressive stretch with a hinged fixator. The difference in arc (78° with no fixator, 89° with fixator) was not significant. There were seven complication related to the use of the fixator and the pins (pin site infection, osteomyelitis, fracture, pin breakage, ulnar nerve irritation). It was viewed that the slight benefit from a hinged fixator did not warrant the increased risks. Sometimes an external fixator is required to maintain stability of the joint post release.

Peden JP, Morrey BF. Total elbow replacement for the management of the ankylosed or fused elbow. J Bone Joint Surg Br. 2008;90(9):1198–204.

Ankylosed elbows are not usually tolerated well. Although the elbow is not painful, patients often have shoulder discomfort. This study reports the use of total elbow replacement for revising ankylosed elbows (mostly post-traumatic). Thirteen patients with spontaneously ankylosed elbows were treated with a linked semi-constrained non-custom total elbow implant (Coonrad-Morrey). Despite good final outcomes with a good mean arc of movement (37° of extension to 118° of flexion) and a high patient satisfaction, there was a high complication rate and re-operation was required in over half of patients. Wound breakdown and infection were more common than expected. There was a high incidence of recurrence of the heterotopic ossification, despite prophylactic measures being used.

Total Elbow Replacement

Gschwend N, Simmen BR, Matejovsky Z. Late complications in elbow arthroplasty. J Shoulder Elbow Surg. 1996;5 (2 Pt 1): 86–96.

Total Elbow Replacement initially had a reputation for a high incidence of perioperative complications. The early literature had a complication rate of approximately 40 %. This important paper from the designing centre of the GSB3 implant (sloppy hinge type) showed a much more acceptable level of complications (15 %). They showed that with careful surgical technique and attention to detail many of the surgical problems could be avoided. They highlighted the importance of releasing the ulnar nerve and removing the medial osteophyte from the bone adjacent to the medial collateral ligament.

Qureshi F, Draviaraj KP, Stanley D. The Kudo 5 total elbow replacement in the treatment of the rheumatoid elbow: results at a minimum of ten years. J Bone Joint Surg Br. 2010;92(10):1416–21.

The Kudo elbow replacement is a stemmed, unlinked replacement, which was commonly used in the UK during the 1990's. The articulating surfaces are relatively cylindrical and therefore this implant does not have much inherent stability. Its use has been superseded by unlinked implants with more modularity and inherent constraint from the articulating surfaces. Implants with 10 year survival rates should be recognized as these are the standard that newer implants must match.

With revision as the endpoint, the mean survival time for the prosthesis was 11.3 years and the estimated survival of the prosthesis at 12 years according to Kaplan-Meier survival analysis was 74 %. Of the 16 surviving implants, 10 were free from pain, 4 had mild pain and 2 moderate.

Little CP, Graham AJ, Carr AJ. Total elbow arthroplasty: a systematic review of the literature in the English language until the end of 2003. J Bone Joint Surg Br. 2005;87(4):437–44.

This systematic review includes the most commonly used implants. It compares the late results of linked and unlinked implants. There was a tendency to find a lower incidence of loosening in the sloppy hinge type of implants compared to the unlinked. The function was regarded as slightly better with the sloppy hinge because of the ability to shorten the humerus and release the soft tissues operatively without the risk of the joint instability that occurs in the unlinked prostheses.

Jeon IH, Morrey BF, Anakwenze OA, Tran NV. Incidence and implications of early postoperative wound complications after total elbow arthroplasty. J Shoulder Elbow Surg. 2011;20(6):857–65.

The Mayo group reviewed 1,749 total elbow replacements, 97 (5.5 %) were found to have wound problems in the early postoperative phase. This group were studied and 24 % of the wound problems had a septic origin (i.e. 1.4 %). Just under a half of these septic cases ultimately required implant removal. Rheumatoid arthritis and previous surgery were identified to be risk factors. Prolonged drainage in the early postoperative phase was associated with a 8.8 % secondary deep infection rate. They suggest that early aggressive surgical management of wound problems is appropriate and especially when a wound haematoma is associated with drainage.

Amirfeyz R, Stanley D. Allograft-prosthesis composite reconstruction for the management of failed elbow replacement with massive structural bone loss: a medium-term follow-up. J Bone Joint Surg Br. 2011;93(10):1382–8.

As revision total elbow replacement (TER) starts to become more common in clinical practice, the incidence of severe bone loss around the elbow is becoming a bigger problem. It is important for clinicians to understand the various salvage techniques that can be used for dealing with these problems. This paper reviews the results of long stemmed prostheses inserted within allograft bone grafts. Good functional results were achieved. Partial resorption of the allograft was noted in 50 % of cases. The incidence of union of the graft to host bone was much higher in ulna grafts than in humeral grafts.

Hand and Wrist

David J. Shewring and Ryan Trickett

Abstract This section deals with the inflammatory and degenerative problems affecting the hand and wrist, with osteoarthritis and rheumatoid disease given special consideration. The urgent condition of hand infection is considered, with up-to-date references on the management of these problems. The soft tissue problems of De Quervain's and carpal tunnel syndrome are covered in detail, with treatment options and outcomes. The pathology underlying Keinbocks and avascular necrosis in the wrist, and the treatment strategies, are dealt with.

Keywords Carpal tunnel syndrome • Carpal instability • Carpo-metacarpal arthritis • Trapeziectomy • Replacement arthroplasty • Radial deficiency/pollicisation • Madelung's deformity • Complex regional pain syndrome • Factitious disorders • De Quervain's disease • Distal radius fractures • Dupuytren's disease • Essex-Lopresti • Flexor tendon repair • Hand infections • Tendon sheath infection • Human bites • Herpetic whitlow • Necrotising fasciitis • Kienbock's disease

D.J. Shewring, FRCSEd (Orth), Dip Hand Surg (Eur) (✉)
R. Trickett, MBBCh, MRCS, MSc, FRCS (Tr & Orth)
Department of Orthopaedic Surgery,
University Hospital of Wales, Heath Park,
Cardiff CF14 4XW, UK
e-mail: davidshewring@me.com

G. Bowyer, A. Cole (eds.), *Selected References in Trauma and Orthopaedics*, DOI 10.1007/978-1-4471-4676-6_13,
© Springer-Verlag London 2014

• Tendon rupture • Thumb deformity • Scaphoid fractures •
Trigger finger • Tumors • Ganglions • Giant cell tumours of
tendon sheath • Enchondromata

Carpal Tunnel Syndrome

Anatomy

**Mackinnon SE, Dellon AL. Anatomic investigations of nerves
at the wrist. I. Orientation of the motor fascicle of the median
nerve in the carpal tunnel. Ann Plast Surg. 1988;21(1):32–5.**

An analysis of the orientation of the motor branch of the
median nerve in the carpal tunnel in dissections of 50 hands.
The motor branch was located on the radial-volar aspect of
the median nerve in 60 % of the hands, the central-volar
aspect in 22 %, and between these two locations in the
remaining 18 %. In 56 % of the hands, the motor branch
passed through a separate distinct fascial tunnel before entering the thenar muscles.

**Lanz U. Anatomic variations of the median nerve in the car-
pal tunnel. J Hand Surg Am. 1977;2(1):44–53.**

Twenty-nine variations in the course of the median nerve
were found in 246 hands explored at operation. The variations
were classified into four groups: I-variation in the course of
the thenar branch; II-accessory branches at the distal portion
of the carpal tunnel; III-high divisions of the median nerve;
and IV-accessory branches proximal to the carpal canal. The
thenar branch variations were extraligamentous in 46 %, sub-
ligamentous in 31 %, and transligamentous in 23 %. The findings emphasize the importance of approaching the median
nerve from the ulnar side when opening the carpal tunnel.

**Leibovic SJ, Hastings H 2nd. Martin-Gruber revisited. J Hand
Surg Am. 1992;17(1):47–53.**

The Martin-Gruber anastomosis is a motor connection
between the median and ulnar nerves in the proximal forearm.

The Riche-Cannieu anomalous connection occurs between the motor branches of the ulnar and median nerves in the hand.

A classification for Martin-Gruber connections is described. There are four types of connection that can theoretically exist. In this meta-analysis the incidence of Martin-Gruber connections was found to be 17 %. In this classification, 60 % are type I, (motor branches from the median to the ulnar nerve to innervate "median" muscles); 35 % are type II, (motor branches from median to ulnar nerves to innervate "ulnar" muscles); 3 % are type III, (motor fibers from the ulnar to the median nerve to innervate "median" muscles); and 1 % are type IV, (motor fibers from the ulnar to the median nerve to innervate "ulnar" muscles).

Diagnosis

Jablecki CK, Andary MT, So YT, Wilkins DE, Williams FH. Literature review of the usefulness of nerve conduction studies and electromyography for the evaluation of patients with carpal tunnel syndrome. AAEM Quality Assurance Committee. Muscle Nerve. 1993;16(12):1392–414.

The sensitivity and specificity of nerve conduction studies and electromyography for the diagnosis of carpal tunnel syndrome were evaluated by a critical review of the literature. 165 articles were identified and reviewed on the basis of six criteria of scientific methodology. The authors conclude that nerve conduction studies (NCS's) are valid and reproducible clinical laboratory studies that confirm a clinical diagnosis of carpal tunnel syndrome (CTS) with a high degree of sensitivity and specificity. Clinical practice recommendations are made based on a comparison of the sensitivities of the several different median nerve conduction study techniques.

Durkan JA. A new diagnostic test for carpal tunnel syndrome. J Bone Joint Surg Am. 1991;73(4):535–8.

Durkan's test consists of application of direct pressure on the carpal tunnel and the underlying median nerve. The results of Tinel's test, Phalen's test, and the new test were evaluated in 31 patients (46 hands) in whom the presence of carpal tunnel syndrome had been proved electrodiagnostically, as well as in a control group of 50 subjects. Durkan's test was found to be more sensitive and specific than the Tinel and Phalen tests for the diagnosis of carpel tunnel.

Treatment

Gelberman RH, Aronson D, Weisman MH. Carpal-tunnel syndrome. Results of a prospective trial of steroid injection and splinting. J Bone Joint Surg Am. 1980;62(7):1181–4.

In order to define the role of steroid injection and splinting as a method of treatment of carpal-tunnel syndrome, a prospective study was performed on 50 hands in 41 consecutive patients. All hands were treated with a single injection and 3 weeks of splinting. Follow-up ranged from a minimum of 6 months to a maximum of 26 months, with a mean of 18 months. Eleven (22 %) of 50 hands were completely free of symptoms at the end of the follow-up period. Hands with mild symptoms of short duration were more likely to respond.

Green DP. Diagnostic and therapeutic value of carpal tunnel injection. J Hand Surg Am. 1984;9(6):850–4.

This retrospective study documents the diagnostic and therapeutic value of steroid injections in patients with carpal tunnel syndrome. There were 281 injections in 233 patients. Eighty-one percent of the patients obtained good or complete relief lasting from 1 day to 45 months. In most of these, symptoms began to recur at an average 3.3 months. In 46 % recurrent symptoms were severe enough to warrant surgical treatment. The study also suggests that carpal tunnel injection is also a reasonably accurate diagnostic test. Correlations between results of injections and subsequent operations indicate that a good response to injection is an excellent diagnostic and prognostic sign. However, the converse is not true; poor relief from injection does not necessarily mean that the patient is a poor candidate for surgery. Injection of the carpal tunnel is an effective, albeit usually transient, therapeutic modality.

Chow JC. Endoscopic carpal tunnel release. Two-portal technique. Hand Clin. 1994;10(4):637–46.

The author describes the history, indications and contraindications and operative technique for the two portal endoscopic carpal ligament release. Also described are the potential complications and how to avoid them. The clinical results of 815 patients (1,154 wrists) are described.

Outcome

Zyluk A, Puchalski P. A comparison of outcomes of carpal tunnel release in diabetic and non-diabetic patients. J Hand Surg Eur Vol. 2013;38(5):485–8.

This retrospective study compared the results of carpal tunnel release in diabetic and non-diabetic patients. No significant differences in any of the measured variables were found at the 6-month assessment. The results of the study show that carpal tunnel release in diabetic and non-diabetic patients are similarly beneficial.

Wilgis EF, Burke FD, Dubin NH, Sinha S, Bradley MJ. A prospective assessment of carpal tunnel surgery with respect to age. J Hand Surg Br. 2006;31(4):401–6.

Six hundred and thirty-five carpal tunnel decompressions in 490 patients were studied prospectively in two hand surgery centres to assess the effect of increasing age on the outcome after surgery. The outcome was assessed using various methods at 2 weeks and 6 months.

Cases were divided into four age groups. Despite a relatively high number of co-morbidities, older patients had an acceptable complication rate and their improvement was comparable to all other age groups.

Zyluk A, Szlosser Z. The results of carpal tunnel release for carpal tunnel syndrome diagnosed on clinical grounds, with or without electrophysiological investigations: a randomized study. J Hand Surg Eur Vol. 2013;38(1):44–9.

The authors compared the results of carpal tunnel release in patients with the diagnosis of carpal tunnel syndrome based on only clinical grounds and those diagnosed on clinical and electrophysiological grounds. Ninety-three patients were randomly assigned to receive carpal tunnel release with (n=45, 48 %) or without (n=48, 52 %) nerve conduction studies. Patients were followed-up at 1 and 6 months, by various assessments. No significant differences were found between the two groups.

Relationship to Work

Dias JJ, Burke FD, Wildin CJ, Heras-Palou C, Bradley MJ. Carpal tunnel syndrome and work. J Hand Surg Br. 2004;29(4): 329–33.

This is a study of 327 consecutive women of working age presenting to a hand unit with carpal tunnel syndrome. Two hundred and seventeen were working, 55 of these in repetitive occupations. One hundred and ten were not in employment. On a population basis more women in non-repetitive occupations presented with carpal tunnel syndrome (220/100,000/year) than those in repetitive work (122/100,000/year) or those not working (129/100,000/year), and more were offered surgery (82 % versus 67 % for those in repetitive work and 58 % for those not working). However, symptoms and disability were less severe in working women. This study suggests that working in repetitive or non-repetitive occupations does not cause, aggravate or accelerate carpal tunnel syndrome. Working women may struggle to accommodate their symptoms compared to women who are not in employment causing more to seek help.

Carpal Instability

Diagnosis

Watson HK, Ashmead D 4th, Makhlouf MV. Examination of the scaphoid. J Hand Surg Am. 1988;13(5):657–60.

In this paper Watson describes his shift test for scapho-lunate instability, as well as the anatomic basis and interpretation of the test.

Classification

Larsen CF, Amadio PC, Gilula LA, Hodge JC. Analysis of carpal instability: I. Description of the scheme. J Hand Surg Am. 1995;20(5):757–64.

Based on a review of the literature the authors suggest a classification of carpal instability with guidelines for treatment and a proposal for standardized analysis. There are six categories describing chronicity, constancy, etiology, location, direction, and pattern of the instability.

Scapholunate Dissociation

Walsh JJ, Berger RA, Cooney WP. Current status of scapholunate interosseous ligament injuries. J Am Acad Orthop Surg. 2002;10(1):32–42.

This is a review article giving an overview of current ideas on biomechanics, investigation and treatment.

Late Repair/Salvage

Elfar JC, Stern PJ. Proximal row carpectomy for scapholunate dissociation. J Hand Surgery Eur Vol. 2011;36(2):111–5.

Thirty-one patients undergoing proximal row carpectomy for static scapholunate dissociation without degenerative arthritis were studied.

Patients were less likely to return to pre-injury occupation and have subjective and objective parameters below values for proximal row carpectomy performed for other conditions. The findings suggest that proximal row carpectomy, when performed for static scapholunate dissociation, results in a stiffened, weakened wrist. Wrist arthrodesis was necessary in four patients for ongoing pain.

Inoue G, Shionoya K. Late treatment of unreduced perilunate dislocations. J Hand Surg Br. 1999;24(2):221–5.

This is a comparison of various treatments for late diagnosed perilunate dislocation, including open reduction, proximal row carpectomy and lunate excision. The former two treatments yielded satisfactory results when performed before or after 2 months post injury respectively. The results of lunate excision were less favourable.

Talwalkar SC, Edwards AT, Hayton MJ, et al. Results of triligament tenodesis: a modified Brunelli procedure in the management of scapholunate instability. J Hand Surg Br. 2006;31(1):110–7.

One hundred and seventeen patients having had a modified Brunelli procedure for scapholunate instability were assessed with a mean follow-up of 4 years. Seventy-nine percent patients were satisfied with the result of the surgery (good to excellent) and 88 % of the patients felt that they would have the same surgery again.

The authors recommend this procedure for dynamic and static scapholunate instability.

Garcia-Elias M, Lluch AL, Stanley JK. Three-ligament tenodesis for the treatment of scapholunate dissociation: indications and surgical technique. J Hand Surg Am. 2006;31(1):125–34.

The authors describe an algorithm of treatment based on a number of prognostic factors to help in deciding treatment for individual cases.

Watson HK, Weinzweig J, Guidera PM, Zeppieri J, Ashmead D. One thousand intercarpal arthrodeses. J Hand Surg Br.1999;24(3):307–15.

This report presents experience with more than 1,000 limited wrist arthrodeses, and provides a review of the indications and technical considerations for specific intercarpal fusions, and subsequent results. The authors claim that the study has demonstrated that these techniques are reliable and effective in dealing with a wide range of wrist disorders including degenerative arthritis, rotary subluxation of the scaphoid, midcarpal instability, scaphoid non-union and Kienbock's disease.

Carpo-metacarpal Arthritis

Prevalence

Armstrong AL, Hunter JB, Davis TR. The prevalence of degenerative arthritis of the base of the thumb in post-menopausal women. J Hand Surg Br. 1994;19(3):340–1.

The authors studied the prevalence of basal thumb arthritis in 143 post-menopausal women. The radiological prevalences of isolated carpometacarpal and scapho-trapezial osteoarthritis were 25 and 2 % respectively. The prevalence of combined carpometacarpal and scapho-trapezial osteoarthritis was 8 %. Twenty-eight percent of women with isolated carpometacarpal osteoarthritis and 55 % with combined carpometacarpal and scapho-trapezial osteoarthritis complained of basal thumb pain.

Treatment: Splintage/Injection

Weiss S, LaStayo P, Mills A, Bramlet D. Prospective analysis of splinting the first carpometacarpal joint: an objective, subjective, and radiographic assessment. J Hand Ther. 2000;13(3): 218–26.

Sillem H, Backman CL, Miller WC, Li LC. Comparison of two carpometacarpal stabilizing splints for individuals with thumb osteoarthritis. J Hand Ther. 2011;24(3):216–25.

These papers both assess the role of splinting in the conservative treatment of 1st carpometacarpal osteoarthritis (CMCOA). The first showed little difference in 26 hands between pain relief and pinch strength between two different splint designs: long and short; but did demonstrate low quality evidence that splinting improved pain scores and activities of daily living. The second paper looked similarly at two splint designs: custom made and "off the shelf"; finding that both improved pain, function as assessed by the Australian Canadian Hand Osteoarthritis Hand Index and grip/pinch strength.

Swindells MG, Logan AJ, Armstrong DJ, Chan P, Burke FD, Lindau TR. The benefit of radiologically-guided steroid injections for trapeziometacarpal osteoarthritis. Ann R Coll Surg Engl. 2010;92(8):680–4.

This paper highlights the difficulties in placement of corticosteroid accurately into the 1st CMC joint and cites this as a potential reason for the variable results seen in the use of injections in these patients. They audited 83 patients undergoing fluoroscopically guided injection of corticosteroid and local anaesthetic. They showed a significant drop in the median visual analogue scale for pain following injection (68–25) and a median perceived effectiveness of 3 months. Some patients reported ongoing relief up to 6 months post injection but the majority (2/3) reported benefit of 2 months.

Trapeziectomy

Davis TR, Brady O, Barton NJ, Lunn PG, Burke FD. Trapeziectomy alone, with tendon interposition or with ligament reconstruction? J Hand Surg Br. 1997;22(6):689–94.

This randomized prospective study compared the results of trapeziectomy alone, or combined with tendon interposition or ligament reconstruction in 76 women with basal thumb osteoarthritis. At 3 month and 1 year follow-up the results of the three procedures were indistinguishable in terms of pain relief, hand function and thumb strength. In the short term at least, tendon interposition and ligament reconstruction do not improve the results of trapeziectomy.

Belcher HJ, Nicholl JE. A comparison of trapeziectomy with and without ligament reconstruction and tendon interposition. J Hand Surg Br. 2000;25(4):350–6.

Forty-three patients were randomly allocated to undergo either trapeziectomy alone or with a ligament reconstruction and tendon interposition (LRTI) using an abductor pollicis longus tendon slip. The patients were reviewed at a median 13 months after surgery. The demographic characteristics, severity of disease and pre-operative clinical measurements of the two study groups were indistinguishable but LRTI lengthened the operation by approximately 15 min. Both groups expressed equal satisfaction with the operation and there were no significant differences between the two treatment groups. Simple trapeziectomy is an effective operation for osteoarthrosis at the base of the thumb and the addition of a ligament reconstruction was not shown to confer any additional benefit.

Davis TR, Pace A. Trapeziectomy for trapeziometacarpal joint osteoarthritis: is ligament reconstruction and temporary stabilisation of the pseudarthrosis with a Kirschner wire important? J Hand Surg Eur Vol. 2009;34(3):312–21.

This randomised prospective study compared two operations for trapeziometacarpal joint osteoarthritis: trapeziectomy with flexor carpi radialis ligament reconstruction, tendon interposition and Kirschner wire insertion followed by splintage for 6 weeks (T+LRTI) and excision of the trapezium with no Kirschner wire and immobilisation of the thumb in a soft bandage for only 3 weeks (T). Sixty-seven thumbs with (T) and 61 with (T+LRTI) were assessed preoperatively and at 3-months and 1-year after surgery. Forty-seven percent and 73 % of patients reported no pain or only aching after use at 3-months and 1-year respectively and the Disabilities of the Arm, Shoulder, and Hand (DASH) and Patient Evaluation Measure (PEM) outcome scores reduced postoperatively indicating improved function. However the pain, DASH and PEM scores, and also key and tip thumb pinch and all the other clinical outcome measures, did not differ significantly between the two groups at either 3-months or 1-year after surgery.

Salem H, Davis TR. Six year outcome excision of the trapezium for trapeziometacarpal joint osteoarthritis: is it improved by ligament reconstruction and temporary Kirschner wire insertion? J Hand Surg Eur Vol. 2012;37(3):211–9.

This randomized prospective study compared the treatment of trapeziometacarpal joint osteoarthritis with (a) trapeziectomy with no ligament reconstruction, no soft tissue interposition and no temporary Kirschner wire stabilization (Group T); (b) trapeziectomy with flexor carpi radialis ligament reconstruction and interposition and temporary K-wire stabilization (Group T + LRTI). Ninety-nine patients were followed with 114 thumbs (59 T and 55 T + LRTI) for a mean of 6.2 (range, 4.2–8.1) years. There were no significant differences between the two treatments in any subjective or objective outcome measure at 6 year follow-up. This study does not provide evidence to support the use of LRTI and temporary K-wire stabilization after trapeziectomy.

Poulter RJ, Davis TR. Management of hyperextension of the metacarpophalangeal joint in association with trapeziometacarpal joint osteoarthritis. J Hand Surg Eur Vol. 2011;36(4):280–4.

This study investigates the management of metacarpophalangeal joint (MCP) hyperextension in patients undergoing trapeziectomy for thumb base osteoarthritis. A total of 297 thumbs with painful trapeziometacarpal osteoarthritis were assessed on pain and thumb key and tip pinch preoperatively and at 1 year. Before surgery 101 had no MCP hyperextension, 168 had hyperextension ≤30° and 28 had hyperextension ≥35°. Of these 157 hyperextension deformities ≤30° and 8 ≥35° were not treated. The others were treated by temporary insertion of a Kirschner wire ($n = 9$), MCP fusion ($n = 6$), sesamoid bone tethering to the MC head ($n = 5$) and palmar capsulodesis using a bone anchor ($n = 11$). Untreated MCP hyperextension deformities <30° did not influence the outcome of trapeziectomy. MCP hyperextension deformities ≥35° can be improved by capsulodesis or MCP fusion but this may not improve the clinical outcome.

Replacement Arthroplasty

Chakrabarti AJ, Robinson AH, Gallagher P. De la Caffinière thumb carpometacarpal replacements.93 cases at 6 to 16 years follow-up. J Hand Surg Br. 1997;22(6):695–8.

The results of 93 de la Caffinière thumb joint replacements in 71 patients were reviewed between 6 and 16 years. The survival rate was 89 % at 16 years. Eleven thumb joints had failed requiring revision. The commonest reason for failure was aseptic loosening of the trapezial component. The failure rate was higher in men of working age than any other group, which possibly reflects the increased demands on the prosthesis of these patients. The authors support the use of this implant for degenerative osteoarthritis, but caution against its use in men under 65 years.

Johnston P, Getgood A, Larson D, Chojnowski AJ, Chakrabarti AJ, Chapman PG. De la Caffinière thumb trapeziometacarpal joint arthroplasty: 16–26 year follow-up. J Hand Surg Eur Vol. 2012;37(7):621–4.

Seventy-one patients (93 implants) had a de la Caffinière prosthesis implanted between 1980 and 1989 and were reviewed and reported in 1997. In this paper the series is reviewed 10 years later. Similar outcome measures were used as in the original study, pinch and grip strength measured and validated outcome scores obtained (DASH and EQ-5D). Radiographic outcome was assessed. Twenty-six patients with 39 implants were available for review at a mean of 19 years (range, 16–26 years). Survivorship at 26 years was 73.9 % (95 % CI, 61.2–86.6) for re-operation and 26.0 % (95 % CI, 0–52.7) for all failure. Patients had satisfactory power and thumb mobility and continued to be satisfied without pain. Registries should log such prostheses and add to implant survival data.

Giddins G. Editorial. J Hand Surg Eur Vol. 2012;37(7): 603–4.

An overview of the published literature to date is presented noting that of the various soft tissue procedures performed to improve the outcome of trapezectomy none had been shown to reliably give a better outcome than trapezectomy alone. Implant arthroplasty has been tried using various materials including silastic and hard-bearing materials, and various designs, including spacers, hemi-arthroplasties, and total arthroplasties. There are very few long-term results and, for some implants, very limited or no obvious published data of good outcomes. Good long-term outcomes for the de la Caffinière implant are reported, but poor outcomes for others, with high complication rates and failure rates. It was recommended that we should stop using implants with known poor outcomes and should continue to be careful about being encouraged into using other new implants until adequate long-term follow-up is available through ethically approved trials.

Congenital

Radial Deficiency/Pollicisation

Lourie GM, Lins RE. Radial longitudinal deficiency. A review and update. Hand Clin. 1998;14(1):85–99.

This article includes a review of the historical background, a discussion of current recommendations for treatment of patients with radial longitudinal deficiency. There is a detailed critical review of recent contributions to the field.

Lister G. Reconstruction of the hypoplastic thumb. Clin Orthop Relat Res. 1985;(195):52–65.

An overview of the subject informed by the author's extensive experience in the field. Blauth has classified congenital hypoplasia of the thumb into five grades. Grade I requires no treatment. Grade II can be reconstructed by widening the first web space with various flaps, stabilizing the metacarpophalangeal joint, and performing an opponensplasty. Grades III, IV, and V require pollicization. Partial aplasia should be treated by phalangization, distraction lengthening with free toe phalanx transfer, on-top plasty, or toe-to-hand transfer. The last is made more complex by the anomalous anatomy frequently present in aplasia. Reconstruction of the infant thumb should be complete before the first birthday.

Buck-Gramcko D. Pollicization of the index finger. Method and results in aplasia and hypoplasia of the thumb. J Bone Joint Surg Am. 1971;53(8):1605–17.

Littler JW. On making a thumb: one hundred years of surgical effort. J Hand Surg Am. 1976;1(1):35–51.

Two classic papers on pollicisation, the second a review article.

Manske PR, McCarroll HR Jr. Index finger pollicization for a congenitally absent or nonfunctioning thumb. J Hand Surg Am.1985;10(5):606–13.

The authors describe 40 pollicizations of index fingers for congenitally absent or nonfunctioning thumbs in patients younger than 16 years old. Twenty-six additional operations were performed after pollicization on 20 transposed digits, including opposition transfer (18), extensor tendon shortening (4), and arthrodesis (4). The operations improved not only the cosmetic appearance of the hand, but also the functional ability of the patients to grasp and handle large objects; preoperative ability to pinch and handle small objects was not impaired by the operative procedure. Additional operative procedures were required most often in patients with radial club hands and/or previous centralization.

Goldfarb CA, Wall L, Manske PR. Radial longitudinal deficiency: the incidence of associated medical and musculoskeletal conditions. J Hand Surg Am. 2006;31(7):1176–82.

The incidence of various syndromes and medical and musculoskeletal conditions in patients with radial longitudinal deficiency (RLD) was investigated. One hundred and sixty-four patients with 245 affected extremities were studied. 138 patients had radius abnormalities and 26 patients had isolated thumb hypoplasia. Twenty-five patients had thrombocytopenia absent radius syndrome; 22 patients had vertebral, anal, cardiac, tracheoesophageal, renal, and limb abnormalities association; 7 patients had Holt-Oram syndrome; and 1 patient had Fanconi anemia. There were 32 patients with cardiac abnormalities and 60 patients with spinal or lower-extremity musculoskeletal abnormalities. The percentage of patients with associated abnormalities increased with an increasing severity of RLD. The high incidence of these conditions in patients with RLD emphasizes the importance of a complete assessment.

Percival NJ, Sykes PJ, Chandraprakasam T. A method of assessment of pollicisation. J Hand Surg Br.1991;16(2):141–3.

The authors describe an assessment for pollicisation based upon tip pinch, opposition, pulp pinch, grasp, mobility, sensitivity and cosmetic appearance which gives a numerical score.

Sykes PJ, Chandraprakasam T, Percival NJ. Pollicisation of the index finger in congenital anomalies. A retrospective analysis. J Hand SurgBr.1991;16(2):144–7.

This paper is a review of 30 pollicisations performed on 22 children with hypoplasia or aplasia of the thumb. Seventy-three percent were graded good or excellent, 17 % fair and 10 % poor. Thirty-six percent required secondary surgery to achieve a satisfactory result. Better results were obtained in Blauth III or IV deformities, with poorer outcomes in Blauth V or patients with associated radial hypoplasia. Good functional and cosmetic results were found in patients operated upon at an early age. The presence of previously unreported bony spikes was a significant cause of poor mobility and was amenable to secondary surgery.

Madelung's Deformity

Dubey A, Fajardo M, Green S, Lee SK. Madelung's deformity: a review. J Hand Surg Eur Vol. 2010;35(3):174–81.

This review paper suggests an algorithm for management of Madelung's deformity based on the literature and the authors' own clinical experience.

Salon A, Serra M, Pouliquen JC. Long-term follow-up of surgical correction of Madelung's deformity with conservation of the distal radioulnar joint in teenagers. J Hand Surg Br. 2000;25(1):22–5.

This paper describes the results of 11 wrists in 7 patients with painful Madelung deformity, corrected during adolescence by a closing wedge osteotomy of the radius and a shortening osteotomy of the ulna, with conservation of the distal radioulnar joint. At late follow-up (9.7 years) function was considerably improved. When the ulnar head was correctly relocated during operation, a new distal radioulnar space developed. Shortening of the ulna must be generous and combined with slight flexion at the osteotomy.

Complex Regional Pain Syndrome/ Factitious Disorders

Field J. Complex Regional Pain Syndrome: a review. J Hand Surg Eur Vol. 2013;38(6):616–26.

This review article elucidates the recent advances in the knowledge of the aetiology, classification and treatment of this condition.

Field J, Warwick D, Bannister GC. Features of algodystrophy ten years after Colles' fracture. J Hand Surg Br. 1992;17(3): 318–20.

This paper describes the long-term outcome of algodystrophy. Ten years after Colles' fracture, 26 % of 55 cases showed features of the syndrome. The finding of poor finger function 3 months following the fracture correlated significantly with the presence of components of algodystrophy after 10 years.

Field J, Protheroe DL, Atkins RM. Algodystrophy after Colles fractures is associated with secondary tightness of casts. J Bone Joint Surg Br. 1994;76(6):901–5.

A method of measuring the tightness of plaster casts is described. Tightness was measured weekly in 23 consecutive patients with Colles' fractures. Six had objective signs of algodystrophy 9 weeks after the fracture. In these patients the plaster cast was significantly tighter during the first 3 weeks than in patients who did not develop algodystrophy. The complex relationship between these findings is discussed.

Puchalski P, Zyluk A. Complex regional pain syndrome type 1 after fractures of the distal radius: a prospective study of the role of psychological factors. J Hand Surg Br. 2005;30(6): 574–80.

A prospective study investigating the role of psychological factors in the development of complex regional pain syndrome (CRPS). Sixty-two patients (mean age 56) with displaced distal radius fractures were operated on by closed reduction and percutaneous fixation with K-wires. Patients were examined psychologically on the day after the operation. Questionnaires was used to assess personality and depression. Fifty of the 62 patients were reassessed at 2 months for symptoms and signs of CRPS Type 1 and a diagnosis of this condition made on clinical grounds. Nine patients (18 %) were diagnosed as having CRPS Type 1. There were no significant differences in scores on any of the personality and depression scales between CRPS Type 1 and non-CRPS Type 1 patients. The authors concluded that patients who eventually developed CRPS Type 1 after radial forearm fracture had neither a unique psychological pattern nor displayed more symptoms of depression than those who recovered uneventfully.

Burke FD. Factitious disorders of the upper limb. J Hand Surg Eur Vol. 2008;33(2):103–9.

This is a review article of factitious disorders of the upper limb. The aetiology, nature and philosophy of treatment of these disorders, which can present a considerable problem, is described and discussed. Recognised specific manifestations such as self mutilation, Secretan's Syndrome, Body Integrity Identity Disorder, Shaft Syndrome and "Malingering" are covered.

De Quervain's Disease

Finklestein H. Stenosing tendovaginitis at the radial styloid process. J Bone Joint Surg Am. 1930;12(3):509–40.

The paper in which Finklestein describes his test for De Quervain's Disease.

Weiss AP, Akelman E, Tabatabai M. Treatment of de Quervain's disease. J Hand Surg Am. 1994;19(4):595–8.

This study compared the use of a mixed steroid/lidocaine injection alone, an immobilization splint alone, and the simultaneous use of both in improving symptoms in de Quervain's disease. Ninety-three wrists were included with an average follow-up of 13 months. Complete relief of symptoms was noted in 28 of 42 wrists receiving an injection alone, 8 of 14 wrists receiving both an injection and splint, and 7 of 37 wrists receiving a splint alone. No significant difference was noted between the injection alone and injection plus splint groups. A significant difference was seen between the injection alone and splint alone groups and the injection/splint and splint alone groups. When the need for operative release was used as an outcome result for treatment failure, the injection alone and splint alone groups demonstrated significance. The authors recommend the use of a mixed steroid/lidocaine injection alone as the initial treatment of choice. No additional benefit is appreciated by the addition of splint immobilization and patients are less restricted with a lower financial burden without its use.

Harvey FJ, Harvey PM, Horsley MW. De Quervain's disease: surgical or nonsurgical treatment. J Hand Surg Am. 1990; 15(1):83–7.

The treatment of 79 wrists in 71 patients who had received their entire treatment from one surgeon is analysed. Uniformity of injection technique is thus ensured. Initial treatment in 63 wrists was an injection of steroids and local anesthetic into the tendon sheath, which gave complete relief in 45 cases. Seven wrists received two injections before the pain abated. Eleven of the 63 injected wrists had an operation. In 10 of these the extensor pollicis brevis tendon was in a separate compartment. The authors conclude that steroid injection is the preferred initial treatment for de Quervain's disease, giving lasting relief in 80 % of cases. If injection fails, it appears likely that the extensor pollicis brevis tendon lies in a separate compartment.

Distal Radius Fractures

Földhazy Z, Törnkvist H, Elmstedt E, Andersson G, Hagsten B, Ahrengart L. Long-term outcome of nonsurgically treated distal radius fractures. J Hand Surg Am. 2007:32(9): 1374–84.

This study reviewed 87 patients between 19 and 78 years old with distal radial fractures who had been treated conservatively. Outcome as assessed by the modified Green and O'Brien score (assessing pain, range of motion, change in occupation, grip strength and radiological changes) was rated as excellent/good for 52 of the 66 unilateral fractures. Patients with more significant displacement scored less well.

Forward DP, Davis TR, Sithole JS. Do young patients with malunited fractures of the distal radius inevitably develop symptomatic post-traumatic osteoarthritis? J Bone Joint Surg Br. 2008;90(5):629–37.

This paper reports unprecedented 38 year mean follow-up of patients sustaining distal radial fractures aged 40 years or less. All patients were treated conservatively with cast immobilisation. There was a 43 % increase in the prevalence of radiological changes of osteoarthritis when compared to the contralateral uninjured side. However, the functional outcome was not deemed clinically significantly different between sides (PEM: 5 % difference extra-articular/9 % difference intra-articular, threshold for clinical significance 10 %; DASH: 0.48 difference extra-articular/0.62 difference intra-articular, threshold for clinical significance 0.8). Only the teardrop angle was deemed to relate significantly to outcome, with a 1 % decrease in PEM for every $1°$ reduction in angle.

Downing ND, Karantana A. A revolution in the management of fractures of the distal radius? J Bone Joint Surg Br. 2008;90(10):1271–5.

This review article summarises the history and development of the distal radial locking plate, highlighting some of the important points associated with its use. Indications, techniques and complications are all discussed. The authors summarise by stating that the optimal treatment of intra-articular distal radial fractures remains debated and further evidence is required before volar locking plates can be universally recommended.

Wei DH, Raizman NM, Bottino CJ, Jobin CM, Strauch RJ, Rosenwasser MP. Unstable distal radial fractures treated with external fixation, a radial column plate, or a volar plate. A prospective randomized trial. J Bone Joint Surg Am. 2009; 91(7):1568–77.

This paper reviewed 46 patients with intra-articular (31) or extra-articular (15) fractures of the distal radius, randomising them for fixation with an augmented external fixator (spanning external fixation with intra-focal/fragment specific K-wiring) or internal fixation, with either a volar locking plate or a radial column locking plate. Outcomes were measured using DASH, visual analog scale [VAS] for pain, grip strength and range of motion [ROM]. The study showed that patients treated with a volar locking plate had a more rapid improvement in DASH score than radial column plating and external fixation. This was evident at the 6 week follow-up visit, with the DASH returning to normative values by 3 months. Patients in the external fixation and radial column groups did not achieve normative values of DASH until 6 months. The DASH was similar between volar locked plate and external fixation at last follow-up of 1 year.

Diaz-Garcia RJ, Oda T, Shauver MJ, Chung KC. A systematic review of outcomes and complications of treating unstable distal radius fractures in the elderly. J Hand Surg Am. 2011; 36(5):824–35.

This well designed systematic review reported on 21 articles (8 randomized controlled trials [RCT], 3 prospective cohort trials and 10 retrospective case series) describing 1,032 patients. The review aimed to determine differences between cast immobilisation (239 patients), percutaneous K-wire fixation

(163 patients), bridging external fixation (249 patients), non-bridging external fixation (83 patients) and volar locking plating (298 patients).

Volar locking plates were utilised in significantly more intra-articular fractures and gave statistically higher DASH scores at 12 months. However, the difference was only 2.5 points on the DASH, this was deemed clinically non-significant. Complications varied between the fixation methods used. In volar locking plate group: 6 % not requiring surgery (including 3 % CRPS and 2 % nerve lesion), 11 % requiring surgery (including 6.2 % tendon rupture/adhesion and 2.75 % hardware failure/loosening/removal). In the percutaneous K-wire fixation group: 7 % not requiring surgery (including 1.5 % CRPS), 2 % requiring surgery (all for tendon rupture/adhesion). In the cast immobilisation group: 7 % not requiring surgery (including 5.1 % CRPS), 1 % requiring surgery (all for tendon rupture/adhesion). Bridging external fixation had higher rates of CRPS (6.6 %) and nerve lesion (4.1 %).

There was a statistically observed difference in the radiological parameters of volar tilt, volar inclination and radial height between the fixation methods. However, this was not reflected in different DASH scores, adding weight to the argument that radiological position has little bearing on function in the elderly distal radial fracture.

The article concluded by highlighting that in the elderly (mean age of patients included = 60) the optimum treatment for unstable distal radius fracture should be individualised for each patient.

Jeudy J, Steiger V, Boyer P, Cronier P, Bizot P, Massin P. Treatment of complex fractures of the distal radius: a prospective randomised comparison of external fixation 'versus' locked volar plating. Injury. 2012;43(2):174–9.

This RCT compared external fixation to volar locked plates in 75 patients. There were no statistically significant differences between the 2 groups when assessed for radiological parameters or clinical outcome (Green and O'Brien score). There was a tendency towards a quicker return to usual activities in the internal fixation group than those treated with external fixation.

Ng CY, McQueen MM. What are the radiological predictors of functional outcome following fractures of the distal radius? J Bone Joint Surg Br. 2011;93(2):145–50.

This paper describes an acceptable position for distal radial fractures after reviewing the published literature. It notes that there are conflicting messages in the literature, importantly that radiological position, particularly articular incongruity can predict subsequent degenerate changes, but these changes are not convincingly linked to functional limitations. Despite this, the paper suggests thresholds of 2 mm articular incongruity (gap or step-off), 2 mm of radial shortening, neutral palmar/volar tilt. The authors also introduce the concept of carpal malalignment (divergence of the long axis of the radius and capitate) and suggest that this is perhaps more important than volar/palmar tilt and if present should be corrected.

Cha SM, Shin HD, Kim KC, Park E. Treatment of unstable distal ulna fractures associated with distal radius fractures in patients 65 years and older. J Hand Surg Am. 2012;37(12):2481–7.

This paper prospectively compared patients over the age of 65 undergoing surgical and non-surgical treatment for unstable distal ulna fractures with associated surgically managed distal radial fractures. Patients were not randomised. There were no differences observed in radiological outcome or functional outcome (VAS, DASH, range of movement, grip strength).

Dupuytren's Disease

Anatomy/Pathology

McFarlane RM. Patterns of the diseased fascia in the fingers in Dupuytren's contracture. Displacement of the neurovascular bundle. Plast Reconstr Surg. 1974;54(1):31–44.

McGrouther DA. The microanatomy of Dupuytren's contracture. Hand. 1982;14(3):215–36.

Strickland JW, Leibovic SJ. Anatomy and pathogenesis of the digital cords and nodules. Hand Clin. 1991;7(4):645–57.

Tubiana R, Leclercq C, Hurst LC, Badalamente MA, Mackin EJ. Dupuytren's Disease. London: Martin Dunitz; 2000. p. 158.

The anatomy of Dupuytren's cords is discussed in these three classic papers and a more recent book. Whilst the references listed largely agree on the common patterns of disease, there remains debate regarding how the micro-anatomy of diseased fascia relates to the normal anatomy of the hand as well as the subtle less common disease variations.

The principle deforming cords are the central or pretendinous cord, the spiral cord (displacing the neurovascular bundles medially and superficially) and the lateral digital cord (extending into the digit causing contracture at any of the joints). Skin pitting is caused by disease occurring in the vertical fascial (Grapow) fibres. Other pathological structures are also described: the retrovascular cord (thought to be important in recurrent cases, distal interphalangeal joint [DIPJ] contracture and uncorrected proximal interphalangeal joint [PIPJ] contracture), the natatory cord (running from the central pretendinous cord of one digit to an adjacent digit across the palmar webspace), the abductor digiti minimi cord and the commissural cords crossing the 1st webspace.

Townley WA, Baker R, Sheppard N, Grobbelaar AO. Dupuytren's contracture unfolded. BMJ. 2006;332(7538): 397–400.

This review article succinctly covers the core features of Dupuytren's Disease. It states that the pathophysiology of Dupuytren's Disease remains poorly understood – variably resembling normal wound healing, malignant processes and keloid scarring. It appears that initially there is marked cellular proliferation with the deposition of type III collagen (similar to normal wound healing). There is also proliferation of the myofibroblast (present in normal granulation tissue). Up-regulation of various growth factors appears to drive the process eventually turning from a proliferative process to deposition of fibrous tissue. It remains unclear why this process occurs in Dupuytren's Disease. It also suggests a simple algorithm of treatment, highlighting that patients with contracture should be referred early to a hand surgeon.

Surgery

Becker GW, Davis TR. The outcome of surgical treatments for primary Dupuytren's disease—a systematic review. J Hand Surg Eur Vol. 2010;35(8):623–6.

Crean SM, Gerber RA, Le Graverand MP, Boyd DM, Cappelleri JC. The efficacy and safety of fasciectomy and fasciotomy for Dupuytren's contracture in European patients: a structured review of published studies. J Hand Surg Eur Vol. 2011;36(5):396–407.

Chen NC, Srinivasan RC, Shauver MJ, Chung KC. A systematic review of outcomes of fasciotomy, aponeurotomy, and collagenase treatments for Dupuytren's contracture. Hand (N Y). 2011;6(3):250–5.

This systematic review looked at English and non-English articles from Medline, EMBASE and the Cochrane databases to compare the complication and recurrence rates between open partial fasciectomy, percutaneous needle aponeurotomy and collagenase injections. Recurrence was greatest for needle aponeurotomy (50–58 %) compared to partial fasciectomy (0–39 %) and collagenase injection (12–31 %). Complications varied between procedures with nerve division more common in partial fasciectomy (0–5 %) compared to aponeurotomy (0.4 %). The review summarised by stating that the quality of data available for long-term follow-up of treated Dupuytren's Disease is variable.

Collagenase

Hurst LC, Badalamente MA, Hentz VR, Hotchkiss RN, Kaplan FT, Meals RA, et al. Injectable collagenase clostridium histolyticum for Dupuytren's contracture. N Engl J Med. 009; 361(10):968–79.

This paper reported the CORD I trial – a prospective, multicentre, phase 3, double blind, placebo controlled RCT. A total of 308 adult patients were enrolled, all with a greater than 20° contracture at either the metacarpophalangeal joint (MCPJ) or PIPJ. Collagenase was used to treat cords affecting both the MCPJ and PIPJ in line with the manufacturer's published guidance and compared to a placebo of the inert buffer tris(hydroxymethyl)aminomethane. Patients were treated with a maximum of 3 injection and manipulations at 30 day intervals. The primary endpoint of resolution of contracture to less than 5° of full extension was obtained in 64.0 % of patients injected with collagenase compared to 6.8 % of those injected with placebo. In addition, clinical improvement was noted in 84.7 % of digits treated with collagenase. In the collagenase group, 96.6 % noted at least one adverse effect of the injection (compared to 21.2 % of the placebo group), the most common being swelling, contusion, haemorrhage and injection site pain.

The following four papers summarise the current evidence about collagenase.

CORD I (USA): Collagenase vs. Placebo

Hurst LC, Badalamente MA, Hentz VR, Hotchkiss RN, Kaplan FT, Meals RA, et al. Injectable collagenase clostridium histolyticum for Dupuytren's contracture. N Engl J Med. 2009;361(10):968–79.

<5° residual deformity 64.0 % v 6.8 %; clinical improvement 84.7 % v 11.7 %

CORD II (Australia): Collagenase v Placebo

Gilpin D, Coleman S, Hall S, Houston A, Karrasch J, Jones N. Injectable collagenase Clostridium histolyticum: a new non-surgical treatment for Dupuytren's disease. J Hand Surg Am. 2010;35(12):2027–38.

<5° residual deformity 44.4 % v 4.8 %; clinical improvement

JOINT I (USA) & JOINT II (Australia & Europe)

Witthaut J, Jones G, Skrepnik N, Kushner H, Houston A, Lindau TR. Efficacy and safety of collagenase clostridium histolyticum injection for Dupuytren contracture: short-term results from 2 open-label studies. J Hand Surg Am. 2013;38(1):2–11.

<5° residual deformity 57 %, after mean 1.2 injections; better results for MCPJ (70 %) than PIPJ (37 %).

CORDLESS: Recurrence of Contracture After Collagenase Injection

Peimer CA, Blazar P, Coleman S, Kaplan FT, Smith T, Tursi JP, et al. Dupuytren contracture recurrence following treatment with collagenase clostridium histolyticum (CORDLESS study): 3-year data. J Hand Surg Am. 2013;38(1):12–22.

This paper reported the planned non-interventional follow-up of patients from the previous collagenase trials (CORD I, CORD II, JOINT I, JOINT II) at 3 years. Of the 950 injected for these trials, 643 patients with 1,080 treated joints were recalled for CORDLESS. Of these, 623 joints had been "successfully" treated to within 5° of full correction during their initial trial. Recurrence of contracture greater than 20° at the same joint occurred in 27 % of MCPJs and 56 % of PIPJs in this subgroup. However, of 7 % of these recurrences had undergone a revision procedure. The 301 patients who had a clinical improvement following injection (residual deformity greater than 5°) were assessed for durability of response, defined as an increase in joint contracture of 20° or need for further intervention. Non-durability occurred in 50 % of joints (38 % of MCPJs and 62 % of PIPJs). Overall, this equated to 38 % of the 924 joints which initially improved with injection developing a 20° or more increase in contracture. Across all studies, 2,600 injections have been administered in 1,082 patients. Overall reported adverse events were rare: flexor tendon rupture (0.3 %), ligament-flexor pulley injury (0.1 %).

Note: Historically there have been a number of retrospective, observational papers published on recurrence and complication following numerous surgical interventions for Dupuytren's Disease. The gold standard remains open partial fasciectomy. This allows adequate visualisation of the neurovascular bundle and results in reliable correction. The CORD, JOINT and CORDLESS trials have set a standard of study design and follow-up that will need to be adopted for future studies.

Essex-Lopresti

Essex-Lopresti P. Fractures of the radial head with distal radio-ulnar dislocation; report of two cases. J Bone Joint Surg Br. 1951;33B(2):244–7.

The original paper in which this injury was described in a case series of two patients.

Marcotte AL, Osterman AL. Longitudinal radioulnar dissociation: identification and treatment of acute and chronic injuries. Hand Clin. 2007;23(2):195–208, vi.

This article explores current concepts in anatomy, biomechanics, diagnosis, and treatment for longitudinal radioulnar dissociation. Encouraging results achieved by bone-ligament-bone reconstruction using a patellar tendon graft are presented with a treatment algorithm to aid in the management of acute and chronic longitudinal radioulnar dissociation.

Hotchkiss RN, An KN, Sowa DT, Basta S, Weiland AJ. An anatomic and mechanical study of the interosseous membrane of the forearm: pathomechanics of proximal migration of the radius. J Hand Surg Am. 1989;14(2 Pt 1):256–61.

The interosseous membrane of the forearm of 12 fresh cadaver specimens was studied anatomically and mechanically to understand its role in stabilization of the radius after radial head excision. A central band of ligamentous tissue, approximately twice the thickness of the membrane on either side was identified in all specimens. Mechanical studies determined the relative contribution to longitudinal stiffness of the forearm. The central band was responsible for 71 % of the longitudinal stiffness of the interosseous membrane after radial head excision. The contribution of the triangular fibrocartilage complex was 8 %. Silicone radial head implants were much less stiff than the intact interosseous membrane. They conclude that injury to the central band of the interosseous membrane may be crucial to the development of proximal migration of the radius after radial head excision.

Flexor Tendon Repair

Basic Science

Matthews P, Richards H. The repair reaction of flexor tendon within the digital sheath. Hand. 1975;7(1):27–9.

A classic paper in which the authors created partial injury to flexor tendons in rabbit forepaws outside the sheath and allowed them to retract back in. No suture/splint/immobilization was used. Sacrifice at intervals showed that the tendons had intrinsic capability for repair and remodeling without need for adhesion formation. It had previously thought that adhesions, created by suture, splints and damage to the synovial sheath, were essential for tendon healing.

Matthews P. The pathology of flexor tendon repair. Hand. 1979;11(3):233–42.

This paper discusses the problems of failure after tendon repair. For a long time the subject has been dominated by the problem of adhesion formation. Recent work had shown that this is not inevitable, and consideration of other factors, particularly the nutrition of tendon tissue was leading to the possibilities of other methods of treatment.

Repair

Savage R. In vitro studies of a new method of flexor tendon repair. J Hand Surg Br. 1985;10(2):135–41.

A new technique of tendon repair was derived and tested in the laboratory. Compared to several well known techniques it has been shown to have three times the tensile strength and to allow one-tenth the gap to form between the tendon ends under load. It has been designed not to constrict the blood supply of the tendon and the tests indicate that it will be strong enough to allow early active mobilisation even after inflammation has caused the tendon to soften.

This technique is still accepted as the strongest method of flexor tendon repair (FTR).

Savage R, Risitano G. Flexor tendon repair using a "six strand" method of repair and early active mobilization. J Hand Surg Br. 1989;14(4):396–9.

The "six-strand" method of tendon repair was used to treat 36 fingers with flexor tendon lacerations. Following surgery, active mobilisation in a protective splint was begun immediately. Sixty-three percent of lacerations were in zone 2 and 27 % in zone 1.

69 % and 100 % respectively achieved an excellent or good result using Buck-Gramcko's assessment method. 81 % of all the fingers were rated excellent or good.

Rehabilitation

Small JO, Brennen MD, Colville J. Early active mobilisation following flexor tendon repair in zone 2. J Hand Surg Br. 1989; 14(4):383–91.

In a prospective study, 114 patients with 138 zone 2 flexor tendon injuries were treated over a 3-year period. Early *active* mobilisation of the injured fingers was commenced within 48 h of surgery. Ninety-eight patients (86 %) were reviewed at least 6 months after operation. Using the grading system recommended by the American Society for Surgery of the Hand, the active range of motion recovered was graded excellent or good in 77 % of digits, fair in 14 % and poor in 9 %. Dehisence of the repair occurred in 11 digits (9.4 %) and in these an immediate re-repair followed by a similar programme of early active mobilisation resulted in an excellent or good outcome in seven digits.

This technique of rehabilitation after FTR has become know as the "Belfast Technique".

Elliot D. Primary flexor tendon repair — operative repair, pulley management and rehabilitation. J Hand Surg Br. 2002;27(6):507–13.

A review article on current techniques.

Infection

Kono M, Stern PJ. The history of hand infections. Hand Clin. 1998;14(4):511–8.

This brief review of the history of hand infections highlights the major contributions that have influenced the contemporary medical and surgical approach to infections of the hand. The current approach to hand infections is a culmination of information gained from centuries of medical teaching by the ancient Greeks, nineteenth-century anatomists, and twentieth-century microbiologists and surgeons.

Tendon Sheath Infection

Kanavel AB. Infections of the hand. 4th ed. Philadelphia: Lea & Febiger; 1921.

Kanavel describes his triad of signs of flexor tendon sheath infection.

Kanavel AB. Infections of the hand. 7th ed. Philadelphia: Lea & Febiger; 1939.

Kanavel adds the fourth and most specific sign; pain on passive extension.

Schnall SB, Vu-Rose T, Holtom P, Doyle B, Stevanovic M. Tissue pressures in pyogenic flexor tenosynovitis of the finger. Compartment syndrome and its management. J Bone Joint Surg Br. 1996;78(5):793–5.

The authors investigated 14 patients with pyogenic flexor tenosynovitis for increased tissue pressures in involved digits. All showed raised pressures, in 8–30 mmHg or more, consistent with a compartment syndrome.

Dailiana ZH, Rigopoulos N, Varitimidis S, Hantes M, Bargiotas K, Malizos KN. Purulent flexor tenosynovitis: factors influencing the functional outcome. J Hand Surg Eur Vol. 2008; 33(3):280–5.

This retrospective study aimed to evaluate the factors that influence the final outcome of treatment of purulent flexor tenosynovitis, viz. delay in treatment, severity of the condition, the infecting pathogen and the method of treatment. Of 41 patients with this condition treated by drainage and irrigation through two small incisions (16) and wide incision (25), 16 were treated after a delay. Continuous postoperative irrigation was applied in 26 patients. Re-operation was necessary in 11 patients. In most cases, *Staphylococcus aureus* was detected. The results were excellent in 32 cases and the mean Disabilities of the Arm, Shoulder and Hand score was 8.1. Irrigation through small incisions and continuous postoperative irrigation decreased the probability of an unfavourable outcome. Delayed treatment and infections with specific pathogens led to a worse outcome. Early diagnosis of purulent flexor tenosynovitis followed by drainage through small incisions and continuous postoperative irrigation appear, from this retrospective review, to lead to the best functional outcome.

Human Bites

Mennen U, Howells CJ. Human fight-bite injuries of the hand. A study of 100 cases within 18 months. J Hand Surg Br. 1991; 16(4):431–5.

100 consecutive patients whose finger had been bitten by another person, or who had cut it on a tooth in a fight were studied. Eighty-two healed completely but 18 eventually needed amputation. Early and thorough debridement is required, plus a suitable mixture of antibiotics. Once infection is established in bone or tendon sheath, amputation is often needed, but most infected joints can be saved.

Goldstein E. Management of human and animal bite wounds. J Am Acad Dermatol. 1989;21(6):1275–9.

The incidence, bacteriology, clinical spectrum, complications, and treatment of animal and human bite wounds is reviewed. The spectrum of pathogenic bacteria causing bite infections was found to be broader than generally appreciated including both aerobic and anaerobic bacteria. Pasteurella multocida was found in 20–25 % of dog bite wounds. Recommendations for choosing empiric antimicrobial therapy were made. Liberal irrigation and elevation of the injured part with early, aggressive medical and surgical management are also cornerstones of therapy.

Herpetic Whitlow

Carter S. Herpetic whitlow: herpetic infections of the digits. Invited comments. J Hand Surg. 1979;4:93–4.

A review article with recommendations for treatment.

Simmons A. Clinical manifestations and treatment considerations of herpes simplex virus infections. J Infect Dis. 2002; 186(Suppl 1):S71–7.

This review article discusses the pathogenesis, diagnosis and management of associated herpes simplex virus (HSV)-related diseases. The article expounds that the sensory nervous system, rather than skin and mucous membranes, is the primary target of HSV infection. It also describes how valacyclovir, as well asacyclovir, is now being used in a number of HSV-related conditions.

Necrotising Fasciitis

Wilson B. Necrotizing fasciitis. Am Surg. 1952;18(4):416–31.

Wilson first used the term "necrotising Fasciitis" recognizing that the condition resulted in fascial necrosis.

Francis KR, Lamaute HR, Davis JM, Pizzi WF. Implications of risk factors in necrotizing fasciitis. Am Surg. 1993;59(5):304–8.

Twenty-five consecutive patients were reviewed and risk factors were identified including diabetes mellitus, intravenous drug abuse, age greater than 50, hypertension, and malnutrition/obesity. The progression of the disease was described and predictors of mortality listed. If more than three identified risk factors were present there was a mortality rate of 50 %. The mainstay of treatment remains aggressive surgical intervention, broad-spectrum antibiotics, and nutrition support.

McHenry CR, Brandt CP, Piotrowski JJ, Jacobs DG, Malangoni MA. Idiopathic necrotizing fasciitis: recognition, incidence, and outcome of therapy. Am Surg. 1994; 60(7):490–4.

Fifty-one patients with necrotizing fasciitis (NF) were reviewed to determine the incidence, clinical features, bacteriology, and results of treatment.

Associated conditions included diabetes mellitus (4), alcoholism (3), remote infection (3), and pregnancy (2). NF affected the lower extremity in eight and the perineum in one patient. Pain and tenderness occurred in all patients, soft tissue gas was recognized in two, and the presence of erythema and edema was variable. The microbiology was variable.

It is important to recognize that NF may occur spontaneously, and it should be suspected in patients with unexplained soft tissue pain and tenderness.

Kienbocks Disease

Kienbock R. Uber traumatische Malazie des Monatbeins und ihre Folgezustande: Entartungsformen und Kompressionsfrakturen. Fortschrit Rontgenstrallen. 1910;16:77.

Robert Kienbock's original paper from Vienna describing the condition.

Watson HK, Guidera PM. Aetiology of Kienböck's disease. J Hand Surg Br. 1997;22(1):5–7.

A leading article outlining a hypothesis drawing together much of what is known of the aetiology in the hope of stimulating further work and insight.

Delaere O, Dury M, Molderez A, Foucher G. Conservative versus operative treatment for Kienböck's disease. A retrospective study. J Hand Surg Br. 1998;23(1):33–36.

In this retrospective study on Kienböck's disease, a comparison was made between 21 cases operated on by various techniques and 22 cases treated conservatively, with a mean follow-up of 65 months. Operative management of the disease did not show any superiority over conservative treatment. Also, surgery was responsible for a loss of mobility of 24 %, and for a change in social activities in about a quarter of the patients, while grip strength was only slightly improved. The authors recommended that surgical indications for Kienböck's disease should be carefully considered, keeping in mind the relatively benign course in some cases.

Dias JJ. Kienböck's disease. J Hand Surg Eur Vol. 2010; 35(7):533.

An editorial summarizing the history of the knowledge of Kienbock's disease.

Dias JJ, Lunn P. Ten questions on Kienböck's disease of the lunate. J Hand Surg Eur Vol. 2010;35(7):538–43.

This paper explores areas of uncertainty of the causes, patterns, natural history, clinical presentation, assessment, differential diagnosis and treatment of Kienbock's disease.

Lichtman DM, Lesley NE, Simmons SP. The classification and treatment of Kienböck's disease: the state of the art and a look at the future. J Hand Surg Eur Vol. 2010;35(7): 549–54.

The authors review the history and rationale for the four-stage step-wise classification system, along with a current treatment algorithm. They also discuss emerging classification systems and speculate on future directions in treatment and research.

Rheumatoid

Tendon Rupture

Vaughan-Jackson OJ. Rupture of extensor tendons by attrition at the inferior radio-ulnar joint; report of two cases. J Bone Joint Surg Br. 1948;30B(3):528–30.

The original paper in which attrition rupture of the extensors at the distal radius was described.

Millender LH, Nalebuff EA, Holdsworth DE. Posterior interosseous-nerve syndrome secondary to rheumatoid synovitis. J Bone Joint Surg Am. 1973;55(4):753–7.

The original paper in which describes paralysis of the common extensor muscle secondary to posterior interosseous nerve compression as a result of elbow synovitis in rheumatoid arthritis (RA).

Mannerfelt LG, Norman O. Attrition ruptures of flexor tendons in rheumatoid arthritis caused by bony spurs in the carpal tunnel. A clinical and radiological study. J Bone Joint Surg Br. 1969;51(2):270–7.

The original paper in which attrition rupture of the flexor pollicis longus at a volar osteophyte on the scaphoid (Mannerfelt lesion) is described.

Thumb Deformity

Nalebuff EA. Diagnosis, classification and management of rheumatoid thumb deformities. Bull Hosp Joint Dis. 1968;29(2): 119–37.

This paper describes Nalebuff's original classification of thumb deformities into four groups. It was later was revised to include a fifth and a sixth group. Type I deformity (boutonnière deformity) is the most common; type III (swan neck deformity) is the second most common. Type IV deformity is seen occasionally, and types II and V are rarer. Type VI is joint destruction and collapse associated with arthritis mutilans.

Management Rationale

Nalebuff EA, Garrod KJ. Present approach to the severely involved rheumatoid wrist. Orthop Clin North Am. 1984;15(2): 369–80.

The authors discuss the treatment modalities available for patients with advanced disease: total wrist fusion, flexible implant arthroplasty and partial wrist fusion. The indications and techniques for each procedure are described.

Taleisnik J. Rheumatoid arthritis of the wrist. Hand Clin. 1989;5(2):257–78.

The author presents a rationale for treatment of the wrist in rheumatoid arthritis. Procedure selection depends on thorough clinical and radiographic evaluations for tendon and joint synovitis, tendon ruptures, nerve compressions, and deformity. Operative treatment varies with the patient's age, handedness, occupation, needs, and expectations. One or more modalities may need to be used: joint and tendon synovectomy, tendon transfer, repair and relocation, ligament repair, ligamentodesis and capsulodesis, limited and total arthrodesis, arthroplasty with and without arthrodesis, and with and without endoprosthesis, and different techniques for the management of the painful distal radioulnar joint.

Burke FD, Miranda SM, Owen VM, Bradley MJ, Sinha S. Rheumatoid hand surgery: differing perceptions amongst surgeons, rheumatologists and therapists in the UK. J Hand Surg Eur Vol. 2011;36(8):632–41.

Rheumatoid arthritis is a systemic disease that requires coordinated management by rheumatologists, surgical specialists and therapists working in a multidisciplinary team. Differences of opinion within the team may adversely affect patient care.

A postal questionnaire was used to assess differences in perception about rheumatoid hand surgery between rheumatologists, hand surgeons and hand therapists in the UK with assessment of commonly performed hand operations. For each procedure, respondents rated the most important indication for surgery and effectiveness at reducing pain, improving function and aesthetics, and preventing deformity. Statistically significant differences were found between all three groups with regards to expected outcome and main indications for surgery. The authors concluded that significant differences do exist in the perceptions of the three groups. More detailed study is needed to clarify indications and outcome to allow consistent advice to patients from all members of the multidisciplinary team.

Reconstruction

Vincent KA, Szabo RM, Agee JM. The Sauve-Kapandji procedure for the reconstruction of the rheumatoid distal radioulnar joint. J Hand Surg Am. 1993;18(6):978–83.

The authors' experience with the Sauve-Kapandji procedure for reconstruction of the rheumatoid distal radioulnar joint is reported. Twenty-one wrists in 17 patients were followed for an average of 39 months post-operatively. Average range of motion at follow-up evaluation was pronation to 78° and supination to 86°. X-ray films demonstrated that significant ulnarward and palmarward translocation of the carpus was prevented. The Sauve-Kapandji procedure provides a stable ulnar side support in the rheumatoid wrist with distal radioulnar degeneration.

Stanley JK. Soft tissue surgery in rheumatoid arthritis of the hand. Clin Orthop Relat Res. 1999;(366):78–90.

This instructional article describes a rationale for surgical treatment of the rheumatoid hand involving careful consideration and planning of the soft tissue component of the disease. The planning must include acknowledgment of the patient's functional requirements and surgical requirements. Multiple surgeries are common in patients with rheumatoid disease and must be planned carefully to avoid conflicting postoperative rehabilitation programs. Joint replacement and other surgery are only an adjunct to the soft tissue treatment. The progressive nature of rheumatoid arthritis is not a barrier to early surgery that may prolong the function of the patient. The logical approach to the surgical requirements is discussed and specific soft tissue surgeries are described. Some details of specific surgical techniques also are included.

Arthroplasty

Swanson AB. Finger joint replacement by silicone rubber implants and the concept of implant fixation by encapsulation. Ann Rheum Dis. 1969;28(5 Suppl):47–55.

Swanson's original paper in which he describes the rationale and early results of his silastic implants for metacarpophalangeal (MCP) joints.

Swanson AB, Maupin BK, Gajjar NV, Swanson GD. Flexible implant arthroplasty in the proximal interphalangeal joint of the hand. J Hand Surg Am. 1985;10(6 Pt 1):796–805.

This paper describes the results of Swanson's silastic prosthesis to treat proximal interphalangeal (PIP) joints.

Wilson YG, Sykes PJ, Niranjan NS. Long-term follow-up of Swanson's silastic arthroplasty of the metacarpophalangeal joints in rheumatoid arthritis. J Hand Surg Br. 1993;18(1): 81–91.

Retrospectively, 48 patients were evaluated by postal questionnaire and 35 of them also underwent objective assessment at intervals ranging from 5 to 14 years postoperatively. Objective variables recorded included range of active motion, recurrence of ulnar drift and radiographic appearances. Both in the early and late stages, the vast majority of patients were satisfied with the outcome, with abolition of pain, correction of deformity and improved range of motion. There was some loss of mobility with time. However, functional improvement was maintained in the majority. Complication rates compare favourably with other reported series and no case of silicone synovitis was diagnosed. The authors found that the procedure is useful for lasting relief of pain and enhancement of a patient's sense of well-being and is associated with few complications.

Scaphoid Fractures

Anatomy

Gelberman RH, Menon J. The vascularity of the scaphoid bone. J Hand Surg Am. 1980;5(5):508–13.

The extraosseous and intraosseous vascularity of the carpal scaphoid was studied in 15 fresh cadaver specimens by injection and clearing techniques. The major blood supply to the scaphoid is via the radial artery. Seventy to eighty percent of the intraosseous vascularity and the entire proximal pole is from branches of the radial artery entering through the dorsal ridge. Twenty to thirty percent of the bone, in the region of the distal tuberosity, receives its blood supply from volar radial artery branches. There is an excellent collateral circulation to the scaphoid by way of the dorsal and volar branches of the anterior interosseous artery. An explanation for the cause of scaphoid necrosis on the basis of the vascular anatomy is proposed. The volar operative approach would be least traumatic to the proximal pole's blood supply.

Diagnosis

Barton NJ. Twenty questions about scaphoid fractures. J Hand Surg Br. 1992;17(3):289–310.

Classic instructional paper in which various controversies are addressed with the then current evidence.

Waizenegger M, Barton NJ, Davis TR, Wastie ML. Clinical signs in scaphoid fractures. J Hand Surg Br. 1994;19(6): 743–7.

In a prospective study 12 clinical features for scaphoid fractures in 52 patients were investigated. In 23 a fracture of the scaphoid was diagnosed radiologically and 29 patients a fracture was clinically suspected but could not be confirmed by radiography or scintigraphy. The signs were tested within a few days of injury and again 2 weeks later. None was reliable in diagnosing a scaphoid fracture.

Barton NJ. Apparent and partial non-union of the scaphoid. J Hand Surg Br. 1996;21(4):496–500.

Ten patients with radiological non-union of the scaphoid and four patients with suspected non-union were explored surgically. At operation, ten scaphoids looked united; five of these went on to definite union but the other five to non-union (in one case, despite a Herbert screw). In another four patients, there appeared at operation to be partial union; all proceeded to complete union. This paper illustrates that even with the scaphoid in front of you, it can be difficult to decide whether it has united or not.

Desai VV, Davis TR, Barton NJ. The prognostic value and reproducibility of the radiological features of the fractured scaphoid. J Hand Surg Br. 1999;24(5):586–90.

This paper investigated whether the radiological features of the fractured scaphoid could be reproducibly measured and used to predict the likelihood of union with conservative plaster cast immobilization. The authors found that the inter- and intra-observer reproducibility of the Compson, Herbert and Russe classification systems were only fair and that none predicted fracture union. Assessments of fracture level, comminution and displacement showed moderate inter- and intra-observer reproducibility but did not predict the likelihood of fracture union. The conclusion was that the radiological features of acute scaphoid fractures cannot be used to predict the likelihood of fracture union.

Singh HP, Forward D, Davis TR, Dawson JS, Oni JA, Downing ND. Partial union of acute scaphoid fractures. J Hand Surg Br. 2005;30(5):440–5.

Sixty-six patients with acute scaphoid fractures were treated non-operatively in a below elbow plaster for 8–12 weeks and underwent computed tomography (CT) scans along the longitudinal axis of the scaphoid at 12–18 weeks. These scans showed that 14 fractures had not united and that 30 had united throughout the whole cross-section of the scaphoid. The other 22 had partially united with bridging trabeculae in some areas of the cross-section. These 22 partial unions were graded as 0–24 % union (0 cases), 25–49 % union (5 cases), 50–74 % union (7 cases), and 75–99 % union (10 cases). The 12 patients who had less than 75 % fracture union were followed-up further and nine underwent another CT scan at 23–40 weeks after the initial injury. These showed union across the whole of the cross-section of the fracture in seven cases and 75–99 % union in the other two cases, who had full and painless wrist function. The authors conclude that partial union of the scaphoid is a common occurrence but, in most cases, it progresses to full union without the need for prolonged plaster immobilization.

Symes TH, Stothard J. A systematic review of the treatment of acute fractures of the scaphoid. J Hand Surg Eur Vol. 2011; 36(9):802–10.

A systematic review of the literature identified eight trials comparing surgery with cast treatment and found no significant difference in pain, tenderness, cost, functional outcome or patient satisfaction. In the group treated surgically, the rate of non-union was three times less, there was a quicker return to function and grip strength and range of movement was also transiently better. There were, however, more complications among those treated surgically. No significant differences were reported in the two trials that compared above and below elbow casts or the trial that compared scaphoid and Colles' casts.

Eastley N, Singh H, Dias JJ, Taub N. Union rates after proximal scaphoid fractures; meta-analyses and review of available evidence. J Hand Surg Eur Vol. 2012 Jun 26.

This paper describes a comprehensive analysis of publications to investigate long-term union rates of acute proximal scaphoid fractures. Of 1,147 acute scaphoid fractures managed non-operatively that were available for analysis, 67 (5.8 %) were proximal. Amalgamating publications revealed that 34 % of acute proximal scaphoid fractures progress to non-union when managed non-operatively. A meta-analysis showed that the relative risk of non-union for these fractures is 7.5 compared with more distal fractures, also managed non-operatively. More trials are needed to allow direct comparison of acute proximal scaphoid fractures managed operatively and non-operatively. Power calculations indicate that 76 cases will need to be recruited for such a study. Currently, the proximal scaphoid is defined inconsistently. To avoid misclassification the authors suggest the region is defined as the proximal fifth of the bone, and computer tomography is used during follow-up.

Fixation

Herbert TJ, Fisher WE. Management of the fractured scaphoid using a new bone screw. J Bone Joint Surg Br. 1984;66(1): 114–23.

The original paper in which Herbert presents the results of treatment with his design of scaphoid screw. In a prospective trial, 158 operations using this technique were carried out between 1977 and 1981. The rate of union was 100 % for acute fractures and 83 % overall. He proposes a classification of scaphoid fractures with indications for surgical treatment.

Filan SL, Herbert TJ. Herbert screw fixation of scaphoid fractures. J Bone Joint Surg Br. 1996;78(4):519–29.

This is a retrospective review of the records of 431 patients who had open reduction and internal fixation of the scaphoid performed by one surgeon (TJH) over a 13-year period. The Herbert bone screw provided adequate internal fixation without the use of plaster immobilisation, promoting a rapid functional recovery. On average, patients returned to work 4.7 weeks after surgery and wrist function was significantly improved, even when the fracture failed to unite. Healing rates for acute fractures were better than those reported for plaster immobilisation and were independent of fracture location. In the case of established non-unions, healing depended on the stage and location of the fracture, but the progress of arthritis was halted and carpal collapse significantly improved. The authors claim that internal fixation of the scaphoid using the Herbert bone screw, although technically demanding, has few complications and appears to offer significant advantages over other methods of treatment.

Vascularised Bone Grafting

Zaidemberg C, Siebert JW, Angrigiani C. A new vascularized bone graft for scaphoid non-union. J Hand Surg Am. 1991;16(3): 474–8.

Using standard latex injection techniques with vascular filling of vessels to less than 0.1 mm diameter in ten fresh cadaver dissections, the authors discovered a consistent vascularized bone graft source from the distal dorsoradial radius. They describe use of this this vascularized bone graft source with good results in 11 patients with long-standing non-union of the scaphoid. It is technically easy and seemingly offers the advantages of a decreased period of immobilization and a higher union rate.

Straw RG, Davis TRC, Dias JJ. Scaphoid non-union: treatment with a pedicled vascularized bone graft based on the 1,2 intercompartmental supraretinacular branch of the radial artery. J Hand Surg Br. 2002;27(5):413–6.

Pedicled vascularized bone grafts (Zaidemberg's technique) were used to treat 22 established scaphoid fracture non-unions, 16 of which were found to have avascular proximal poles at surgery. After a follow-up of 1–3 years, only 6 (27 %) of the 22 fracture non-unions had united. Only 2 of the 16 non-unions with avascular proximal poles united, compared with 4 of the 6 non-unions with vascular proximal poles. The authors conclude that this technique of pedicled vascularized bone grafting may not improve the union rate for scaphoid fracture non-unions with avascular proximal pole fragments.

Kapoor AK, Thompson NW, Rafiq I, Hayton MJ, Stillwell J, Trail IA. Vascularised bone grafting in the management of scaphoid non-union – a review of 34 cases. J Hand Surg Eur Vol. 2008;33(5):628–31.

This paper documents the outcomes of 34 patients who had undergone vascularised bone grafting for a chronic scaphoid non-union. Mean age was 27 years (range 16–46 years). The dominant hand was involved in 17 cases. Eleven patients were smokers. In 18 cases the fracture involved the proximal and in 16 cases the middle third of the scaphoid. In 26 patients the proximal scaphoid fragment was deemed avascular. Sixteen patients had previously undergone scaphoid fixation and non-vascularised bone grafting. At a follow-up of 1–3 years (mean 1.6 years), 15 of the 34 scaphoid non-unions had united. Injury to the dominant hand and duration of the non-union significantly increased the risk of failure. Persistent non-union was more common in proximal third fractures and in the presence of an avascular proximal pole but these findings did not reach statistical significance.

Salvage

Malerich MM, Clifford J, Eaton B, Eaton R, Littler JW. Distal scaphoid resection arthroplasty for the treatment of degenerative arthritis secondary to scaphoid non-union. J Hand Surg Am. 1999;24(6):1196–205.

Nineteen patients with chronic scaphoid non-union and associated degenerative arthritis between the distal fragment and the radial styloid were treated by resection of the distal fragment. All patients had a dorsal intercalated segment instability wrist collapse. The duration of the non-union averaged 12 years and the follow-up period averaged 49 months. Range of motion improved 85 % and grip improved 134 %. Thirteen of the patients experienced complete pain relief. One patient required additional surgery and elected wrist arthrodesis. Resection of the distal fragment is not recommended for patients with capitolunate arthritis. Two of the 4 patients with capitolunate arthritis had persistent symptoms; 3 had progressive degenerative changes.

Imbriglia JE, Broudy AS, Hagberg WC, McKernan D. Proximal row carpectomy: clinical evaluation. J Hand Surg Am. 1990;15(3):426–30.

Proximal row carpectomy as a treatment of disorders of the radiocarpal joint remains controversial despite numerous reports documenting clinically successful outcomes. Criticism includes postoperative loss of grip strength, unsatisfactory range of motion, prolonged rehabilitation time, and the potential for progressive painful arthritis. Twenty-seven patients were studied to address these concerns. The average length of follow-up was 4 years. Postoperative pain relief was achieved in 26 patients, allowing 24 of the 27 patients to return to their previous activity status within an average of 4.5 months after surgery. In all cases, range of motion matched or surpassed preoperative values. Grip strength improved to an average of 80 % of the contralateral side. A detailed radiographic analysis of the radii of curvature of the lunate fossa and the capitate showed that the radius of curvature of the capitate is approximately two-thirds of the corresponding value of the lunate. Motion between the capitate and the radius is translational with a moving center of motion, which may dissipate load on the radius and explain the relative success of the procedure.

Trigger Finger

Aetiology

Hueston JT, Wilson WF. The aetiology of trigger finger explained on the basis of intratendinous architecture. Hand 1972;4(3):257–60.

In this paper, Hueston and Wilson suggested that "bunching" of the interwoven tendon fibers occurs, akin to the effect of pulling a multifilament strand through the eye of a needle.

Treatment

Newport ML, Lane LB, Stuchin SA. Treatment of trigger finger by steroid injection. J Hand Surg Am. 1990;15(5):748–50.

A retrospective study of 235 patients with 338 primary trigger fingers determined the efficacy and safety of steroid injection. Initial treatment consisted of one to three injections of corticosteroid mixed with local anesthetic. Those fingers that failed injection therapy had conventional release of the first annular pulley. Seventy-seven percent of all fingers showed resolution or improvement; 49 % after a single injection, 23 % after two injections, and 5 % after three injections.

Stothard J, Kumar A. A safe percutaneous procedure for trigger finger release. J R Coll Surg Edinb. 1994;39(2):116–7.

A safe and easily performed method for percutaneous release of trigger digits is described which is performed in the outpatient clinic within a few minutes, without requiring any special instrument. Results in terms of abolishing triggering immediately and patient acceptance are excellent. No important complications were observed in the first 38 procedures.

Turowski GA, Zdankiewicz PD, Thomson JG. The results of surgical treatment of trigger finger. J Hand Surg Am. 1997; 22(1):145–9.

A three-part retrospective study was undertaken to review the long-term results of surgical treatment of trigger finger. Seventy-five patients were identified by chart review. Fifty-nine of these were assessed by a telephone survey, with a mean follow-up period of 48 months. Forty-six patients (78 %) underwent follow-up physical examination. Surgical treatment was successful in all patients. Ninety-seven percent of patients had complete resolution of triggering, and the rest had significant improvement of symptoms. The recurrence rate was 3 %, with only a single patient requiring reoperation. Complications were infrequent and resulted in minimal morbidity. No nerve injuries, tendon bowstringing, or ulnar deviation of the digits were observed. There were no wound infections. Although steroid injections should remain the initial remedy for most trigger fingers, surgical intervention is highly successful for conservative treatment failures and should be considered for patients desiring quick and definitive relief from this disability.

Griggs SM, Weiss AP, Lane LB, Schwenker C, Akelman E, Sachar K. Treatment of trigger finger in patients with diabetes mellitus. J Hand Surg Am. 1995;20(5):787–9.

This is a retrospective study of 54 diabetic patients with 121 trigger digits treated over a 3-year period by one to three injections of corticosteroid mixed with local anesthetic. As a group, diabetic patients responded less favourably to treatment by steroid injection (50 % symptom resolution) when compared to reported outcomes of steroid injection treatment for stenosing tenosynovitis in the general population. Insulin-dependent diabetic patients have a higher incidence of multiple digit involvement (59 % of patients) and of requiring surgical release for relief of symptoms (56 % of digits) when compared to non-insulin-dependent diabetic patients (28 % of patients with multiple digit involvement; 28 % of digits requiring surgery).

Trigger Thumb in Children

Dinham JM, Meggitt BF. Trigger thumbs in children. A review of the natural history and indications for treatment in 105 patients. J Bone Joint Surg Br. 1974;56(1):153–5.

The authors report that approximately 30 % of trigger thumbs diagnosed before 1 year of age resolved and about 10 % diagnosed between the ages of 6 months and 1 year of age resolved spontaneously.

Slakey JB, Hennrikus WL. Acquired thumb flexion contracture in children: congenital trigger thumb. J Bone Joint Surg Br. 1996;78(3):481–3.

Four thousand seven hundred and nineteen newborn infants were examined prospectively to determine the congenital incidence of trigger thumb. No cases were found. Fifteen other children aged from 15 to 51 months had surgery for this condition. The anomaly had not been seen at birth and all thumbs presented with a flexion contracture without triggering. The condition is usually seen after birth as a flexion contracture of the interphalangeal joint. The term 'congenital' is a misnomer because patients acquire the deformity after birth. The term 'trigger' is inaccurate as most thumbs show a fixed-flexion contracture without triggering. The authors suggest suggest that rather than 'congenital trigger thumb' a more appropriate description of this disorder is 'acquired thumb flexion contracture in children'. If the contracture persists after 1 year of age, treatment by dividing the A-1 pulley is simple and effective.

Tumours

Baumhoer D, Jundt G. Tumours of the hand: a review on histology of bone malignancies. J Hand Surg Eur Vol. 2010;35(5):354–61.

This review article focuses on the histology of malignant bone tumours of the hand, which are uncommon, and gives an overview of the main differential diagnoses. Close correlation to radiologic and clinical features usually leads to the correct diagnosis.

Ganglions

Angelides AC, Wallace PF. The dorsal ganglion of the wrist: its pathogenesis, gross and microscopic anatomy, and surgical treatment. J Hand Surg Am. 1976;1(3):228–35.

During a period of 25 years, 500 dorsal ganglions of the wrist were treated surgically. Three hundred and forty-six were followed for a minimum of 9 months; there were three recurrences. Dissection of the cysts under magnification of 6–25 times and serial microscopic studies showed evidence of a one way, valve-like system between the scapholunate joint and the ganglion. Stress, as a cause of ganglions, is suggested. Operative treatment involved excising all attachments to the scapholunate ligament.

Dias J, Buch K. Palmar wrist ganglion: does intervention improve outcome? A prospective study of the natural history and patient-reported treatment outcomes. J Hand Surg Br. 2003;28(2):172–6.

A prospective cohort study observing the long-term outcome of different treatments for palmar wrist ganglia. One hundred and eighty-two patients participated in the study. One hundred and fifty-five patients (88 %) responded at 2 or 5 years. Seventy-nine had been treated by surgical excision, 39 by aspiration and 38 by reassurance alone. At 5 years no significant differences were observed in the recurrence rates, which were 42 % after excision and 47 % (19 of 39) after aspiration. Twenty of the 39 untreated ganglia had disappeared spontaneously. Eighty-five per cent of the patients were satisfied irrespective of treatment.

Patients having surgery had a complication rate of 20 % and took more time off work (14 days). Significantly more patients in the untreated group felt the persistent ganglion was unsightly. The patient evaluation measure scores were similar. At 2 and 5 year follow-up, regardless of treatment, no difference in symptoms was found, regardless of whether the palmar wrist ganglion was excised, aspirated or left alone. One in four wrists remained weak regardless of treatment or disappearance of the ganglion.

Dias JJ, Dhukaram V, Kumar P. The natural history of untreated dorsal wrist ganglia and patient reported outcome 6 years after intervention. J Hand Surg Eur Vol. 2007; 32(5):502–8.

The authors evaluated long-term outcome of excision, aspiration and no treatment of dorsal wrist ganglia prospectively in 236 (83 %) of 283 patients who responded to a postal questionnaire at a mean of 70 months. The resolution of symptoms was similar between the treatment groups ($p > 0.3$). Pain and unsightliness improved in all three treatment groups. The prevalence of weakness and stiffness altered only slightly in all three treatment groups. More patients with a recurrent, or persistent ganglion complained of pain, stiffness and unsightliness ($p < 0.0001$). Patient satisfaction was higher after surgical excision ($p < 0.0001$), even if the ganglion recurred. Twenty-three of 55 (58 %) untreated ganglia resolved spontaneously. The recurrence rate was 58 % (45/78) and 39 % (40/103) following aspiration and excision, respectively. Eight out of 103 patients had complications following surgery. In this study, neither excision nor aspiration provided significant long-term benefit over no treatment.

Crawford RJ, Gupta A, Risitano G, Burke FD. Mucous cyst of the distal interphalangeal joint: treatment by simple excision or excision and rotation flap. J Hand Surg Br. 1990;15(1): 113–4.

In this paper 35 patients who had 37 mucous cysts excised from the distal interphalangeal joints were reviewed not less than 1 year later. Seven out of 25 which had been treated by simple excision recurred, whereas only 1 out of 12 treated by excision and skin closure with a rotation flap recurred.

Giant Cell Tumours of Tendon Sheath

Glowacki KA, Weiss APC. Giant cell tumors of tendon sheath. Hand Clin. 1995;11(2):245–53.

This review article discusses the clinical, histologic, and treatment options for giant cell tumours of tendon sheath and the technique of excision with a review of the literature.

Enchondromata

Bauer RD, Lewis MM, Posner MA. Treatment of enchondromas of the hand with allograft bone. J Hand Surg Am. 1988;13(6): 908–16.

The authors investigated whether cortico-cancellous allograft obtained from cadaveric banked bone is effective in the treatment of enchondroma of the hand. Twelve patients had 15 operations on 19 enchondromas using allograft bone. These patients were compared with 16 patients with enchondroma treated with autogenous iliac cancellous bone. The distribution of tumors was similar in both groups. There was no significant difference in the patient's age, their occupations, or whether the operation involved the dominant hand. In both groups, immobilization was maintained until clinical union was obtained. The duration of immobilization for both groups was identical. There were no recurrences, refractures, or complications in patients treated with allograft bone. The grafts incorporated and remodeled in all patients. The authors concluded that allograft cortico-cancellous bone can be used effectively in the treatment of enchondromas of the hand.

Kuur E, Hansen SL, Lindequist S. Treatment of solitary enchondromas in fingers. J Hand Surg Br. 1989;14(1): 109–12.

The results after operative treatment of 21 solitary enchondromas of finger bones are described. Fifteen cases were treated by curettage and cancellous bone grafting, five by curettage alone, and one with amputation. One case did not heal after curettage and grafting. When symptoms are present or the cortical strength is decreased, the authors recommend operation. They found that the eccentric type of enchondroma can be treated adequately by curettage alone, while curettage and filling of the cavity with cancellous bone should be preferred in the central and polycentric forms. It is important that all material is removed from the cyst, which has to be packed completely with bone chips. The possibility of malignant change in enchondromas should be borne in mind, but this was not seen.

Wulle C. On the treatment of enchondroma. J Hand Surg Br. 1990;15(3):320–30.

The author recommends simply removing an enchondroma without filling the cavity with cancellous bone or plaster-of-Paris. This method can also be applied to other benign bone conditions, such as aseptic necrosis.

Tordai P, Hoglund M, Lugengård H. Is the treatment of enchondroma in the hand by simple curettage a rewarding method? J Hand Surg Br. 1990;15(3):331–4.

Forty-six enchondromata of the hand were treated by simple curettage without bone grafting. Eighty-two percent healed and 16 % were left with only small bone defects. Only one patient had a recurrence requiring re-operation. This simple method is recommended.

Hasselgren G, Forssblad P, Törnvall A. Bone grafting unnecessary in the treatment of enchondromas in the hand. J Hand Surg Am. 1991;16(1):139–42.

Twenty-eight consecutive patients with enchondromas in the hand had simple curettage of the tumor without bone grafting. The patients were followed-up with a radiologic examination mean 6 years (range from 0.5 to 16 years) after operation. There were no recurrences or postoperative fractures in this series. The authors conclude that simple curettage without bone grafting is a safe and effective treatment of enchondromas in the hand.

Part V
Applied Basic Science

Applied Basic Science

James Gibbs and Stephen Bendall

Abstract There is a broad range of topics that can be considered as Applied Basic Science. These include an understanding of the musculo-skeletal tissues and their responses to trauma, the mechanical and engineering sciences behind orthopaedic implants, and the forces that act on them. The design of the operating theatre and the prevention of infection are covered here. Osteoporosis, Paget's disease, thrombo-embolic complications and genetic diseases are key topics where basic science has an important application in clinical practice. An understanding of statistics is important in assessing the orthopaedic literature, so some focused updates are provided.

Keywords Gait cycle • Biomechanics • Articular cartilage • Fracture healing • Paget's disease of bone • Biomaterials • Nerve injury • Antibiotics in joint replacement • Operating

J. Gibbs, MBBS, MSc, FRCS (Tr & Orth)
Department of Trauma and Orthopaedics,
Brighton and Sussex University Hospitals,
NHS Trust, Eastern Road, Brighton, UK

S. Bendall, MBBS, FRCS (Orth) (✉)
Department of Orthopaedics,
Brighton and Sussex University Hospitals,
Princess Royal Hospital, Lewes Road,
Haywards Heath, West Sussex RH16 4FX, UK
e-mail: stephen.bendall@btinternet.com

G. Bowyer, A. Cole (eds.), *Selected References in Trauma and Orthopaedics*, DOI 10.1007/978-1-4471-4676-6_14,
© Springer-Verlag London 2014

theatre design • Orthopaedic implants • Osteoporosis • Thromboprophylaxis in trauma and orthopaedics • Tourniquets • Gene therapy

Gait Cycle

Shetty N, Bendall S. Understanding the gait cycle, as it relates to the foot. Orthopaedics and Trauma. 2011;25(4):236–40.

The gait cycle is outwardly something complex, which seems difficult to grasp. This really isn't the case and with a few relatively simple facts to understand it can be easily understood. The purpose of this article is to try and break this complex process into a series of comprehensible steps. The gait cycle is defined and its major components are then described. The key is understanding how the foot can be both a flexible and then a rigid structure in different parts of the gait cycle. This is a function of the subtalar and especially the midtarsal joints. The authors also look at how the plantar fascia plays a part. Finally they look at how the cycle may be altered in various clinical scenarios.

Chambers HG, Sutherland DH. A practical guide to gait analysis. J Am Acad Orthop Surg. 2002;10(3):222–31.

A comprehensive review paper on gait, the gait cycle and gait analysis. Clarifies some of the recent changes in nomenclature and discusses determinants of normal gait.

Biomechanics

Ramachandran M, editor. Basic orthopaedic sciences: the stanmore guide. London: Hodder Arnold; 2007.

Papers specific to orthopaedics with regard to biomechanics are few and far between. The chapters on basic concepts in biomechanics and biomaterial behaviour in *The Stanmore Guide* are well written for the orthopaedic surgeon with an interest in this topic.

Nordin M, Frankel VH, editors. Basic biomechanics of the musculoskeletal system. 2nd ed. Philadelphia: Lea &Febiger; 1989.

This is a readable text and covers just about everything in terms of musculoskeletal biomechanics. Free body diagrams are well covered in the knee and hip sections.

Sariali E, Veysi V, Stewart T. Biomechanics of the human hip—consequences for total hip replacement. Curr Orthop. 2008;22(6):371–5.

This is a review/instructional paper which is clearly written.

Byrne DP, Mulhall KJ, Baker JF. Anatomy & biomechanics of the hip. Open Sports Med J. 2010;(4):51–7.

The anatomy section of this paper starts simply, but the sections on biomechanics and 2-D analysis is particularly clear with a good explanation of the forces acting on the hip and how to resolve these to calculate the joint reaction force. There are details about the forces going through the hip in a variety of day to day activities. It also explains the effect of using a walking stick.

Articular Cartilage

Ulrich-Vinther M, Maloney MD, Schwarz EM, Rosier R, O'Keefe RJ. Articular cartilage biology. J Am Acad Orthop Surg. 2003;11(6):421–30.

This paper looks at the structure and biology of articular cartilage. It goes on to examine the developments in the understanding of cellular and molecular processes had how research is seeking to clarify the effects of agents such as glucosamine, chondroitin, hyaluronic acid and nonsteroidal anti-inflammatory drugs (NSAIDs) on the symptoms and the course of osteoarthritis. It goes on to discuss techniques for stimulating repair or replacing damaged cartilage through enzymes and bio-active molecules such as growth factors and cytokine inhibitors, gene therapy. The potential roles of artificial cartilage substitutes and tissue engineering are also covered.

Mow VC, Holmes MH, Lai WM. Fluid transport and mechanical properties of articular cartilage: a review. J Biomech. 1984;17(5):377–94.

This review brings together the concepts of cartilage's visco-elastic properties in compression and its compression dependent permeability, controlling the interstitial fluid flow.

Armstrong CG, Mow VC. Variations in the intrinsic mechanical properties of human articular cartilage with age, degeneration, and water content. J Bone Joint Surg. 1982;64(1):88–94.

This paper described the compression creep characteristics of 103 cartilage specimens from the lateral patellar facet. As water content of the tissue increased, so matrix became softer and more permeable – the permeability of the matrix was not significantly correlated with age or degeneration.

Minas T. A primer in cartilage repair. J Bone Joint Surg Br. 2012;94(11 Suppl A):141–6.

This review looks at the basic science of articular cartilage structure and function. It examines the techniques which are currently being used to attempt repair of this challenging tissue. The introduction of autologous chondrocyte implantation raised hopes for cartilage repair and regeneration.

Fortier LA, Barker JU, Strauss EJ, McCarrel TM, Cole BJ. The role of growth factors in cartilage repair. Clin Orthop Relat Res. 2011;469(10):2706–15.

This literature review looks at the role of bioactive factors from the transforming growth factor-β superfamily, fibroblast growth factor family, insulin-like growth factor-I, and platelet-derived growth factor in the management of chondral injury, defects and early arthritis. The anabolic and anticatabolic effects of a variety of growth factors have demonstrated potential in both in vitro and animal studies of cartilage injury and repair, but the authors conclude that further research is needed at both the basic science and clinical levels before routine application of these factors.

Steadman JR, Rodkey WG, Rodrigo JJ. Microfracture: surgical technique and rehabilitation to treat chondral defects. Clin Orthop Relat Res. 2001;(391 Suppl):S362–9.

This report looks at the microfracture technique used in more than 1,800 patients in a single unit. Specially designed awls are used to make multiple perforations, or microfractures, into the subchondral bone plate. The released marrow elements (including mesenchymal stem cells, growth factors, and other healing proteins) form a surgically induced super clot that provides an enriched environment for new tissue formation, leading to durable repair cartilage. The rehabilitation program is crucial to optimize the results of the surgery.

Fracture Healing

McKibbin B. The biology of fracture healing in long bones. J Bone Joint Surg Br. 1978;60-B(2):150 62.

A review paper but accessible and readable. It covers the basics of fracture repair, healing by external callus and primary bone healing which was at the time of writing a relatively new concept.

Perren S. Physical and biological aspects of fracture healing with special reference to internal fixation. Clin Orthop. 1979;(138):175–96.

A classic paper outlining the scientific basis that underpinned the AO Group philosophy.

Perren SM. Evolution of the internal fixation of long bone fractures. The scientific basis of biological internal fixation: choosing a new balance between stability and biology. J Bone Joint Surg Br. 2002;84(8):1093–110.

This paper marks the change in understanding and emphasis with the introduction of the concept of 'biological internal fixation'. It presents the scientific basis of the fixation and function of more flexible implants such as the "internal fixator" plates, as well as the advantages of minimising surgical damage to the blood supply of the bone and related tissues. The strain theory offers an explanation for the maximum instability which will be tolerated and the minimal degree required for induction of callus formation.

Claes L, Recknagel S, Ignatius A. Fracture healing under healthy and inflammatory conditions. Nat Rev Rheumatol. 2012;8(3):133–43.

This review looks at the factors influencing fracture healing, emphasising the role of inflammation in the overall process. Inflammation is important in the initial phase in response to fracture, with immune cells and molecular factors activated by the tissue damage, and then in the repair phase where immune cells interact with bone cells. The paper discusses the way in which systemic inflammation in conditions such as sepsis, diabetes and rheumatoid arthritis can adversely affect fracture healing.

Simpson AH, Mills L, Noble B. The role of growth factors and related agents in accelerating fracture healing. J Bone Joint Surg Br. 2006;88(6):701–5.

This excellent review article looks at the Bone Morphogenetic Proteins BMP-2 and BMP-7, their potential indications and mode of action, as well as advantages and disadvantages. It goes on to look at other bio-active molecules such as the range of Growth Factors, Growth Hormone and Parathyroid Hormone. The clinical studies and levels of research are set out, and the need for further research is acknowledged.

Alsousou J, Thompson M, Hulley P, Noble A, Willett K. The biology of platelet-rich plasma and its application in trauma and orthopaedic surgery: a review of the literature. J Bone Joint Surg Br. 2009;91(8):987–96.

This paper looks at the new "orthobiologic" factors which now have a role in fracture healing. Platelet-rich plasma (PRP) is derived from autologous blood; the platelet alpha granules are rich in growth factors that play an essential role in tissue healing. The paper looks at techniques for preparing PRP as well as looking at the studies evaluating its efficacy.

Macey LR, Kana SM, Jingushi S, Terek RM, Borretos J, Bolander ME. Defects of early fracture-healing in experimental diabetes. J Bone Joint Surg Am. 1989;71(5):722-33.

Rat model findings were that diabetes had an effect to decrease callus volume, tensile strength, callus stiffness & collagen content.

Funk JR, Hale JE, Carmines D, GoochHL, Hurwitz SR. Biomechanical evaluation of early fracture healing in normal and diabetic rats. J Orthop Res. 2000;18(1):126-32.

A rat study examining fracture healing at 3 and 4 weeks. Diabetic rats versus controls. Standard fractures allowed to heal and tested biomechanically (failure torque, failure stress, structural stiffness material stiffness). Findings were that diabetic rats were a week slower than controls in healing.

Al-Hadithy N, Sewell MD, Bhavikatti M, Gikas PD. The effect of smoking on fracture healing and on various orthopaedic procedures. Acta Orthop Belg. 2012;78(3):285-90.

Smoking is said to be a cause of impaired fracture healing. There are 13.5 million smokers in the U.K. Healing of tibial fractures, for instance, requires 2 more months in smokers. Nicotine, carbon monoxide and hydrogen cyanide are most often seen as the offenders, among the 4,000 chemicals found in cigarettes. Many studies plead for the negative effect of smoking in general, yet there is uncertainty as to the precise role of nicotine. The authors recommend that patients should attempt smoking cessation therapy before elective orthopaedic treatment.

Moghaddam A, Weiss S, Wölfl CG, Schmeckenbecher K, Wentzensen A, Grützner PA, et al. Cigarette smoking decreases TGF-b1 serum concentrations after long bone fracture. Injury. 2010;41(10):1020-5.

TGF Beta 1 serum concentrations are considered to be one of the most promising markers of fracture healing. This study demonstrated that, after fracture, TGF-b1 serum concentrations are reduced by smoking, and this reduction is statistically significant during the fourth week after surgery.

Raikin SM, Landsman JC, Alexander VA, Froimson MI, Plaxton NA. Effect of nicotine on the rate and strength of long bone fracture healing. Clin Orthop Relat Res. 1998;(353): 231–7.

Empirical clinical observation suggests that cigarette smoking has an inhibitory effect on long bone fracture healing, but this has not been proven scientifically. Forty female New Zealand White rabbits had midshafttibial osteotomies performed and plated. These were divided randomly into two groups receiving either systemic nicotine or saline (placebo). The rabbits were sacrificed 8 weeks after fracture, and healing was compared biomechanically. Three (13 %) fractures showed no clinical evidence of union in the nicotine group, whereas all fractures in the control group healed. Biomechanical testing showed the nicotine exposed bones to be 26 % weaker in three-point bending than were those exposed to placebo.

Strube P, Sentuerk U, Riha T, Kaspar K, Mueller M, Kasper G, et al. Influence of age and mechanical stability on bone defect healing: age reverses mechanical effects. Bone. 2008;42(4):758–64.

An animal model (rat femur) matching fixator stiffness in young and elderly rats. Rats sacrificed at 6 weeks and callus tested for torsional stiffness and maximum torque at failure. Study showed significant differences between young and old with both fixator configurations semi rigid and stiff. The mechanism by which age-related changes in callus occur is not clear.

Khan SN, Cammisa FP Jr, Sandhu HS, Diwan AD, Girardi FP, Lane JM. The biology of bone grafting. J Am Acad Orthop Surg. 2005;13(1):77–86.

This paper considers the biological characteristics of bone graft. Autogenouscancellous graft is osteogenic, osteoconductive and osteoinductive and remains the "gold standard"; there are, however, potential problems with the harvest site morbidity. The paper discusses the graft's structural, mechanical and biological features, autogenous versus allogeneic graft, vascularized or not, site of transplant and host bed preparation.

Hak DJ. The use of osteoconductive bone graft substitutes in orthopaedic trauma. J Am Acad Orthop Surg. 2007;15(9): 525–36.

Bone graft substitutes to augment fracture healing are principally osteoconductive. There is a wide range of materials that will act in this mode, from coralline hydroxyapatite, calcium phosphate, calcium sulphate, tricalcium phosphate and collagen-based matrices. The paper sets out the factors that make these osteoconductive and the material properties that differ between them.

Paget's Disease of Bone

Hadjipavlou AG, Gaitanis IN, Kontakis GM. Paget's disease of bone and its management. J Bone Joint Surg. 2002;84(2):160–9.

A useful and well-referenced review. Focus is on spine and general management.

Lewallen DG. Hip arthroplasty in patients with Paget's disease. Clin Orthop Relat Res. 1999;(369):243–50.

Paget's disease may present unique problems during the preoperative assessment, intraoperative treatment, and postoperative follow-up. Preoperative determination of disease activity and assessment of the cause of hip symptoms is important. Intraoperatively, deformity such as coxavara, femoral bowing, acetabular protrusio, and bony enlargement may cause alterations in implant choice or fixation method used and the patient may even require corrective osteotomy. Excessive bleeding and bone quality changes may complicate these efforts additionally. Postoperative problems include heterotopic bone formation, and in those patients in whom the underlying disease is highly active or poorly controlled, rapid postoperative bone resorption is possible.

Lusty PJ, Walter WL, Walter WK, Zicat B. Cementless hip arthroplasty in Paget's disease at medium-term follow-up (average of 6.7 years). J Arthroplasty. 2007;22(5):692–6.

Thirty-three cementless total hip arthroplasties for arthritis in 27 patients with an established diagnosis of Paget's disease on the acetabular or femoral side of the hip. There were 3 revisions. One stem for aseptic loosening at 55 months, and 2 stems after periprosthetic fractures at 9 and 70 months. Twenty-three cases were available for follow-up at an average of 6.7 years (range, 2–14 years). Harris hip score improved from 56/100 preoperatively (16–98/100) to 90/100 postoperatively (78–100/100). All surviving components were radiographically bone ingrown. Based on our findings, it appears that a cementless total hip arthroplasty can have a good outcome in Paget's disease.

Biomaterials

Jones LC, Hungerford DS. Cement disease. Clin Orthop Relat Res. 1987;(225):192–206.

A classic paper which in retrospect directed orthopaedics in two directions, the first down the route of uncemented devices on the basis of the properties of methylmethacrylate cement and second towards a deeper understanding of tribiology and failure of implants from the effects of wear debris.

Horowitz SM, Doty SB, Lane JM, Burstein AH. Studies of the mechanism by which the mechanical failure of polymethylmethacrylate leads to bone resorption. J Bone Joint Surg Am. 1993;75(6):802–13.

An in vitro study where macrophages phagocytosed particles of less than 12 microns and then released tumor necrosis factor (TNF).

Jiranek WA, Machado M, Jasty M, Jevsavar D, Wolfe HJ, Goldring SR, et al. Production of cytokines around loosened cemented acetabular components. Analysis with immunohistochemical techniques and in situ hybridization. J Bone Joint Surg Am. 1993;75(6):863–79.

A tissue retrieval type study looking at membrane behind failed polyethylene cups. It showed the presence of macrophages and fibroblasts. Debris was noted and present within macrophages and giant cells. Marrophages were demonstrated to produce cytokines (IL-1B). This then gave a basis to the particle based paradigm causing implant failure.

Nerve Injury

Seddon HJ. Three types of nerve injury. Brain. 1943;66(4): 237–88.

Sunderland S. A classification of peripheral nerve injuries producing loss of function. Brain. 1951;74(4):491–516.

These two classic papers look at types of nerve injury, as studied during and after the Second World War.

Hall S. The response to injury in the peripheral nervous system. J Bone Joint Surg Br. 2005;87(10):1309–19.

This paper offers a thorough and up-to-date description of the biological and physical responses following peripheral nerve injury. It is very clearly written and illustrated, and goes on to include work on repair with autograft, conduits and stem cells as well as looking ahead to the potential role of tissue engineering. The full text is available free on-line.

British Orthopaedic Association. The management of nerve injuries: a guide to good practice. London: British Orthopaedic Association; 2011.

This small handbook offers advice across three main areas: the management of nerve injury complicating skeletal injury, the prevention of nerve injury in orthopaedic surgery, the importance of rehabilitation following nerve injury. It provides advice and guidance on the management of nerve injury at early and delayed presentation. It considers specific anatomic nerve injuries in the upper and lower limb, nerve injuries related to compartment syndrome and military type injuries. Advice is given on the appropriate investigations and the role of surgical repair.

Antibiotics in Joint Replacement

Pollard JP, Hughes SP, Scott JE, Evans MJ, Benson MK. Antibiotic prophylaxis in total hip replacement. Br Med J. 1979; 1(6165):707–9.

A controlled prospective trial to compare the efficacy of the antibiotics cephaloridine and flucloxacillin. The antibiotic regimens began before surgery, cephaloridine being continued for 12 h and flucloxacillin for 14 days afterwards. Three hundred and ten hip replacements were entered into the trial and randomly allocated to one of the regimens. The follow-up period ranged from 1 to 2½ years. All operations were performed in conventional operating theatres; at two of the hospitals these were also used by various other surgical disciplines. Four patients developed deep infection, two having received the cephaloridine and two the flucloxacillin regimen. The overall rate of deep infection was therefore 1.3 %. Thus three doses of cephaloridine proved to be as effective as a 2-week regimen of flucloxacillin.

Tang WM, Chiu KY, Ng TP, Yau WP, Ching PT, Seto WH. Efficacy of a single dose of cefazolin as a prophylactic antibiotic in primary arthroplasty. J Arthroplasty. 2003;18(6):714–8.

Two hundred and fifteen arthroplasties were performed with three doses (3×750 mg) of cefuroxime, and 1,152 arthroplasties were performed with a single preoperative dose (1×1 g) of cefazolin as antimicrobial prophylaxis. All wound infections that occurred within 2 years of the index surgery were analyzed. The deep wound infection rate of total hip arthroplasty was 1.1 % (95 % confidence interval [CI], 0–3.3 %) in the cefuroxime group and 1.1 % (95 % CI, 0–2.2 %) in the cefazolin group (Fisher's exact test, $P = 1.0$). The deep wound infection rate of total knee arthroplasty in the cefuroxime group (1.6 %; 95 % CI, 0–3.8 %) was not significantly different from the cefazolin group (1.0 %; 95 % CI, 0.3–1.7 %) (Fisher's exact test, $P = .63$). It was concluded that a single dose (1 g) of cefazolin given at anesthetic induction offered similar protection to 3 doses (3×750 mg) of cefuroxime in preventing infection in primary total joint arthroplasty.

Operating Theatre Design

Lidwell OM, Lowbury EJ, Whyte W, Blowers R, Stanley SJ, Lowe D. Effect of ultraclean air in operating rooms on deep sepsis in the joint after total hip or knee replacement: a randomised study. Br Med J (Clin Res Ed).1982;285(6334): 10–4.

Lidwell OM. Air, antibiotics and sepsis in replacement joints. J Hosp Infect. 1988;11 Suppl C:18–40.

Lidwell OM. The cost implications of clean air systems and antibiotic prophylaxis in operations for total joint replacement. Infect Control. 1984;5(1):36–7.

The well known Lidwell studies demonstrated that laminar flow ventilation reduces the number of airborne bacteria present in operating theatres. Some criticism has been directed towards this study, in that although the trial was randomised, it was not well-controlled, involving a large number of sites, surgeons, treatment regimes and types of ventilation. Whether laminar flow ventilation continues to have a significant impact on reducing post-operative wound infection is a matter for some clinical debate, given that most patients receive modern prophylactic antibiotics.

Hooper GJ, Rothwell AG, Frampton C, Wyatt MC. Does the use of laminar flow and space suits reduce early deep infection after total hip and knee replacement?: the ten-year results of the New Zealand Joint Registry. J Bone Joint Surg Br. 2011;93(1):85–90.

51,485 primary total hip replacements (THRs) and 36,826 primary total knee replacements (TKRs) were analysed. The rate of revision for early deep infection was not been reduced by using laminar flow and space suits. The results question the rationale for their increasing use in routine joint replacement, where the added cost to the health system seems to be unjustified.

Evans RP. Current concepts for clean air and total joint arthroplasty: laminar airflow and ultraviolet light: a systemic review. Clin Orthop Relat Res. 2011;469(4):945–53.

The conclusion is that there is an absence of high level data that shows that these measures reduce infection around protheses. That in itself is not proof of ineffectiveness. Ultraviolet light (UVL), it is pointed out, poses health risks to personnel but laminar air flow (LAF) is much cheaper to install and is widely recommended for orthopaedic implant surgery.

Orthopaedic Implants

DeCoster TA, Heetderks DB, Downey DJ, Ferries JS, Jones W. Optimizing bone screw pullout force. J Orthop Trauma. 1990;4(2):169–174.

Good article on screw design and also how design properties influence pull out strength. The major diameter was an important determinant of pullout force in a roughly linear manner. Pitch was important with a finer thread giving greater purchase. Minor (core) diameter and the ratio of major to minor diameter had a small but significant effect on pullout force.

Bong MR, Kummer FJ, Koval KJ, Egol KA. Intramedullary nailing of the lower extremity: biomechanics and biology. J Am Acad Orthop Surg. 2007;15(2):97–106.

This article looks at intramedullary (IM) nails in terms of biomechanics and biology. It looks at the intrinsic features of the nail materials and design which determine its strength and potential mode of failure. It also looks at extrinsic factors such as reaming and fracture configuration.

Kessler SB, Hallfeldt KK, Perren SM, Schweiberer L. The effects of reaming and intramedullary nailing on fracture healing. Clin Orthop Relat Res. 1986;(212):18–25.

A description of the effects of reaming along bone. The effect on blood flow is noteworthy and concern about that stimulated interest in the use of fixators and the development of unreamed nailing systems.

Osteoporosis

Hippisley-Cox J, Coupland C. Predicting risk of osteoporotic fracture in men and women in England and Wales: prospective derivation and validation of QFractureScores. BMJ. 2009; 339:b4229.

This was the first of two papers published by the authors developing and validating two new fracture risk algorithms (QFractureScores) for estimating the individual risk of osteoporotic fracture or hip fracture over 10 years. It involved a prospective cohort study with routinely collected data from 357 general practices to develop the scores (derivation cohort) and data from another 178 practices to validate the scores. There were 1,183,663 women and 1,174,232 men aged 30–85 in the derivation cohort. There were 24,350 incident diagnoses of osteoporotic fracture in women and 7,934 in men, and 9,302 incident diagnoses of hip fracture in women and 5,424 in men. The authors identified a comprehensive list of the risk factors for the development of osteoporotic fractures. They then identified that the hip fracture algorithm had the best performance among men and women. The algorithms were well calibrated with predicted risks closely matching observed risks. The QFractureScore for hip fracture also had good performance for discrimination and calibration compared with the FRAX (fracture risk assessment) algorithm. The study concluded that these new algorithms can predict risk of fracture in primary care populations in the UK without laboratory measurements and are also suitable for self assessment (www.qfracture.org). QFractureScores could be used to identify patients at high risk of fracture who might benefit from interventions to reduce their risk.

Collins GS, Mallett S, Altman DG. Predicting risk of osteoporotic and hip fracture in the United Kingdom: prospective independent and external validation of QFractureScores. BMJ. 2011;342:d3651.

This paper aimed to evaluate the performance of the QFractureScores for predicting the 10 year risk of osteoporotic and hip fractures in an independent UK cohort of patients from general practice records. Involving 2.2 million adults registered with a general practice between 27 June 1994 and 30 June 2008, aged 30–85 (13 million person years), with 25,208 osteoporotic fractures and 12,188 hip fractures.

Results from this independent and external validation of QFractureScores indicated good performance data for both osteoporotic and hip fracture end points. QFractureScores are useful tools for predicting the 10 year risk of osteoporotic and hip fractures in patients in the United Kingdom.

Hippisley-Cox J, Coupland C. Derivation and validation of updated QFracture algorithm to predict risk of osteoporotic fracture in primary care in the United Kingdom: prospective open cohort study. BMJ. 2012;344:e3427.

This study and the second *BMJ* paper aimed to develop and validate the updated version of the QFracture algorithm for estimating the risk of osteoporotic fracture in the primary care setting. It was a prospective open cohort study using routinely collected data from 420 general practices in the UK. It was used to develop updated QFracture scores. Two hundred and seven practices were used to validate the scores. The study involved 3,142,673 patients in the derivation cohort and 1,583,373 in the validation cohort, aged 30–100 years. The study identified 59,772 osteoporotic fractures in the derivation cohort and 28,685 in the validation cohort. Significant independent associations with fracture risk were identified in women and included, age, body mass index (BMI), ethnic origin, alcohol, smoking chronic obstructive pulmonary disease (COPD), any cancer, cardiovascular disease, dementia, epilepsy, history of falls, parkinson's disease, rheumatoid arthritis (RA), systemic lupus erythematosus (SLE),Chronic renal disease, diabetes endocrine disorders, gastrointestinal malabsorption, any antidepressants, corticosteroids, unopposed hormone replacement therapy, and parental history of osteoporosis. Risk factors for hip fracture in women were similar except for gastrointestinal malabsorption and parental history of hip fracture. Risk factors for men were similar. This allowed update of the QFracture algorithms. The QFracture algorithm can be found at http://www.qfracture.org/

National Clinical Guideline Centre. Osteoporosis: fragility fracture risk [updated 2012 Jan; cited 2013 May 29]. Available from: http://www.nice.org.uk/nicemedia/live/13281/58077/58077.pdf

This is a comprehensive document detailing the evidence and recommendations for the management of osteoporosis. It details who needs assessment, the risk assessment tools such as FRAX, QFracture, bone mineral density (BMD) and has made specific recommendations with regards to treatment. The document also details a health economic review with regards osteoporosis. The recommendations made are:

- Consider assessment of fracture risk in women of 65 years and over and men of 75 years and over.
- Consider assessment of fracture risk in women under 65 years and men under 75 years if they have any of the following risk factors, previous fragility fracture current use or frequent past use of oral glucocorticoids history of falls

family history of hip fracture other secondary causes of osteoporosis, low body mass index (BMI) (less than 18.5 kg/m^2) smoking more than ten cigarettes per day alcohol intake of more than four units per day.

- Do not routinely assess fracture risk in people under 50 years unless they have major risk factors (for example, current or regular oral glucocorticoid use, untreated premature menopause or previous fragility fracture) because they are unlikely to be at high risk.
- Calculate absolute risk when assessing risk of fracture (for example, the percentage predicted risk of major osteoporotic fracture over 10 years).
- Use either FRAX (without a bone mineral density [BMD] value) or QFracture to calculate 10-year 21 predicted absolute fracture risk when assessing risk of fracture in people of between 40 and 84 years.
- Use clinical judgment when assessing fracture risk in people of 85 years and over, because predicted 10-year fracture risk may underestimate their short-term fracture risk.
- Do not routinely measure BMD to assess fracture risk without prior assessment using FRAX (without a BMD value) or QFracture.

Thromboprophylaxis in Trauma and Orthopaedics

National Institute for Health and Care Excellence. Venous thromboembolism – reducing the risk (CG92), Jan 2010 [updated 2013 May 02; cited 2013 May 29]. Available from: http://www.nice.org.uk/CG092

This is a thorough document dealing with both different modes of prophylaxis but also the various types of surgery involved in orthopaedics. It sets out the risks for thromboembolism in major joint replacements and in femoral neck fractures, with various forms of prophylaxis such as Low Molecular Weight Heparin with and without graduated compression stockings, Fondaparinux and Rivaroxaban. It also considers the bleeding risks associated with these therapies.

Warwick D, Friedman RJ, Agnelli G, Gil-Garay E, Johnson K, Fitzgerald G, et al. Insufficient duration of venous thromboembolism prophylaxis after total hip or knee replacement when compared with the time course of thromboembolic events: findings from the Global Orthopaedic Registry. J Bone Joint Surg. 2007;89(6):799–807.

This paper took data from the multinational registry pooling 6639 THR and 8326 TKR. The cumulative incidence of venous thromboembolism within 3 months of surgery were 1.7 and 2.3 % respectively. Approximately 25 % of patients were not receiving chemical prophylaxis 7-days after surgery, whereas the demonstrable risk was longer than that.

Ploumis A, Ponnappan RK, Maltenfort MG, Patel RX, Bessey JT, Albert TJ, et al. Thromboprophylaxis in patients with acute spinal injuries: an evidence-based analysis. J Bone Joint Surg Am. 2009;91(11):2568–76.

This literature review found 21 appropriate studies. The major conclusions were that thromboembolic events were significantly lower in those whose spinal injury did not involve the spinal cord. Commencing chemical thrombo-prophylaxis within 2 weeks of injury resulted in fewer episodes of pulmonary embolism (PE). Low molecular weight heparin was better than unfractionated heparin, in terms of thrombo-prophylaxis and risk of bleeding. The authors conclude that pharmaco-prophylaxis should commence as soon as the bleeding risk allows.

Sheth NP, Lieberman JR, Della Valle CJ. DVT prophylaxis in total joint reconstruction. Orthop Clin North Am. 2010;41(2): 273–80.

This North American paper looks at the evidence around thrombo-prophylaxis in hip and knee arthroplasty. It addresses the controversy of bleeding risk versus efficacy of prophylaxis and outlines two guidelines based on the currently available literature.

Kakkos SK, Warwick D, Nicolaides AN, Stansby GP, Tsolakis IA. Combined (mechanical and pharmacological) modalities for the prevention of venous thromboembolism in joint replacement surgery. J Bone Joint Surg Br. 2012;94(6):729–34.

This systematic review found six randomized controlled trials (RCTs) which were suitable for pooling and meta-analysis. In TKR the rate of deep vein thrombosis (DVT) was reduced from 18.7 % with anticoagulation alone to 3.7 % with combined modalities (pharmaco-prophylaxis and mechanical compression). In hip replacement, there was a non-significant reduction in DVT from 8.7 % with mechanical compression alone to 7.2 % with additional pharmacological prophylaxis (RR 0.84) and a significant reduction in DVT from 9.7 % with anticoagulation alone to 0.9 % with additional mechanical compression. The authors conclude that the addition of intermittent mechanical leg compression augments the efficacy of anticoagulation in preventing DVT in THR and TKR.

Cohen AT, Skinner JA, Warwick D, Brenkel I. The use of graduated compression stockings in association with fondaparinux in surgery of the hip. A multicentre, multinational, randomised, open-label, parallel-group comparative study. J Bone Joint Surg Br. 2007;89(7):887–92.

This prospective, randomised single-blind study looked at whether the addition of compression stockings to fondaparinux conferred any additional benefit. The study included 874 patients, of whom 795 could be evaluated. Fondaparinux was given post-operatively for 5–9 days, either alone or combined with wearing stockings, which were worn for a mean 6-weeks. The study outcomes were venous thromboembolism, or sudden death before day 42. Duplex scanning was scheduled around day 42. Safety outcomes were bleeding and death from venous thromboembolism. The prevalence of deep-vein thrombosis was similar in the two groups 5.5 % in the fondaparinux group and 4.8 % in the fondaparinux plus stocking group, so the addition of graduated compression stockings to fondaparinux appears to offer no additional benefit over the use of fondaparinux alone.

Tourniquets

Kam PC, Kavanagh R, Yoong FF. The arterial tourniquet: pathophysiological consequences and anaesthetic implications. Anaesthesia. 2001;56(6):534–45.

This paper reviews the local and systemic physiological effects and the anaesthetic implications of tourniquet use. Localised complications result from either tissue compression beneath the cuff or tissue ischaemia distal to the tourniquet. Systemic effects are related to the inflation or deflation of the tourniquet.

Smith TO, Hing CB. The efficacy of the tourniquet in foot and ankle surgery? A systematic review and meta-analysis. Foot Ankle Surg. 2010;16(1):3–8.

This study looks at the outcomes of tourniquet assisted or tourniquet free foot surgery, by examining the orthopaedic literature. Only four studies were identified. The findings suggest that hospital length of stay was significantly shorter, and that the post-operative period was less painful, with reduced swelling from the fifth post-operative day, in surgeries undertaken without a tourniquet, compared to tourniquet-assisted procedures. There may be a greater incidence of wound infection and deep vein thrombosis in tourniquet-assisted foot and ankle procedures. The authors point out that the methodological quality of the evidence base is limited.

Smith TO, Hing CB. Is a tourniquet beneficial in total knee replacement surgery? A meta-analysis and systematic review. Knee. 2010;17(2):141–7.

This systematic review compared the outcomes of tourniquet assisted to tourniquet-free TKR. Fifteen studies were identified evaluating 16 outcome measures and parameters of 1040 TKRs in 991 patients. There was a significantly greater intra-operative blood loss in non-tourniquet compared to tourniquet assisted surgery. There was no significant difference between the groups for total blood loss or transfusion rate. There was a trend for greater complications in tourniquet compared to non-tourniquet patients. There was no difference between the groups for any other outcome measure assessed.

Olivecrona C, Blomfeldt R, Ponzer S, Stanford BR, Nilsson BY. Tourniquet cuff pressure and nerve injury in knee arthroplasty in a bloodless field. Acta Orthop. 2013;84(2):159–64.

This study reports neurophysiological examinations and the incidence of nerve injuries after total knee arthroplasty (TKA) in a bloodless field. It is a prospective study of just 20 patients for whom Electroneurography and quantitative sensory testing of thermal thresholds were performed on day 3 and repeated at 2 months after surgery, looking at the operated and non-operated legs. The mean tourniquet cuff pressure was 237 (SD 33) mmHg. Electromyographic signs of denervation were found in 1 patient, who also had the highest cuff pressure in the study population (294 mmHg). The sensory nerve response amplitudes were lower in the operated leg on day 3; otherwise, the neurophysiological examinations showed no differences between the legs. The authors conclude that with low tourniquet pressures the risk of nerve injury is minor.

Oragui E, Parsons A, White T, Longo UG, Khan WS. Tourniquet use in upper limb surgery. Hand (N Y). 2011;6(2):165–73.

This review examines the designs, principles, and practical considerations associated with the use of tourniquets in the upper limb. The literature suggests that the risk of tourniquet-related complications can be significantly reduced by selecting cuff inflation pressures based on the limb occlusion pressure, and by a better understanding of the actual level of pressure within the soft tissue, and the effects of cuff width and contour. The evidence behind tourniquet time, placement, and limb exsanguination is also discussed as well as special considerations in patients with diabetes mellitus, hypertension, vascular calcification, sickle cell disease and obesity. The evidence in the literature suggests that upper limb tourniquets are beneficial in promoting optimum surgical conditions and modern tourniquet use is associated with a low rate of adverse events.

Gene Therapy

Musgrave DS, Fu FH, Huard J. Gene therapy and tissue engineering in orthopaedic surgery. J Am Acad Orthop Surg. 2002; 10(1):6–15.

A new biologic era of orthopaedic surgery has been initiated by basic scientific advances that have resulted in the development of gene therapy and tissue engineering approaches for treating musculoskeletal disorders. The terminology, fundamental concepts, and current research in this burgeoning field must be understood by practicing orthopaedic surgeons. Different gene therapy approaches, multiple gene vectors, a multitude of cytokines, a growing list of potential scaffolds, and putative stem cells are being studied. Gene therapy and tissue engineering applications for bone healing, articular disorders, intervertebral disk pathology, and skeletal muscle injuries are being explored. Innovative methodologies that ensure patient safety can potentially lead to many new treatment strategies for musculoskeletal conditions.

Index